Home-Based Care for a New Century

Home-Based Care for a New Century

Edited by

Daniel M. Fox

and

Carol Raphael

A Copublication with the Milbank Memorial Fund

BLACKWELL *Publishers*

Copyright © Milbank Memorial Fund 1997

First published 1997
2 4 6 8 10 9 7 5 3 1

Blackwell Publishers Inc.
350 Main Street
Malden, MA 02148
USA

Blackwell Publishers Ltd
108 Cowley Road
Oxford OX4 1JF
UK

All rights reserved. Except for the quotation of short passages for the purposes of criticism and review, no part of this publicaton may be reproduced, stored in a retrieval system, or transmitted, in any form or by any means, electronic, mechanical, photocopying, recording or otherwise, without the prior permission of the publisher.

Except in the United States of America, this book is sold subject to the condition that it shall not, by way of trade or otherwise, be lent, resold, hired out, or otherwise circulated without the publisher's prior consent in any form of binding or cover other than that in which it is published and without a similar condition including this condition being imposed on the subsequent purchaser.

Library of Congress Cataloging-in-Publication Data
Home-based care for a new century / edited by Daniel M. Fox and Carol Raphael.
    p. cm.
  "A co-publication with the Milbank Memorial Fund."
  Includes bibliographical references and index.
  ISBN 1-57718-040-2
  1. Home care services. 2. Hospitals—Home care programs.
I. Fox, Daniel M. II. Raphael, Carol. III. Milbank Memorial Fund.
RA645.35.H637   1996
362.1'4—dc20   96-29240
                                                                                   CIP

British Library Cataloguing in Publication Data
A CIP catalogue record for this book is available from the British Library.

Copublished by the Milbank Memorial Fund
Printed in Great Britain by Hartnolls Limited, Bodmin, Cornwall.

This book is printed on acid-free paper

Contents

	Contributors	vii
	Foreword *Samuel L. Milbank and Carl H. Pforzheimer III*	ix
	Acknowledgments	xi
	Introduction *Daniel M. Fox and Carol Raphael*	1
1	The Restructuring of Home Care *Carroll L. Estes and Elizabeth A. Binney*	5
2	Boundaries of Home Care: Can a Home-Care Approach Transform LTC Institutions *Rosalie A. Kane*	23
3	Home-Care Politics in the 1990s *A. E. Benjamin*	47
4	Integration of Home- and Community-Based Services: Issues for the 1990s *Robyn I. Stone*	71

Contents

5 Home Health Services in a Managed-Care System:
   Policy Recommendations from a Program of Research   99
   Merwyn R. Greenlick and Kathleen K. Brody

6 Home-Care Dollars and Sense: A Prescription for Policy 121
   William G. Weissert

7 Financing Long-Term Care   135
   Robert B. Friedland

8 Labor Market Issues in Home Care   155
   Penny Hollander Feldman

9 Housing Policy and Home-Based Care   185
   Sandra J. Newman

10 Care at Home for Children with Chronic Illness:
   Program and Policy Implications   219
   James M. Perrin, Ute Thyen, and Sheila Bloom

11 AIDS and Home Care: Lessons for Policy and Practice   245
   David A. Gould

12 Home Care for Persons with Serious Mental Illnesses   269
   Allan V. Horwitz and Susan Reinhard

Index   293

Contributors

A. E. Benjamin is professor in the Department of Social Welfare, School of Public Policy and Social Research at the University of California at Los Angeles.

Elizabeth A. Binney is a post-doctoral fellow at Rutgers University.

Sheila Bloom is research associate in general pediatrics research at the Massachusetts General Hospital.

Kathleen K. Brody is a research associate at the Kaiser Permanente Centre for Health Research.

Carroll L. Estes is director of the Institute for Health and Aging, University of California at San Francisco.

Penny Hollander Feldman is director of the Center for Home Care Policy and Research at the Visiting Nurse Service of New York.

Robert B. Friedland is director of research at the National Academy on Aging in Washington, D.C.

David A. Gould is vice-president for program at the United Hospital Fund in New York City.

Merwyn R. Greenlick is professor and chair of the Department of

Public Health and Preventive Medicine, School of Medicine at the Oregon Health Sciences University.

Allan V. Horwitz is professor of sociology in the Department of Sociology and the Institute for Health, Health Care Policy, and Aging Research at Rutgers University.

Rosalie A. Kane is professor in the Institute for Health Services Research, School of Public Health, at the University of Minnesota. She is also on the faculty of the Center for Biomedical Ethics and the School of Social Work at the University of Minnesota, and she directs the National Long-Term Care Resource Center at the University of Minnesota.

Sandra J. Newman is associate director for research and research professor in the Institute for Policy Studies at the Johns Hopkins University.

James M. Perrin is associate professor of pediatrics at the Harvard Medical School, and director of ambulatory care programs and general pediatrics at the Massachusetts General Hospital.

Susan Reinhard is deputy commissioner of the New Jersey Department of Health and Senior Services.

Robyn I. Stone is acting assistant secretary, Administration on Aging, US Department of Health and Human Services.

Ute Thyen is clinical and research fellow in general pediatrics at the Massachusetts General Hospital.

William G. Weissert is professor of health management and policy, School of Public Health, and research scientist in the Institute of Gerontology at the University of Michigan.

Foreword

The Milbank Memorial Fund and the Visiting Nurse Service (VNS) of New York have long been involved in making and implementing health policy. In 1992 and 1993, in anticipation of VNS's centennial, the two institutions began a series of activities to discuss appropriate policy for home health care in the current period of enormous change in how health services are organized and financed.

The Milbank Memorial Fund is an endowed national foundation that supports nonpartisan analysis, study, and research on significant issues in health policy. The Fund often makes available the results of its work in pamphlets and books, and it publishes as well the *Milbank Quarterly*, a peer-reviewed journal of public health and health-care policy.

Most of the Fund's work is collaborative with decision makers in the public and private sectors. The Fund currently emphasizes work in clinical policy (caring for patients), organization and financing policy (governing the health system and paying for care), and public health policy (community responsibility for health).

The Visiting Nurse Service of New York is a not-for-profit healthcare organization that provides comprehensive home-care services to individuals in the greater New York area. Established in 1883, VNS is the largest nonprofit provider of home health care in the United States and is recognized nationally for the scope and innovation of its programs. Through its subsidiaries, VNS Home Care, VNS Family Care Services, and Partners in Care, the agency manages more than 20,000 patients each week.

VNS provides professional and paraprofessional care and offers

Foreword

programs and clinical expertise in adult care, pediatric and maternal/child health care, respite services, home-infusion therapy, AIDS home care, hospice, community mental health services and long-term home health care. In addition, VNS is active in helping to shape public policy regarding home health care on a federal, state, and city level. The VNS Center for Home-Care Policy and Research, established in 1993, conducts research on key issues affecting the cost, quality, and outcomes of home and community-based services, and provides information on issues of national significance.

Samuel L. Milbank
Chairman
Milbank Memorial Fund

Carl H. Pforzheimer III
President, Board of Directors
Visiting Nurse Service of New York

Acknowledgments

In addition to the contributors, a number of persons assisted the joint project that led to this book by participating in a planning meeting and/or serving as a reviewer of the papers. They are as follows, listed in the positions they held at the time of their participation in this project:

Nancy Barhydt, director, Bureau of Home Health Care Services, New York State Department of Health, Office of Health Systems Management; Rachel Block, executive director, Health Care Authority, State of Vermont; Robert N. Butler, Brookdale professor of Geriatrics and Adult Development, The Mount Sinai Medical Center; John A. Capitman, research professor, director of Long-Term Care Studies, Brandeis University; Mary Lou Carraher, vice president for Operations, Visiting Nurse Service of New York; Lyle Churchill, vice president, Development, Visiting Nurse Service of New York; Pamela Doty, senior policy analyst, Office of the assistant secretary for Planning and Evaluation, Department of Health and Human Services; Caswell A. Evans, Jr., director, Public Health Programs and Services, Los Angeles County Department of Health Services; Theresa M. Forster, staff director, Senate Special Committee on Aging; Jonathan M. Fuchs, vice president, Managed Care, Employers Health Insurance; Lee Greenfield, chair, Health and Human Services Appropriations Subcommittee, Minnesota House of Representatives; Joseph H. Hafkenschiel, president, California Association for Health Services at Home; Robert J. Haggerty, professor of Pediatrics, emeritus, University of Rochester School of

Acknowledgments

Medicine; David Harris, vice president, Medical Affairs, Visiting Nurse Service of New York; Kathryn Hyer, vice president, Business Development and Research, Visiting Nurse Service of New York; Richard C. Ladd, commissioner, Texas Health and Human Services Commission; Joan Marren, vice president, Clinical Services, Visiting Nurse Service of New York; Lorna McBarnette, dean, School of Health Technology and Management, SUNY at Stony Brook; Mathy Mezey, Independence Foundation professor of Nursing Education, New York University; Joseph M. Millstone, director, Medical Care Policy Administration, Maryland Department of Health and Mental Hygiene; Marilyn Moon, senior research associate, The Urban Institute; Vincent Mor, director, Center for Gerontology and Health Care Research, Brown University; Christine H. Nye, director, Geriatrics Health Services Networking for the Johns Hopkins Health System; Jon Pynoos, director, Program in Policy and Service Research, Andrus Gerontology Center, University of Southern California; Donald L. Redfoot, legislative representative, Federal Affairs, American Association of Retired Persons; David E. Rogers, The Walsh McDermott University professor of Medicine, The New York Hospital-Cornell Medical Center; Thomas D. Romeo, executive in residence, College of Human Science and Services, University of Rhode Island; Charlene Rydell, member, Appropriations Committee, Maine House of Representatives; Timothy M. Smeeding, professor of Economics and Public Administration, Syracuse University; Mary E. Stuart, director, Policy and Health Statistics Administration, Department of Health and Mental Hygiene, State of Maryland; Jane Tilly, senior coordinator, Center on Elderly People Living Alone, American Association of Retired Persons; Peter Ungvarski, clinical nurse specialist HIV, Visiting Nurse Service of New York Home Care; Joan Wagnon, member, Taxation Committee, Kansas House of Representatives; and Arthur Y. Webb, chief executive officer, Village Care of New York.

Introduction

Home-based care is rapidly becoming more important to individuals, families, providers and payers. On any given day over 1.5 million Americans are using health and supportive services at home. These services range from "high tech" home-infusion therapy through skilled nursing and rehabilitative care to management of chronic conditions and assistance with activities of daily living. Over 8,000 agencies are providing home-based care, and the industry employs a professional and paraprofessional workforce of approximately 650,000. Home-care spending grew nearly twelve-fold between 1980 and 1993 – from $2.1 billion to $24.9 billion – and home-care expenditures have been the fastest growing category of personal health expenditures for four of the past five years.

With expansion, the home-care market is becoming more diverse and more competitive. For-profit agencies are multiplying. Nursing homes and hospital systems are moving beyond their institutional walls to provide an array of home- and community-based services. Managed care organizations are enrolling record numbers of individuals and families. They and other third-party payers are aggressively shopping among home-care providers, seeking better value for their money.

As the goals of home care evolve and proliferate, so do the models for providing it. Home-care *patients* and *clients* are transforming themselves into *consumers* and *customers*, demanding greater choice and control over service delivery. With support from government coffers and private foundations, Social HMOs, Programs of All-Inclusive Care for the Elderly (PACE Demonstrations), and other

2   Introduction

health-care organizations are experimenting with new models of acute and long-term care designed to be better integrated and more responsive to consumer needs. Assisted-living centers, continuing-care retirement communities and "naturally occurring retirement communities" are developing innovative combinations of housing plus health and supportive services.

Despite – or perhaps because of – its phenomenal growth and change, the home-care system faces a new century that is likely to be marked by shrinking public resources to support escalating service demand. On the one hand, the use of home-based care is on the rise. Driven in part by technological advances, in part by financial incentives for shrinking the hospital and nursing-home sectors, and in part by population aging and consumer preferences, both the number of home-care users and the number of visits per user have grown dramatically in recent years. On the other hand, rising use – and rising expenditures – have generated the demand for tighter management of home-care cost, quality, and outcomes. Cost-containment pressures, steadily building since the late 1980s, have intensified as a result of the 1994 elections and the Congressional pledge to cut Medicare alone by some $500 billion over the next seven years. Given its extraordinary rate of growth, home-based care has become a visible target for budget cuts at both the federal and state level.

How will future resource allocation decisions affect the availability of home-based services to individuals in need of care? What public and private-sector choices will have the greatest impact on the availability, use, quality, and cost of home-care services in the coming century? What can be done to ensure that home-based care in the future will be appropriate, compassionate, and affordable? These are the broad questions addressed in this book. The chapters synthesize the knowledge of experts in home-based care and project that knowledge into the future.

This book results from the collaboration of the Visiting Nurse Service of New York (VNS) and the Milbank Memorial Fund. The book marks the Centennial Celebration of the VNS and the completion of Milbank's health-policy review on households and health services. We commissioned the chapters and submitted them to the review of decision makers as well as researchers. Their ideas and recommendations were the focus of a conference on the future of home- and community-based care, which was also part of the VNS Centennial Celebration.

The book begins with five chapters that offer provocative overviews of home-based care. Estes and Binney argue that popu-

Introduction 3

lation dynamics, technological advances and cost-containment initiatives have transformed and weakened the community-care system, exacerbating access problems. Benjamin, writing before the demise of Clinton's health reform plan, cautions that the national mood is hostile to expanded human service programs and that the imminent prospect of long-term care reform may be a "false hope." Kane describes the "blurring" of distinctions between home-based and institutional care as providers deliver personal assistance services not only in traditional home settings but also in adult day-care centers, assisted-living complexes and other congregate settings. Greenlick and Brody suggest that the evolution of the Medicare home health benefit and its concomitant regulations has impeded the creative development and full integration of home-care models within HMOs, while Stone examines the broader meaning of integration in the context of home and community-based care. She describes four dimensions of integration that need to be elaborated and evaluated lest integration become a buzzword rather than a reality. Weissert calls for more realistic goals for home-based care and proposes five principles for altering the incentive structure, task definition, risk factors and training which must be put into place to encourage appropriate behavior by providers and consumers.

Three chapters focus on major challenges for public and private-sector policymakers. Friedland attacks the issue of long-term care financing, outlining a variety of options ranging from tax credits for the purchase of private LTC insurance to the expansion of public LTC coverage through Medicaid, Medicare or a completely new program. Feldman examines home-care labor market issues, arguing that the avoidance of recurrent or persistent labor shortages in the face of rising service demand will require public payment and regulatory policies that allow employers significant control over the compensation, skills, and deployment of professional and paraprofessional workers. Newman moves beyond traditional health-policy concerns to consider the impact of housing policies on the use of home-based care. She notes that US housing policy over the past five years has taken significant steps toward accommodating individuals in need of in-home assistance, although the system as a whole lacks formal mechanisms for coordinating the arenas of housing and health policy and practice.

Finally, because most discussions of home-based care focus on the needs of the elderly or the priorities of young disabled adults, three chapters emphasize what is particular to three special populations (and offer lessons for all home-based care from the experiences of caring for these populations). Perrin, Thyen and Bloom describe the evolution of in-home care for children with chronic illnesses and recommend a system of ongoing care that is generic, comprehensive, and designed to promote integration with schools and other community programs. Gould describes the emergence of home-care services for people with AIDS, pointing to problems of care planning, care management and care financing that affect elder care as well. Horwitz and Reinhard explore the meaning of home-based care for individuals with serious mental illnesses, who reside not only with families but also in a variety of community-based residential treatment settings (e.g., board and care facilities, group homes, halfway houses) as well as in shelters. Their chapter, like others in this volume, emphasizes that effective home-based care depends on the availability of suitable housing, the integration of housing with other therapeutic and support services, and the availability of a stable and adequate funding base.

In our efforts to expand this book beyond the range of issues, venues, and populations typically included in works on home-based care, we realize that we have omitted certain prominent topics. For these omissions we apologize. As for the chapters we have included, we hope and trust that they will stimulate further discussion and policy development aimed at preserving the strengths of our existing home-based service system while accommodating the (sometimes conflicting) dictates of individual choice and responsibility, fiscal prudence, and accountability to public and private purchasers of care.

Daniel M. Fox
President, Milbank Memorial Fund

Carol Raphael
Chief Executive Officer, Visiting Nurse
Service of New York

1

The Restructuring of Home Care

Carroll L. Estes and Elizabeth A. Binney

Profound changes in health policy during the 1980s and 1990s contributed to what became a major restructuring of the health-care industry in general and of the home health-care industry in particular.

Policy Context

The passage of Medicare in 1965 was the first major federal legislative stimulus to the development of formal home health care. Title XVIII of the Social Security Act authorized home health agencies (HHAs) and required them to provide nursing service and at least one additional service. In the same year, Title XIX of the Social Security Act authorized home health as an optional service at the state level. The federal government then became the major payer for home health care. Since 1965, policy changes in Medicare and Medicaid have influenced the growth, organization, and delivery of home health care.

Federal restrictions initially allowed only public and nonprofit home health agencies to participate in Medicare. Although home health benefits were optional under Medicaid from 1965, home health was not a mandated Medicaid benefit until 1971. The 1970s brought the inclusion of two new eligibility groups under Medicare – the disabled in 1972 and end-stage renal disease patients for home dialysis in 1978 – greatly expanding the population covered by home health benefits. Other policies, such as Title XX of the Social Security Act (1974) and the Older Americans Act (1978), included provisions for in-home personal care and nonmedical in-home services, respectively.

Market Growth

Public policy, hospital cost containment, and the expansion of technology stimulated rapid growth in all types of home-care providers. Most of the recent dynamic changes in the structure and operation of the home health-care industry can be traced to: (a) deregulation beginning in 1980; (b) the Reagan administration's policy of promoting competition; (c) changes in Medicare certification policy, benefits, and coverage; (d) new technology; and (e) the Medicare prospective payment system (PPS) for hospital reimbursement and the resultant decline in hospital lengths of stay (Estes, Swan, and Associates 1993).

The most significant policy changes in home health since Medicare occurred with passage of the Omnibus Reconciliation Act (ORA) in 1980 and Medicare prospective hospital payment in the Omnibus Budget Reconciliation Act (OBRA) of 1981. ORA eliminated the Medicare Part A prior-hospitalization requirements; removed limitations on the number of visits under Medicare Parts A and B; eliminated the Part B deductible; and removed Medicare's certification restrictions on for-profit home health agencies in states without licensure of home health agencies. This latter change is credited with stimulating much of the boom in for-profit HHAs as well as a number of other changes in the industry (Bergthold, Estes, and Villanueva 1990).

Between 1972 and 1986, the number of certified for-profit HHAs mushroomed, growing 4,251 percent (from 43 to 1,871) compared with 105 percent in the number of nonprofit HHAs (from 665 to 1,361) and a 7 percent decline in the number of public HHAs (down from 1,255 to 1,165) (Estes et al. 1992). For-profit HHAs doubled the proportion of their billings under Medicare between 1982 and

1984, accounting for over one-fourth of Medicare home health billings (Waldo, Levit, and Lazenby 1986).

The trend toward for-profit ownership has been accompanied by a transformation in the structure of home health agencies of all types, signaled by growing numbers of chains and multifacility systems and complex organizational arrangements, some combining nonprofit and for-profit entities in mixed forms (Estes et al. 1992). In fact, the most significant change in the home health industry has been the emergence of proprietary agencies, particularly chains, as the largest single form of organization. Studies indicate that home health agency (HHA) chains, perceiving home health to be a lucrative market, have been growing rapidly (Waldo, Levit, and Lazenby 1986, p. 11).

One of the most significant elements of the structured changes in home care is toward greater organizational linkage and system affiliation. Industry changes have fueled concern about access to and utilization of home health services. In question is the effect of the growth of for-profit HHAs and HHAs as part of larger chains and multifacility systems on patients served and services provided. Both tax status and system membership have been shown to be consequential for various dimensions of organizational performance in home health, including access to care (Estes et al. 1992; Swan and Estes 1993; Estes and Swan 1994; Estes and Linkins 1994). Past studies of ownership and access to health care, particularly in the hospital sector, suggest that for-profit organizations may cream and skim or select clients to avoid serving patients who cannot pay (Marmor, Schlesinger, and Smithey 1987). More recent research on access to certified home health care (Estes and Swan 1994) generally supports the contentions regarding differences between for-profit and nonprofit agencies. When both agency types are independent and freestanding agencies, for-profit agencies are more likely than nonprofit agencies to refuse services to some types of clients. Within multifacility systems or chains, however, for-profit and nonprofit agencies are equally likely to refuse services to certain types of clients. The differences vanish when home health organizations are part of large rationalized systems.

Similarly, research on uncertified home-care organizations also found that for-profit tax status and high reliance on out-of-pocket revenue increase the likelihood that clients are refused service for financial reasons (Estes and Linkins 1994). However, in comparison to certified agencies, uncertified agencies were less likely to refuse clients for financial reasons, perhaps indicating that Medicare-certified agencies are subjected to increasingly stringent regulatory and fiscal conditions that affect the types of clients the agencies are able to serve. Given their impact on service delivery and the cost of care, the effects of structural changes in the industry warrant continuing research.

Spectacular growth in the number and proportion of for-profit HHAs in the 1980s (from 471 in 1982 to 2,674 in 1992) reversed a 20-year pattern of dominance, first by government and VNA agencies in the 1960s, and then by nonprofit and VNA agencies in the 1970s. By 1986, for-profit HHAs comprised nearly one-third of the total home health agency market, and by 1992, "about the same percent of HHAs were privately owned as were nonprofit" (Strahan 1993, p. 2). Of the 7,000 home health agencies in the US in 1992, 38.2 percent were proprietary, 41.7 percent were voluntary nonprofit, and 20.1 percent were government and other (Strahan 1993). Since 1987, proprietary and hospital-based agencies "have grown faster than any other type of [Medicare] certified agency" (National Association for Home Care 1993, p. 1). In 1991, proprietary agencies accounted for 64 percent of the industry growth (Marion, Merrell, and Dow 1993).

The strength of the proprietary sector in home care is underestimated by these statistics because a substantial industry of both high-tech and low-tech providers is not accounted for in the recent National Survey of Home and Hospice Care. An unknown number of home-care providers that do not require Medicare certification to be reimbursed have chosen not to be Medicare certified (Hughes 1992; Miller 1991). Very little is known about these providers, although both the National Association of Home Care and a recent study by the Institute for Health and Aging (Estes and Linkins 1994) report that the number of uncertified home-care agencies is roughly equal to the number of Medicare certified home health agencies. The Institute study, conducted in three states and localities, also found that the majority (more than 60 percent) of uncertified providers (both low tech and high tech) are proprietary. Low-tech services, such as homemaker and chore or personal services, are largely maintenance or custodial and are often provided by home health aides.

The National Association of Home Care estimates that in 1993 there were 13,951 home-care agencies (including 1,223 hospices), of which slightly more than half (55 percent) were Medicare certified (46.6 percent of HHAs and 8.7 percent of hospices) (table 1.1). Forty-five percent were not certified (NAHC 1993). Other estimates are that there are as many as 30,000 to 45,000 uncertified home-care agencies in the United States (Hughes 1992). These data do not include a substantial number of additional independent providers of home care, largely in the category of attendant care.

Table 1.1 Home-care agencies

Year	Total	HHAs	Hospices	Other
1989	11,097	5,676	597	4,824
1990	11,765	5,695	774	5,296
1991	12,433	5,780	898	5,755
1992	12,497	6,004	1,039	5,454
1993	13,951	6,497	1,223	6,231

Source: National Association of Home Care inventory of home-care agencies.

In the only known study investigating the effects of policy changes on both certified and uncertified home-care providers, more than half of both types of providers reported that their agency service budgets grew and that they added services between 1987 and 1990 (Estes and Linkins 1994). Public policy and, specifically, implementation of the Medicare PPS in 1983 to contain hospital costs raised home health-care utilization by the elderly because patients were discharged from hospitals earlier than before (Spohn, Bergthold, and Estes 1987/1988). Overall, home health utilization rose 55 percent between 1981 and 1985, a pattern that was consistent across all age groups and all states (Guterman et al. 1988). In the two-year period following implementation of the PPS, the proportion of Medicare beneficiaries using home health care increased more than 9 percent and the number of home health visits per user of home health care increased 19 percent (Kinney 1991). The percentage of discharges using home health care rose from 8.5 to 13.3 percent between 1981 and 1984/5, as did the average number of home health visits per user (from 12.8 to 14.1) (Neu and Harrison 1988, p. vii). Declines in hospital lengths of stay were "more pronounced for those patients who actually used . . . home health care than for the general population of Medicare hospital patients" (Neu and Harrison 1988, p. vi). The recent growth in Medicare home health-care utilization has been attributed to increases in visits per home-care user since the average number of visits per user increased from 24 in 1988 to 44.5 in 1991 and the percentage of users receiving over 100 visits rose from 4 to 12 percent in the same period (Bishop and Skwara 1993). Skilled nursing and home health aide services represented the largest proportion of the increased number of Medicare home health visits per user (Bishop and Skwara 1993).

Cost, Quality, and Access

With declining lengths of hospital stays, hospital care shifted to outpatient, sub-acute, in-home, and other settings, raising the salience of issues of cost, quality, and access to home health care.

In addition to industry-wide medical and home-care organizational transformations and changes in demand due to the PPS, HHAs experienced multiple coterminous regulatory changes. For example, the waiver-of-liability provisions designed to protect HHA service claims were threatened. Shortly after the PPS was implemented, claims denial rates quadrupled (US General Accounting Office 1990), creating disincentives for some HHAs to serve Medicare patients and contributing to the decision of others to leave the business altogether. To curtail costs, the Health Care Financing Administration (HCFA) adopted additional aggressive cost-containment strategies: policy and procedural changes, new paperwork requirements, and redefinitions and reinterpretations of eligibility. A 1987 lawsuit successfully challenged HCFA's interpretation that care needed to be "part-time *and* intermittent" rather than "part-time *or* intermittent," limiting Medicare home health reimbursement to those requiring care less than eight hours daily and less than four days weekly. Medicare regulatory changes (HIM-11) followed, which reinterpreted "medical necessity" provisions, adding management of unskilled care (Helbing, Sangl, and Silverman 1992) and opening the way for more coverage for chronic-care services (Bishop and Skwara 1993).

The National Medical Expenditures Survey (NMES) provides comprehensive estimates of national home-care spending, including that for uncertified providers and hospital-based agencies. The home-care market is estimated to have grown at an annual rate of 10 percent between 1986 and 1991 and 12 percent from 1991 to 1996 (NAHC 1993; FIND/SVP 1992). Updated expenditure estimates (FIND/SVP 1992; Lewin-VHI 1993; Levit et al. 1994) are between a range of $16.7 to $21.8 billion and $21.2 to $26.2 billion in total home-care spending for 1993 (NAHC 1993; Lewin-VHI 1993; Levit et al. 1994). Home-care expenditures comprise 3 percent of national home-care expenditures (NAHC 1993).

Medicare has always been the single biggest payer of home care. Indeed, Medicare funding initially created the market incentives that transformed home health care from a cottage industry into a large corporate enterprise (Marmor, Schlesinger, and Smithey 1987;

Spohn, Bergthold, and Estes 1987/1988). Medicare pays 37.8 percent of all home-care costs. In rank order, other sources of payment for home care are out-of-pocket (31.4 percent), Medicaid (24.7 percent), and private insurance (5.5 percent) (NAHC 1993, p. 3) (table 1.2). 1993 national health expenditures (1994) for home care were paid by four sources: Medicare (38 percent), Medicaid (15 percent), out-of-pocket (21 percent) and private insurance (24 percent) (Levit et al. 1994).

Table 1.2   Sources of payment for home care, 1992

Source of Payment	1992
Total	100.0%
Medicare	37.8
Medicaid	24.7
Private Insurance	5.5
Out-of-pocket	31.4
Other	0.6

Changes in Medicare policy and regulations generated corresponding changes in utilization during the post-PPS period and heightened the stakes in the already-dynamic organizational restructuring of the industry. The combination of rising numbers of HHAs and the modest growth in the number of home health users illustrates that "competition for referrals [is] . . . intense and at times, desperate" (Benjamin 1986, p. 484). Added to the competition generated by rapid growth in the proprietary and hospital-based sectors of the home-care industry, competition for clients stimulated many of the organizational changes and interorganizational linkages (including vertical and horizontal integration) that occurred (Estes et al. 1992).

Medicare and other policy and health delivery system changes have pressured HHAs to make increasingly creative home-care industry adaptations. Organizational and structural changes were widespread among HHAs by the mid-1980s. Agencies divided like cells, forming new and more complex configurations to merge into hybrid and multidivisional entities; HHAs added non-Medicare branches and divisions, sometimes comprised of multiple entities of varying tax status; spun off new product lines; established formal relationships with complementary organizations; and bought and sold other health entities (Estes et al. 1992).

In a recent study, a number of HHAs reported themselves in considerable jeopardy; others characterized their situation as one of great organizational stress and change (Estes et al. 1992). Public policy changes and restrictions in the form of service and eligibility requirements placed on hospitals, nursing homes, and HHAs contributed to the rapid rate of organizational change in the industry. Agency reactions appear to be defensive efforts to mitigate or avoid the adverse effects of Medicare policy and a rapidly changing health-policy environment.

Mega-Trends Driving Home Care

Three major trends are fueling the expansion of home care – the imposition of cost containment in various forms (discussed above), population dynamics, and technological advances that have made ambulatory surgery and reduced hospital stays commonplace.

Demographics

The over-65 population grew 22 percent in the 1980s, more than double the growth of the nation as a whole. This older population will at least double in the next 40 years; and 50 years from now, the nation is expected to have more people over age 65 than are 20 years of age and younger. The population 85 years and older is the fastest growing age group in the United States and will increase more than five-fold (from 3 to 15 million) between 1990 and 2050 (Tauber 1992). Even these startling figures may be a gross underestimate. If the Bureau of the Census assumptions of low mortality and high fertility are used, the estimated number of persons 85 and over rises to 24 million by 2050.

In all scenarios, including Manton's most recent projections of lower levels of disability than formerly expected, there will be absolute increases in the need for long-term care (Manton, Stallard, and Liu 1993). In addition, significant high-risk elderly subgroups remain, particularly among low socioeconomic classes, minority groups, and women. To the extent that there are increases in the proportion of the nondisabled elderly, there will be a need for changes in the mix of long-term care services, increasing the need for community-based care (e.g., in-home and adult day care) and equipment use (Manton 1992).

Technology

High technology has been the fastest growing segment of home care over the past decade (US Special Committee on Aging 1988) and represents not only a sizable volume of care that is provided in the home, but a segment of the industry that creates new challenges for both providers and policymakers alike. In fact, three of the major policy issues that face the industry as a whole (de Lissovoy and Feustle 1991) also apply specifically to the arena of high-tech home care. First, the organization of the home-care industry and the development of models of provision of care could both be profoundly affected by changes in high-tech home care. De Lissovoy and Feustle's (1991) model, which differentiates between a clinical service and a supply service, is a useful example of the increasing diversification between the certified home health agencies that provide skilled labor and the durable medical equipment (DME) companies with material inputs. In addition, uncertified providers may be increasingly entering the equation by supplying a specialized labor force trained specifically in the provision of high-tech services such as infusion therapy and home renal dialysis. These "niche" providers are changing the organizational structure of the home-care market by fragmenting service provision and potentially affecting overall access by creaming potentially high-profit patients from more general service providers (Estes, Swan, and Associates 1993). Currently, DME represents one of the fastest growing segments of home care, with a 31 percent increase in Medicare "allowable amounts" for DME from 1989 to 1991.

Second, policy interest in quality assurance standards is especially pertinent to a discussion of high-tech home care. Traditionally, quality assurance in home health care has focused on structure and process measures such as the qualifications of accreditation bodies and staffs, provision standards, and recordkeeping (de Lissovoy and Feustle 1991). The fragmentation of the delivery process and the inherently risky nature of these services, many of which would have been provided only in an acute hospital setting a few years ago, mandate that quality assurance standards for home care need to enforce increasingly strict labor training regulations and move from process to outcome measures.

Third, the extent and degree of coverage for specific services under proposed health-care reform legislation is currently uncertain and may be limited to very impaired patients. However, it is likely that, given its highly medical nature and potential for decreasing costly inpatient hospitalization, there will be substantial growth in high-tech home care as a result of health-care reform. The growth in DME is almost certain to continue, particularly in light of the propensity of state and private payers to favor medical equipment and devices over more labor-intensive procedures. The implications are far-reaching, including the impact of the provision of high-tech home technologies on informal caregivers (often with limited training), and the legal implications of the provision of such care in unsupervised settings.

Transformation of the industry
Research at the community level documents the occurrence of a series of important changes in local health and social service delivery during the 1980s and 1990s (Estes, Swan, and Associates 1993). Included are the weeding out of weak, less competitive nonprofit community-based agencies; consolidation and concentration within and across large provider entities and industries through vertical and horizontal integration with a significant decline of single free-standing provider organizations; dramatic growth in the number and influence of for-profit providers; and blurred boundaries between nonprofits and proprietaries.

Changes at the System Level

Dramatic and rapid changes have occurred in home health-care service provision in the 1980s and 1990s. Changes in the structure and organization of the local delivery system and the health industry at large have numerous consequences for the recipients of home- and community-based long-term care. Policy changes, budget cuts, cost containment, and deepening fiscal austerity in the states and localities have challenged the capacity of both formal and informal caregivers to address the community-care needs of elderly persons. The magnitude and profundity of these changes are tantamount to a restructuring and transformation of the community care system including:

1 An increase in privatization, as measured by increases in the number and proportion of for-profit providers relative to nonprofits and a decline in public providers of home health care;
2 The bureaucratization and rationalization of care reflected in organizational restructuring, industry consolidation and concentration, and increased management and control strategies;
3 Increased competition between for-profit and nonprofit providers vying for patients, market share and profits;
4 A decline in the proportion of social and supportive services that

home health agencies provide relative to the medical or medically related ancillary services (Binney and Estes 1990; Goldberg and Estes 1990, 1993);
5 Labor restructuring including the increased use of part-time and contract labor;
6 The fragmentation of service delivery by unbundling and selling single procedures and services to increase reimbursement;
7 The informalization of care with the transfer of services and work from the formal (e.g., hospital) to the informal delivery system (i.e., home) and an increase in women's informal work; and
8 A deepening stratification in care provision between those who can and cannot pay for services, extending class divisions in access to care.

Commodification and the Culture of Caring

The political and ideological climate that provided the context for this restructuring of care delivery contributed to a reshaping of the culture of caring. A cultural revolution in nonprofit service delivery has imposed a new set of values on community services: the conversion of health care from a "merit good" into a "market good"; winning in price competition; quick turnover of clientele; the provision of the highest number of reimbursable service units at the lowest cost; the unbundling of services; the elimination of unprofitable services (regardless of need); and attracting private-pay clients while avoiding the "adverse selection" of no-pay and low-pay clients. Simultaneously, increased care management and other control mechanisms have been imposed over both consumers and providers.

The culture of caring has been commodified and bureaucratized, reflecting a shift away from norms of charity that initially guided traditional community voluntary social service agencies and toward goals that are more consistent with the market-oriented medical industry. As a result of these changes, the 1990s opened with a challenged, weakened, and transformed system of community care. The inadequacy of the existing system has created problems for elders living in the community and their families, for the public, for business, and for government. These problems are exacerbated by the policy approach that has generously financed acute medical care and starved social and chronic care, fostering the dependency of elders by paying for nursing-home care only after forcing them to spend down their assets to poverty.

Implications for the Future

With the advent of the Medicare prospective payment system, attention turned to posthospital care and the adequacy of the community-based delivery system. Many older patients being discharged from the hospital with lower levels of functioning and greater needs for ongoing care find inadequate and strained community resources.

While difficulties have plagued providers and communities in the past, the critical nature of the long-term care problem today is both unprecedented and unlikely to be remedied without significant policy change. In particular, there is no assurance that an older person who is denied access to one type of service will necessarily be referred to, or served by, another. The most important conclusion is that access to community-based care has become an issue for all elements of the delivery system. For example, both the hospital and the home health agency need to be able to refer patients to other more appropriate levels of services such as adult day care or assisted living.

Research demonstrates that virtually all components of the delivery system have experienced ripple or domino effects of the Medicare hospital PPS as well as other policy changes in the past decade, and each has been influenced by the restructuring of the US health-care system. The more "social" forms of care – social and supportive services – have also experienced the greatest of these effects, as well as the most serious spending constraints in US domestic expenditures (Goldberg et al. 1993). It is not surprising that home- and community-based long-term care services are consistently identified by state and local policymakers in current studies as the most important areas of unmet need (Carrell and Estes 1993). Recent data underscore the need for more and better organized and targeted in-home and community-based noninstitutional services, backed by appropriate financing mechanisms to support the total package of care for disabled persons of all age groups.

Health and Long-Term Care Reform and Home Care

The future of home care will be dramatically shaped by the events to follow on the health and long-term care reform front – now to be decided primarily by the results of private market reform, Medicare policy changes, and decision making and resource allocations at the state level. Although President Clinton's health reform effort failed, major changes in the market are profoundly altering the organization, financing, and delivery of medical care, including home care as multiple new organizational and interorganizational arrangements and alliances are forged to increase market share, lower costs, and increase profits. There is extensive growth in the care-management industry as insurers attempt to make their competing plans more cost efficient. There is no surety about the magnitude of the role of home care in the health plans, but there is certainty that there will be at least a two-fold impact: both the demand for home care and the supply of home-care services are expected to increase.

The support of attendant care and other home- and community-based long-term care services are highly dependent on policy developments at the state level. Other relevant developments are the anticipated growth in the durable medical equipment (DME) and pharmaceutical industries, as well as in the hospice and rehabilitation-related industries.

It is safe to project, overall, that pressures on the supply of home care will be accelerated by the private market-driven health-care restructuring that is occurring as well as increases in demand resulting from population dynamics. It has been argued that the supply of home care is not as constrained as that of nursing-home care because market entry does not require a high capital investment (Mundinger 1983; Swan and Estes 1993). Nevertheless, a serious constraint on home care and its quality is the supply, retention, and training of staff, which may limit the availability of services and/or their quality (Canalis 1987; Jones 1988).

The future of home care remains fraught with a series of continuing and crucial issues with regard to access, cost, and the quality of services. The failure of health-care reform and the uncertainty of long-term care reform advance these issues with a new sense of urgency.

The present state of knowledge only taps the surface of the nature and consequences of changes in the home-care industry. Research is required to understand the effects of organizational characteristics (e.g., tax status and vertically and horizontally integrated systems) and of broader environmental and market forces on multiple facets of home-care delivery. Research is also needed to delineate the effects of health-care reform and the effects of tax status and plan affiliation on dimensions of access, quality, and cost of home care, as well as responsiveness to community need. Significant but unexplicated policy implications are inherent in the likelihood that organizational restructuring affects micro policy-making within home-care organizations in unknown ways and that it will create profound, but as yet unanticipated changes in organizational orientation (Alexander, Morlock, and Gifford 1988; Friedman and Shortell 1988). For organizational theory, such work promises to contribute to a much-needed theory of institutional change (Winship and Rosen 1988).

Given the influence of Medicare policy on the growth and fabric of home health care, policymakers must attend to the ways in which Medicare policy changes may affect home care in the future. Public policies have a way of fostering organizational changes, changes that may become a goal in and of themselves, while the effects on the recipients of services may neither be thoroughly anticipated nor investigated. Whether or not specific types of home-care agencies thrive or survive is not the most important policy question. It is whether or not those in need receive the services they require.

References

Alexander, J.A., L.L. Morlock, and B.D. Gifford. 1988. The Effects of Corporate Restructuring on Hospital Policy Making. *Health Services Research* 23: 311–37.

Altman, B., and D. Walden. 1993. Home Health Care: Use, Expenditures and Sources of Payment. National Medical Expenditure Survey Research Findings 15, Agency for Health Care Policy and Research. AHCPR Pub. No. 93-0040. Rockville, MD.

Applebaum, R., and P. Philips. 1990. Assuring the Quality of In-Home Care: The "Other" Challenge for Long Term Care *The Gerontologist* 30(4): 444–50.

Benjamin, A.E. 1986. Trends and Issues in the Provision of Home Health Care: Local Governments in a Competitive Environment. *Health* 7(4): 480–94.

Bergthold, L.A., C.L. Estes, and A.M. Villanueva. 1990. Public Light and Private Dark: The Privatization of Home Health Services for the Elderly in the US *Home Health Care Services Quarterly* 11(3/4): 7–33.

Binney, E.A., and C.L. Estes. 1990. *Setting the Wrong Limits: Class Biases and the Biographical Standard. In A Good Old Age? The Paradox of Setting Limits,*

ed. P. Homer and M. Holstein, 240–57. New York: Simon and Schuster.
Bishop, C., and K. Skwara. 1993. Recent Growth of Medicare Home Health. *Health Affairs* 12(3): 95–110.
Canalis, D.M. 1987. Homemaker-Home Health Aide Attrition: Methods of Prevention. *Caring* 6(4): 84–9.
Carrell, D.S., and C.L. Estes with C. Douglas. 1993. Policy Elites and Fiscal Crisis. In *Long Term Care Crisis: Elders Trapped in the No-Care Zone*, ed. C.L. Estes, J.H. Swan, and Associates, 225–40. Newbury Park, CA: Sage.
De Lissovoy, G., and J.A. Feustle. 1991. Advanced Home Health Care. *Health Policy* 17: 227–42.
DesHarnais, S.I., E.J. Kobrinski, J.D. Chesney, M.J. Long, R.P. Ament, and S.T. Fleming. 1987. The Early Effects of the Prospective Payment System on Inpatient Utilization and the Quality of Care. *Inquiry* 24: 7–16.
Estes, C.L., and K. Linkins. 1994. Unpublished Data on Uncertified and Certified Home-Care Providers: Agency Characteristics by Tax Status. Institute for Health and Aging, University of California, San Francisco.
Estes, C.L., and J.H. Swan. 1994. Privatization, System Membership and Access to Home Health Care for the Elderly. *Milbank Quarterly*, 72: 277–98.
Estes, C.L., J.H. Swan, and Associates. 1993. *The Long Term Care Crisis: Elders Trapped in the No-Care Zone*. Newbury Park, CA: Sage.
Estes, C.L., J.H. Swan, L.A. Bergthold, and P.H. Spohn. 1992. Running as Fast as They Can: Organizational Changes in Home Health Care. *Home Health Care Services Quarterly* 12(1): 35–69.
FIND/SVP. 1992. The Market for Home Care Services. New York: FIND/SVP, Inc.
Friedman, B., and S. Shortell. 1988. The Financial Performance of Selected Investor-Owned and Not-For-Profit System Hospitals Before and After Medicare Prospective Payment. *Health Services Research* 23: 237–67.
Goldberg, S.C., and C.L. Estes. 1990. Medicare DRGs and Post-Hospital Care for the Elderly: Does Out of the Hospital Mean Out of Luck? *Journal of Applied Gerontology* 9: 20–35.
Goldberg, S.C., and C.L. Estes. 1993. Does Out of the Hospital Mean Out of Luck? In *Long Term Care Crisis: Elders Trapped in the No-Care Zone*, ed. C.L. Estes, J.H. Swan, and Associates, 64–73. Newbury Park, CA: Sage.
Goldberg, S.C., C.C. McKetty, J.H. Swan, et al. 1993. Access in Peril. In *Long Term Care Crisis: Elders Trapped in the No-Care Zone*, ed. C.L. Estes, J.H. Swan, and Associates, 171–84. Newbury Park, CA: Sage.
Guterman, S., P.W. Eggers, G. Riley, T.F. Greene, and S.A. Terrell. 1988. The First Three Years of Medicare Prospective Payment: An Overview. *Health Care Financing Review* 9(3): 67–77.
Helbing, C., J.A. Sangl, and H.A. Silverman. 1992. Home Health Agency Benefits. *Health Care Financing Review* (annual supplement): 125–48.
Hughes, S. 1992. Home Care: Where Are We and Where We Need to Go. In *Home Care for Older People*, ed. M.G. Ory and A.P. Duncker, 53–74. Newbury Park, CA: Sage.

Jones, P.A. 1988. The Home Care Personnel Shortage Crisis: Preliminary Results of a NAHC Survey. *Caring* 7(5): 6–9.

Kane, M. 1989. The Home Care Crisis of the Nineties. *The Gerontologist* 22: 24–41.

Kinney, G.M. 1991. Understanding the Effects of PPS on Medicare Home Health Use. *Inquiry* 28: 129–39.

Levit, K.R., A.L. Sensenig, C.A. Cowan, et al. 1994. National health expenditures, 1993. *Health Care Financing Review* 16(1): 247–94.

Lewin-VHI. 1993. *The Heavy Burden of Home Care*. Washington, D.C.: Families USA.

Manton, K.G. 1992. The Dynamics of Population Aging: Demography and Policy Analysis. *Milbank Quarterly* 69: 309–38.

Manton, K.G., E. Stallard, and K. Liu. 1993. Forecasts of Active Life Expectancy: Policy and Fiscal Implications. *Journal of Gerontology* 48 (Special Issue): 11–26.

Marion Merrell Dow. 1993. Nursing home and home care industry report. *Managed Care Digest: Long Term Care Edition*. Kansas City, Missouri.

Marmor, T.R., M. Schlesinger, and R.W. Smithey. 1987. Nonprofit Organizations and Health Care. In *The Nonprofit Sector: A Research Handbook*, ed. W. W. Powell, 221–39. New Haven: Yale University Press.

Miller, J.A. 1991. *Comunity-Based Long Term Care: Innovative Models*. Newbury Park, CA: Sage Publications.

Miller, N. 1992. Medicaid 2176 Home and Community-Based Care Waivers: The First 10 Years. *Health Affairs*. 162–71.

Mundinger, M.O. 1983. *Home Care Controversy: Too Little, Too Late*. Rockville, MD: Aspen.

National Association for Home Care (NAHC). 1993. Basic Statistics about Home Care 1993. Washington, D.C.: NAHC.

National Health Policy Forum (NHPF). 1993. Adding to the Continuum: Emerging New Markets for Subacute Care: Issue Brief No. 626. D.L. Zimmerman, Author, National Health Policy Forum. Washington, D.C.: The George Washington University.

Neu, C.R., and S.C. Harrison. 1988. *Posthospital Care Before and After the Medicare Prospective Payment System*. Santa Monica, CA: Rand.

Spillman, B.C., and P. Kemper. 1993. Community-Dwelling Elders Would Benefit the Most from Expanding Long-Term Care Benefits. Research Activities, Agency for Health Care Policy and Research, No. 167, August, 1993, 13–14. See also, *Home Health Care Services Quarterly* 13: 5–34.

Spohn, P.H., L.A. Bergthold, and C.L. Estes. 1987/88. From Cottages to Condos: The Expansion of the Home Health Care Industry Under Medicare. *Home Health Care Services Quarterly* 8(4): 25–55.

Strahan, G.W. 1993. Overview of Home Health and Hospice Care Patients. Advance Data, No. 235, July 28: 1–9. Washington, D.C.: US DHHS/NCHS/CDC.

Swan, J.H., and C.L. Estes. 1993. Access to Nursing Home and Home Health Services. In *Long Term Care Crisis: Elders Trapped in the No-Care Zone*, ed.

C.L. Estes, J.H. Swan, and Associates, 143–54. Newbury Park, CA: Sage.
Tauber, C.M. 1992. *Sixty-Five Plus in America*. Washington, D.C.: US Bureau of the Census.
US General Accounting Office. 1990. Medicare: Increased Denials of Home Health Claims during 1986 and 1987. Washington, D.C.: Government Printing Office (Jan. 24).
US Senate Special Committee on Aging. 1988. Home Care at the Crossroads: An Information Paper. No. 100-H-April. Washington, D.C.: US GPO.
US Senate Special Committee on Aging. 1990. *Developments in Aging: 1990*. Vol. 1: 188. Washington, D.C.: US GPO.
Waldo, D.R., K.R. Levit, and H. Lazenby. 1986. National Health Expenditures, 1985. *Health Care Financing Review* 8(1): 1–21.
Winship, C., and S. Rosen. 1988. Introduction: Sociological and Economic Approaches to the Analysis of Social Structure. *American Journal of Sociology* 94(Suppl.): 1–16.

2

Boundaries of Home Care: Can a Home-Care Approach Transform LTC Institutions?

Rosalie A. Kane

Introduction

The definition of home care appears obvious; indeed, it seems to be contained in the very term. Home care seems to refer to care given to people with disabilities or diseases in their homes. In the United States, home care also refers to a series of programs that are licensed and reimbursed in specific ways and that have been contrasted to nursing-home care as a way of serving people with chronic illnesses and functional impairments.

This chapter identifies several trends that, if allowed to continue, blur the definitions of home care and institutional care, change the cast of characters providing both types of care, and even challenge the definition of home. Taken to logical conclusions, this redefinition of home care could result in a sharply different conceptualization of both home care and nursing homes. The chapter begins with a discussion of trends for some home-care providers to deliver personal assistance services (PAS) in the community to people who are not homebound and also of the trend to provide home-care services to people whose "homes" are apartment units in organized assisted-living complexes. The chapter next discusses features associated with a "home-care model" for long-term care (LTC), and then turns to factors that facilitate or impede these trends. The conclusion summarizes the challenges to policy makers that stem from the blurring of boundaries between home-care and other LTC services.

Home-care and residential-care providers may decide either to welcome this boundary blurring or to fight to maintain programmatic distinctions. Arguably, widespread confusion about the definition of home and home care could be a positive development, bringing new possibilities to home-care providers, reconceptualizing the work done by staff of residential settings, and, most important, bringing new options to disabled people of all ages. The trends toward clouding distinctions between home care and institutional care particularly promise to improve the lives of elderly disabled people – the largest population in need of care and the people whose care presently is most formula driven, owing to the regulatory and reimbursement provisions in Medicare and in state Medicaid policies.

Thematically interwoven are arguments for the policy of developing and financing a flexible array of home-care services that achieve the following:

- Eliminate arbitrary distinctions between home health care and other in-home service.
- Encourage a PAS model of home care, which provides service to persons with functional impairments in the places where they live and at any community locations where they wish to go for vocational, business, or recreational reasons.
- Encourage a PAS model of group residential care where people who have relocated into the setting because of functional impairments receive their care in, at a minimum, small, self-contained apartments with full baths and kitchenettes, and where they can experience the privacy, individualization, dignity, and normal lifestyles that are absent from the dominant nursing-home model.
- Change the balance of power for both home care and residential care (now nursing-home care) so that the clients or, when applicable, their agents (usually family members) have more control.
- In group residential LTC settings, separate the mechanisms for

financing the housing and hotel-like functions from those for the care functions (the former include housekeeping, laundry, and restaurant services; the latter include personal care, nursing, and other professional services).

Trends toward Blurring Boundaries

In the past decade, "home care" has assumed a wider meaning than care in self-contained private homes. On the one hand, home-care providers are following clients into the community; on the other, home-care providers are following people into group-living situations. Both these directions were accentuated in the community LTC entitlement proposed by President Clinton in 1993 as part of the Health Security Act. Although the specific proposed health-care reforms expired in 1994, the principles enunciated for home- and community-based care were derived from experiences at the state level, and states are continuing to develop their LTC programs along those lines (Kane and Kane 1994).

Home care moves out of the private home

Increasingly, home-care workers are assisting home-care clients, including some elderly clients, in settings other than their own homes. For example, home-care workers may assist clients to travel about the community, participate in the labor force, go shopping, and perform errands. This development has been heralded by some spokespersons for younger disabled people, who advocate for PAS under the direction of the consumer rather than, or as a supplement to, home health care under a medical model. Arguably, PAS maximize overall functioning of people with disabilities (Sabatino and Litvak 1992).

Spokespersons for young disabled people often object to both words of the term "home care." Some prefer to reserve the term "care" for intimate relationships characterized by affection, maintaining that disabled people who need concrete help or assistance should be able to choose whether or not to have that help provided by family members or others in caring relationships with them (Asch 1993). Furthermore, they argue that disabled people need assistance not only when they are in their homes, but also to function and flourish at work and at leisure in the larger community. Most certainly this model is incompatible with the requirement that clients must be homebound to receive assistance. Personal care attendants are viewed as enabling clients to go where they wish whenever they wish (Litvak, Zukas, and Heumann 1987).

Most of the public dollars for financing home care for the elderly come from Medicare, a program that requires the beneficiary of services to be homebound, to have rehabilitation potential, and to have a medically identified need for skilled care on an intermittent basis. Medicaid programs in most states mimic this model, which has become ingrained after almost three decades as practice orthodoxy in the thinking of staffs of thousands of home health agencies. Thus, home care for the elderly in the United States has a dynamic that differs markedly from PAS. On the other hand, by 1991, statewide PAS benefits ordered by physicians were available in 28 state Medicaid programs. These programs largely serve younger recipients, and tasks requiring professional skill are explicitly excluded from the benefit (Lewis-Idema, Falik, and Ginsburg 1991). However, the boundaries between the services of a PAS worker and of a home health aide, or even a licensed professional under home health funding, are less clear cut than the program descriptions would suggest.

Recent developments in state-funded and Medicaid-waiver-funded programs, moreover, have allowed an end-run around Medicare definitions of home health care for the elderly. For example, most waiver programs emphasize PAS rather than home health care, and they make eligibility for benefits contingent on measurable functional impairment rather than medically endorsed "need" for specific services (e.g., skilled nursing, physical therapy, speech therapy, occupational therapy, medical social work, and home health aide services, as in the Medicare rules).

Thus, care plans under Medicaid waiver and state programs tend to endorse and authorize an amount of help (measured in hours) and enumerate the tasks for which help is required rather than order services from particular professionals. In some jurisdictions, home-care personnel assist elderly clients by taking them on walks and accompanying them to the doctor, the grocery store, and other destinations where they have business. Depending on the program, the home-care provider's duties may include chauffeuring the client in their own or the worker's cars and assisting the client in participating in activities that might be viewed as social. Well-to-do elderly people with functional impairments have purchased such assistance for centuries; what is new in the United States is the gradual and somewhat grudging recognition that people requiring public subsidy for their care should also have access to this model of service. Of course, when the person is eligible for Medicare coverage, the

Medicaid program seeks to utilize the federal dollars, and the Medicare regulations and conventions apply. The relation between services under the two forms of funding is typically poorly articulated.

The trends toward PAS were reflected in the 1993 Health Security Act, which called for a new community LTC entitlement with the following features:

1   Program eligibility is not based on age.
2   Program eligibility is based on measurable impairments (the measures differing somewhat for different target groups) rather than on medically prescribed services.
3   Personal care is at the heart of the benefit.
4   States are required to make available client-directed home care (where the client is responsible for selecting, training, supervising, and evaluating the worker) and care purchased from agencies.

Home-care workers follow clients into group residential settings

In some jurisdictions home-care agencies and workers provide service to people living in group residential settings such as board and care homes (Hawes, Wildfire, and Lux 1993) and adult foster homes (Kane et al. 1991b). In such instances, a person who receives room and board and housekeeping help from staff of a residential setting also may receive personal care and/or home health care from an outside agency. This clearly stretches the definition of home. Such patterns are familiar in Canada (Kane and Kane 1985) and in Europe (Jamieson 1991), but are relatively new in the United States.

Recent trends in the United States have encouraged a group residential model, often called assisted living (Mollica et al. 1992; Kane and Wilson 1993). There, people disabled enough to be found in nursing homes live and receive service in self-contained, unfurnished apartments in complexes that offer a full range of personal care, nursing services, housekeeping, and congregate meals. In these settings, the residents (or tenants, as they may be called) are likely to have units with full baths, kitchenettes with stoves and refrigerators, and keys to lock their doors. Attendants bring care and service to the apartments according to individual plans. One could argue that such settings should be construed as the clients' own homes, analogous to apartments anywhere, rather than as upscale institutions, resembling nursing homes. If viewed as a home, then the services constitute a form of home care, whether they are provided by staff in the complex, by home health workers from an outside agency, or some combination of these.

Currently, state regulation of assisted-living settings has resulted in substantial intrastate and interstate variation (Kane and Wilson 1993). Among the standards that may be in place are environmental standards, which refer to the settings themselves; staffing and services standards, which refer to type and ratio of staff; and admission and retention standards, which refer to the characteristics of the clientele who may be admitted to, or retained in, the setting (Kane and Wilson 1993). Some states have forms of assisted living that are literally licensed as types of home care, which means that operators must take out a separate home-care license if they provide personal care services to their tenants. In other jurisdictions, operators of assisted-living complexes have been precluded from delivering hands-on personal care or nursing services directly; they may, however, help their tenants gain access to services from certified home health agencies or from other home-care agencies. Some states require no licensure for assisted-living complexes at all if the complexes are composed of individual apartments with cooking facilities. In these states, no governmental subsidy is requested for the shelter or the service, arrangements can be made for tenants to receive care from staff of the program, staff of outside agencies, or both. The charges and the location of the care coordination role vary in such programs.

In some state jurisdictions, state-funded or Medicaid-waiver-funded clients have been able to receive subsidized care in assisted-living programs as authorized by a case manager who controls access to the subsidies. In such schemes, the tenants pay for the housing, housekeeping, and congregate meals from their incomes, and the service component is fully or partly funded by the public program (if these tenant clients meet the pertinent income requirements). If an older person has a very low income, the housing component may also be subsidized by SSI supplements, and public assistance may be used to furnish the apartment unit. In some states, notably Oregon, most of the services are purchased directly from the operator of the licensed assisted-living setting, although the case manager or the private-pay client may purchase additional assistance from outside agencies or consultants, say, home health agencies or licensed health-care personnel as needed.

Again, some federal reform proposals and a few existing state policies recognize and encourage assisted living by making people eligible for the new community-care service regardless of where they reside as long as they are not in a licensed nursing home.

Credibility for the role blurring in the definition of home is also found in a recent monograph on home care for the elderly, designed to provide an overview of the field:

> The concept of "home" also requires comment. In the current context, this includes any residential setting in which formal medical services are not provided as part of the housing component, although supportive services may be. In other words, nursing homes are excluded but board and care homes are included. "Home" may mean a detached home, an apartment in a family member's home or a large complex, or a unit in a congregate housing arrangement with supportive services. (Benjamin 1992, 13).

For practical purposes, some states have defined a home by the presence of a kitchen with cooking facilities (or at least a microwave and small refrigerator) and a bathroom within the unit rather than off a common corridor. Market analysts assert that older people and their families much prefer this design even when they are so disabled that their use of the kitchen will be minimal and when they require the three daily served meals in a congregate dining room, which could be viewed as a restaurant.

Features of a Home-Care Model of LTC

A home-care model, in this discussion, refers to a model of care that shifts the balance of power from professionals to consumers and views the client's living space as his or her home, where he or she can expect to exercise control. This chapter argues for such a model, which in turn has minimum requirements. The residential setting must be sufficiently private and self-contained to coincide with a reasonable definition of home; and the providers of service, whether they are home-care agency personnel or staff of the residential program, must treat clients as tenants in their homes rather than residents of an institution.

A hospital or a nursing home is the turf of paid staff, both professional and paraprofessional. A person's home, according to the proverb, is his or her castle. The very circumstances that render quality assurance difficult in home care (Kane et al. 1991a) give consumers a chance to make the ultimate decisions about their lives. Elderly and disabled people in their own homes have the opportunity to set their schedules, eat their choice of food, maintain their lifestyles, and reject medical and nursing advice from time to time (Kane et al. 1994). Elderly and disabled people in nursing homes live according to care plans, presumably crafted for their benefit. These care plans shape the clients' daily lives, and exceptions require specific permission from professionals. Nursing-home residents have little opportunity to set their own schedules or reject professional advice (Kane and Caplan 1990).

Thus, clients receiving home care, in contrast to those with equivalent disability receiving nursing-home care, are more likely to have individualized care, to exercise choice, to maintain privacy, and to experience "normal" lifestyles. Some would argue that values of individualization, dignity, privacy, autonomy, and "normalization" should also apply to nursing-home residents. However, the design of the space, with its doubled-bedded rooms and lack of privacy, and the conventions of care (driven by regulation, interpretation of regulation, fear of liability, and efforts at efficiency) stand in the way (Kane and Caplan 1990).

Arguably, therefore, settings where elderly or disabled people relocate in order to receive LTC services at affordable prices should be designed to feel like a private home, and the service model should foster a balance of power between client and care provider that resembles home more than it does nursing-home care. With some conceptual rearrangement, policymakers and regulators could begin to consider complexes that would serve disabled persons as a collection of individual homes, avoiding the sparse and uniform physical settings and the forced sharing of quarters with strangers that would belie the concept of home.

Home tenancy (whether ownership or rental) does not carry unbridled license. The mortgage or rent must be paid. The property must be kept in reasonable condition to protect the investment of mortgage holders or owners. The tenant's personal habits must not constitute a public nuisance or health hazard for the others in the building or neighborhood. Short of these kinds of problems, however, public authorities cannot remove people from their own homes against their will just because of a view that they would be safer or better served somewhere else. In contrast, a resident may be removed from a licensed board-and-care home, foster home, or assisted-living setting in many states because his or her disabilities exceed the legal capacity for service licensed for that setting. A person living in an apartment, however, cannot easily be removed to a "higher" level of institutional care because, for example, he or she cannot transfer in and out of bed, or because a professional has judged that he or she is unsafe in the setting. Such removals are only possible in the wake of draconian legal steps to assert that the person is incompetent, and to strip him or her of legal rights. When an entity is construed as a private home, its inhabitants have rights that do not apply in a health-related facility.

To summarize, consumers who experience a home-care model for LTC control its arrangements, the activities that take place there, and the timing and intensity of the health- and personal-care services brought to them there. The living space must meet minimum prerequisites for privacy and autonomous living: single occupancy, a full bathroom inside the unit, a kitchenette, and a locking door. The tenant (or the tenant's agent, in the case of those who are cognitively impaired) bears ordinary responsibility for upkeep of the premises and payment of the rent. The rent and the service arrangements are priced separately, and may be subsidized through either public or private insurance.

Forces Accelerating and Impeding Boundary Breakdown

Various factors contribute to the blurring between home- and community-based services and institutional services. These factors largely provide opportunities for expanded home care and for more flexible, normal, dignified approaches to the care of people of all ages with functional impairments. However, forces in the public policy arena at both the state and the federal level threaten to undermine the best features – tenant autonomy and reasonable pricing – inherent in the assisted-living movement.

Cost-effective alternatives to nursing homes

Starting from the assumption of a dichotomy between home- and community-based care, on the one hand, and nursing-home care, on the other, policymakers and researchers have labored for at least two decades to identify the circumstances under which home care can be a cost-effective alternative (Applebaum, Harrigan, and Kemper 1986; Weissert, Cready, and Pawelak 1988). A series of controlled demonstration projects has shown that, under current pricing structures and service models, home care will be more expensive than nursing-home care for people with substantial disabilities, unless they receive the bulk of their care from unpaid family members. The economies of scale attained by caring for people with substantial disability under a single roof, rather than at far-flung individual locations, and the current pricing structures for Medicaid payment in both sectors have foreordained that nursing homes will be more cost-effective than community care for identical clientele with severe functional impairments.

Such studies, of course, are done in the context of reimbursement rates established for nursing homes by state Medicaid programs (often artificially low) and rules governing home-care frequency and type. Ironically, given the below-subsistence low wages typically paid the line paraprofessional home-care worker, the cost of home care has often been kept relatively high by the amounts of service deemed necessary, the high costs of the legally required visits of professional nurses either to supervise the workers at established intervals or, sometimes, to render services that only licensed nurses can provide, and the front-end costs of professional (often team) assessment and care planning. Care for very disabled persons in group settings should be cheaper than care at home because of absence of travel costs, joint production functions, and economies of scale.

There is a break-even point below which the cost of home care is the same or less than the cost of nursing-home care, and after which home care will exceed the cost of nursing-home care. Obviously that break-even point is more likely to be reached if the home-care client has high levels of disability, has little or no family help, and lives in a home that is inaccessible or difficult to maintain. It is less often recognized that people with substantial disabilities will be likely to receive care at home under the break-even point if nursing-home reimbursement rates are relatively high, if home-care rates are relatively low, if plans for home care are relatively parsimonious, and if home-care providers can organize their services to achieve economies of scale. Such an eventuality can be achieved by eliminating requirements for minimum hours of service and by assigning workers or teams to particular buildings and geographic areas where many clients reside.

Nursing homes are billed as 24-hour care. In a typical scenario, a doctor explains to a family that the discharge planner will look for a nursing home because their mother needs 24-hour care. In reality, these settings provide remarkably little nursing care. A recent study of a large sample of nursing homes and nursing-home residents in six states uncovered the following facts: about 39 percent of the sample received no care from a registered nurse (RN) during the 24-hour study period; the average RN time per resident was 7.9 minutes, the average LPN time 15.5 minutes; and the average nursing-assistance time 76.9 minutes (Friedlob 1993). Yet this modest amount of care cannot be replicated at home for the same price because the nursing home efficiently provides stand-by assistance and can meet unscheduled, quickly arising needs.

The need to re-examine the way housing and ongoing care needs are met is illustrated by the experience of On Lok, a capitated program in San Francisco's Chinatown, where low-income enrollees with nursing-home levels of disability are served by an organization that receives a capitated rate from Medicare and Medicaid and is at financial risk for all the enrollees' acute-care and LTC needs. The program and its replication programs, known as Programs for All-Inclusive Care for the Elderly (PACE), rely on adult day health care to monitor and serve the clientele. They have found that highly disabled clients who need care at night and on weekends, and who have no relatives able to provide this assistance, cannot be cared for cost-effectively or kept out of nursing homes unless their housing and services are rearranged. Thus, On Lok has invested in housing developments that have created communities of elderly apartment dwellers. On Lok has also enabled its enrollees to obtain assistance from live-in personal care attendants. In some arrangements, one such attendant provides service to several On Lok clients who live in the same apartment (Kane, Illston, and Miller 1992).

Thus, capitated programs like On Lok and PACE (so far feasible only to low-income persons dually eligible for Medicare and Medicaid) had to innovate in order to cut through the barriers between home care and nursing-home care and to provide practical assistance to people in settings they could consider as home. This same principle applies to services that are pieced together by, and on behalf of, functionally impaired elderly people whose incomes exceed Medicaid eligibility and who can afford to pay for much of their care. At present, rigid licensing definitions for group residential settings, for home-care agencies, and even for home-care workers may prohibit their purchase of the kind of help consumers want at prices they can afford. Developments in assisted living can cut through those barriers.

Some state officials still think in strict dichotomies between nursing homes and their "alternatives." Indeed, such distinctions are embedded in the home- and community-based Medicaid-waiver program, in which those served must have a medical "need" for nursing-home care according to some operational definition. Unfortunately, several states acknowledge a catch-22 attached to the use of waivers for assisted living. Licensure for group residential homes may prohibit admitting or retaining anyone who needs routine nursing service, yet the waiver requires that clients need a nursing home before their care can be reimbursed.

Other states, impelled partly by safety concerns and partly by pressure from the nursing-home industry, are setting new thresholds for nursing-home admission, construing that some "nursing-home eligible" people can be served in assisted living, which permits them to be financed under the waiver, whereas others are classified as too disabled. A state using case-mix designations for Medicaid nursing-home reimbursement may target assisted living to the lower acuity levels of the nursing-home clientele. Or, a state may determine that some procedures or some client disabilities are incompatible with assisted living. Some states, notably Oregon, have made a commitment that Medicaid-waiver- and state-funded LTC programs will provide true alternatives to nursing homes for people with high levels of disability. They have accordingly created a range of flexible home-care options, some linked to housing alternatives. In a review of such programs in Oregon, Washington, and Wisconsin, the US General Accounting Office (1994) substantiated the widely held perception of Oregon's programs as both cost-effective and user-friendly.

Such steps still vastly expand the home-care-like possibilities in assisted living. However, the policies just described cling to the idea of a continuum that suggests that professionals can determine how different disability levels dictate different care arrangements and that rates the nursing-home model as the most appropriate for some. The goal of a continuum of care can be critiqued insofar as a continuum requires professionals to judge the best "placement" for clients (Kane 1993a). On these grounds, continuing-care retirement communities are vulnerable to criticism. Although designed to offer older people the security of a full spectrum of care from home care to nursing homes, typically the consumer does not retain the right to decide where in the community to live, and fixed levels of care are linked to residential arrangements along the continuum.

Nurse delegation

Many nurse practice statutes have been interpreted to mean that only an RN or licensed practical nurse (LPN) can do a wide range of tasks (e.g., administer oral or injectable medications, care for wounds, monitor vital signs, change catheters, monitor ostomies, monitor people on respirators). Of course, in practice, family members carry out these tasks for their relatives of all ages. In fact, the home-care field has a long literature and tradition of instructing

Boundaries of Home Care   35

patients in self care and family members in the care of patients who cannot care for themselves. Although some strict interpretations of nurse practice acts state that even unpaid relatives cannot legally perform functions defined as nursing practice (Kapp 1993), home health nurses themselves have included the transmission of skills to family members in the definition of their functions. It is only when individuals unrelated to the client perform tasks and receive compensation for them that the boundaries are drawn between the responsibilities of a nurse and those of other personnel, and the conditions under which the latter are carried out receive scrutiny.

In the late 1980s, Oregon modified its nurse practice act explicitly to permit people who are not nurses to perform nursing functions if they have been taught by a nurse on a patient-specific and procedure-specific basis and have been certified as able to do the task. Thus, paraprofessional home-care workers, adult foster-care staff, and assisted-living staff may be instructed in the specific nursing procedure for a particular patient. Records of tenants in assisted-living settings in Oregon typically contain documentation for each person who has been delegated as capable of performing a list of nursing functions for each tenant. Assisted-living settings in Oregon typically hire a nurse directly if they serve more than 50 tenants, and typically contract with a nurse for part-time service if they are smaller, but any and all nursing procedures can be delegated to people who are not nurses. Indeed, the nurse on the staff or on contract may spend considerable time preparing others for their delegated duties. Sometimes staff of certified home-care agencies provide the delegation instruction to staff of adult foster-care homes while delivering Medicare-reimbursed home health service. Oregon case-management programs also employ or contract with nurses who can provide the delegation training to persons who deliver home care under the client-directed home-care program. Some adult foster-care homes also have their own contractual arrangements with a nurse who provides this function. Contrast this to rules in some states (e.g. Washington) that require licensed nursing personnel for assisted living, thus driving up the costs and also making small programs economically inviable.

Oregon authorities believe that their nurse-delegation provisions opened the way for the state's well-known cost-effective community programs (US General Accounting Office 1994) for people who are as disabled as nursing-home residents in other states. Kansas also has nurse-delegation provisions in its nurse practice act, although these do not extend to injectable medications. Texas enacted such a provision in 1992, and Colorado also has made changes that permit greater delegation of nursing functions. Some informants suggest that the current nurse practice acts in their states do not really prohibit an Oregon-style delegation, although, in practice, it might not occur. For example, Minnesota's nurse practice act explicitly states that licensed personnel may delegate their tasks. It is left to the nurse, however, to interpret what tasks may be safely delegated and how much ongoing supervision would be expected of the nurse, who is responsible for any untoward events. Conservative interpretations are most likely under these conditions, especially since home health nurses are schooled by Medicare regulations that require frequent supervision of home health aides. Minnesota's home-care licensing statute is more restrictive than nurse practice statutes because it exacts requirements that all personnel delivering more than 40 hours of assistance a year to a functionally impaired person in their own homes must receive training and supervision from a licensed agency (Kane, O'Connor, and Baker 1995).

One nursing task ripe for delegation is dispensing of oral medications. This task is performed by outpatients on their own behalf as part of regular medical practice and by parents on behalf of their outpatient children. Performance is not particularly monitored and is known to vary markedly from the specifications for dosage, timing, and other conditions on the prescriptions. Yet current regulations and practice conventions that allow the patient and the family to assume this responsibility do not allow nonlicensed paid caregivers to dispense medications, even if they have been taught how, and even though one would expect accuracy standards to be at least as good as those observed by the patient and family. Because medication management is one of the services that assisted-living tenants most frequently need, elaborate rules are built around a system that is often a charade. Assisted-living staff are allowed to provide assistance with self-administration of medications. In some states (e.g., New York) self-administration of medicines is construed so broadly that it can describe a staff member selecting the medication from a locked cabinet, delivering it to the tenant in unit doses, or opening the bottle, removing the medicine, and placing the pill on the tenant's tongue. This liberal definition of self-administration of medications avoids grappling with the real issue, which is whether a nurse must administer medications or provide frequent surveillance of paraprofessionals who administer medications when clients are incapable of administering the medications themselves. So far, a number of states find it easier to create a fiction that many clients – even those with dementia – are self-administering drugs rather than to face this issue head-on.

The National Council of State Boards of Nursing (1990) and the American Nurses Association (1992) have addressed the issue of delegation directly. Neither organization is opposed to nurse delegation as long as authority to delegate is at the discretion of the nurse and nurses are not forced to delegate tasks. In general, nursing assessment, diagnosis, and planning require professional judgment and are viewed as inappropriate to delegate to unlicensed personnel. A review of this topic (Kane, O'Connor, and Baker 1995) suggests that considerable training and support services are needed before nurses generally will be comfortable with exercising delegation.

ADA and fair housing

The Americans with Disabilities Act (ADA) is new enough that regulations have not been fully promulgated for housing settings, nor has much case law been developed. It is plausible, however, for the ADA to be evoked to prohibit insistence that people be evicted from assisted-living settings where they, in fact, have their home because of increasing disability. In some instances where this has occurred, the argument has been successfully made that persons with dementia need not leave a particular assisted-living setting just because the state had approved for the setting only people who could summon help and preserve themselves against danger. The Fair Housing Act (FHA) prohibits discrimination in housing because of disability, and may also be invoked to establish the right of disabled people to live in homes of their own choosing (Redfoot 1993). Although the terms "eviction" and "transfer to a higher level of care" denote very different acts, their effects may appear identical to the person being moved.

ADA and FHA introduce untraveled roads in law. Clearly, a hospital "discriminates" on the basis of health and disability; such distinctions form the basis for diagnosis and treatment recommendations. Nursing homes make such discriminations, and case-mix reimbursement systems employ fine gradations of payment based on configurations of measurable functional and cognitive disability and prescriptions for measurable service.

Thus, a health-care facility is expected to make distinctions based on disability. A hotel or a housing development is not. This leaves open possible legal interpretations regarding assisted-living complexes where tenants rent self-contained apartments, however small, and receive hotel-like services from the complex (e.g., meals in a dining room and housekeeping). Some developers and managers of assisted-living programs interviewed in a recent study (Kane and Wilson 1993) frankly preferred that their product be construed as a health-care setting because they wished to be exempted from ADA and Fair Housing requirements; those who prefer assisted living to be an option that replaces nursing homes for many residents rather than a niche on a continuum expressed the hope that ADA requirements would undermine the state licensing rules that force discharge of people at specified levels of disability.

At present, requirements for assisted living are murky and sometimes contradictory. For instance, the assisted-living accommodations may be in private apartments with kitchens, but the state may require a higher standard of fire safety for retention of persons who cannot transfer in such assisted-living settings than it does for hotels or high-rise residential structures that may well be housing people with the identical physical limitations. Another contradiction may occur if the state takes no notice of the situations that prevail in the private market (often because the residences themselves are unlicensed), but imposes strict admission, retention, and service-level standards on persons who receive public subsidy for the service. This introduces the inequity that well-to-do people can live in apartments that provide service and can purchase private-duty care to supplement what the complex provides when they have reached a level of disability that would prohibit a home-care agency or management of assisted living from billing the state for their care.

Pressures for state governments
It is axiomatic that LTC is a large part of state expenditure, and states have many pressures that influence their stance about the emerging phenomenon of assisted living. Most states feel impelled to curtail the growth of LTC budgets, and are willing to invest in assisted living only if they believe it really can reduce total fiscal liability for LTC. States are also concerned about quality issues; state officials dread the specter of a major board-and-care quality scandal on their watch. Officials may fear that the delegation of nursing functions and the increased personal autonomy for tenants associated with some assisted-living settings are formulas for disaster, and that the cost of doing it any other way would be the same or more than nursing-home costs.

States also combine an interest in system reform with a need to utilize existing state resources. In many states, the licensed entities providing board and care are sharply bifurcated into relatively luxurious entities for private-pay clientele and lower-amenity settings that accept SSI as payment in full for the room-and-board function. Clients and workers in the latter "SSI-settings" are already marginalized (Eckert and Lyon 1992). Some states doubt that they can mandate the kind of minimal environmental standards for private occupancy, kitchens, and baths to pertain to programs serving low-income clientele and justify costs. Oregon, in contrast, does require single occupancy, full bath, kitchenettes, and many other features that enhance autonomy and dignity for its licensed assisted-living facilities and expects the requirement to be met regardless of the clientele payment source. Oregon, however, has few staffing standards (largely the requirement that at least one person be on duty and awake at any time) or service standards (three meals must be served congregate style), trusting to internal and external case-management and market forces to maintain quality. External case-management is provided by the case managers who allocate the service for low-income people and, therefore, have a presence in the setting. The state also expects providers to have an internal capacity for case management and to have developed specific plans with and for each tenant. Market forces act in the sense that privately paying consumers seem to prefer foster care (Kane et al. 1991b) and assisted living to nursing homes. Finally, nurse delegation and regulatory relief keep costs within bounds.

Most other states have proliferated staffing and service standards that drive up costs and have failed to establish the minimal environmental standards that would make assisted living fit common definitions of home. (Despite the rhetoric that promotes the view of a nursing home or board-and-care home as the resident's home, when staff can enter at will, when residents are told not to expect their possessions to be safe, when hospital beds and small amounts of furniture are arranged according to regulation and staff convenience, and when the mathematics of room assignment preclude true choice of roommates or of single rooms for most people, residents and their families are not fooled. They know they are living in an institution.)

In wending their way through the problems created by a genuine wish to improve quality, an urgent need to contain costs, and a desire to get a proactive handle on planning by building on the existing housing stock, state governments are also subject to multiple interest-group pressures. Nursing homes may lobby against rules that allow alternative housing settings to serve any but the least disabled of the LTC clientele – i.e. those who do not "need" nursing-home care. Existing board-and-care homes may lobby against enhanced environmental standards for new payment programs that would eliminate them as vendors. Professional groups like nursing and pharmacy boards may argue that flexibility reduces quality. Ombudsmen and advocates for LTC clients may also argue for increased protections. Sometimes consumer groups convey the double message to state officials that they want increased personal autonomy for their constituency while still holding the state responsible for accidents that occur to clients who are receiving care with public dollars or from publicly licensed programs. Most federal and state home-care organizations have not yet formulated policy on the issue of assisted living (Kane and Wilson 1993).

Policy Challenges

At present, organized home care (especially organized home *health* care) has paid little attention to assisted living or other developments that may change the very shape of home-care provision. A key informant study of assisted living (Kane and Wilson 1993) showed that, with some exceptions, state and federal home health or home-care organizations had not developed policy on the topic and were not particularly monitoring developments. At some point, however, home-care organizations will be jolted into taking a stand on the topics discussed here. Their positions will either move service systems in the direction of more flexible, individualized provision of care to persons with functional disabilities regardless of where they live or reaffirm rigid service categories of home care, board and care, and nursing-home care. Arguably, the way of thinking about the "customer" that has necessarily been reflected by home-care agencies, who realize their staff cannot ultimately control the consumer's behavior, would benefit workers in other locations of care. The agencies and individuals who provide home care could, with reorganization and different ground rules, work in settings that are not exactly private homes, but are their clients' homes nonetheless. For this to occur, the home-care industry needs to consider the following issues.

Distinguishing type of care from place of care
The place of care should not be confused with the type of care. Public policies are dysfunctional if they insist that people who are "appropriate" for care in a nursing-home setting because of their disability levels, therefore must receive care either in a nursing home or not at all (at least under public expense). As an intermediate step, home-care providers and case managers for home-care programs should reconsider their criteria for determining that a client can no longer be cared for safely in the community.

The interchangeability of various care arrangements for persons needing LTC should be recognized. It is a fallacy to suggest that a single best arrangement can be designed for an individual based on his or her health needs. Personal choice and resources can suggest different ways for services to be mixed and matched.

Delegation
Serious attention must be given to determining what care can be safely delegated to non-professionals and under what circumstances. Rather than supporting rules that require certain increments of professional supervision (which are based on professional orthodoxy), the home health industry should support and participate in studies that test the efficacy of arrangements where nurses provide training and backup support rather than ongoing supervision at fixed intervals.

Personal assistant services (PAS) models
Flexible home care and PAS that are under the control of the consumer of care to the extent of that consumer's desire and capability are goals that disabled people of all ages are likely to support. Policymakers will confront a number of decisions, however, as they move toward this model. One issue requires disentangling the concept of PAS and consumer direction from that of the consumer as employer. For in-home workers to receive adequate protection as employees, it may be impractical to expect each disabled individual to manage the benefits of a small group of employees. Perhaps different kinds of home-care agencies can emerge that serve as low-cost finders, screeners, and fiscal intermediaries for such workers. Another issue concerns whether the public mood will tolerate an approach to serving disabled people that emphasizes PAS and facilitating their functioning in the community. Although unit costs of PAS are lower than those of home health, some critics might view it as frivolous to use public dollars to assist older people to navigate in the community, although they may be willing to use such money to enable younger people to remain in the workforce. Subsidized services should be linked to clear, and probably stringent, eligibility criteria. Moreover, it will be important to explore ways of ensuring that the technical health-care needs of those receiving PAS are met.

Assisted living with services
Home-care organizations should welcome the opportunity to provide service in group residential settings (here called assisted living). They should also be open to arrangements where assisted-

living staff become a de facto home-care agency that provides most of the service to the clients. The latter is obviously a more efficient model for meeting unscheduled need. Nurses and other professional therapists from outside agencies may have to visit tenants of assisted living when they have specialized needs that cannot be met internally. They may also be engaged to teach and delegate tasks to unlicensed personnel. The effects and costs of various ways of mingling staff-delivered and externally contracted services in programs of various sizes and in environments with varying service availability should be studied.

This chapter has argued for a minimum environmental standard that emphasizes privacy, space, and autonomy-enhancing features like bathrooms and kitchenettes, even for people who are very disabled and may seldom use the kitchens. These features may be criticized as either an expensive indulgence or a dangerous innovation that combines more opportunity for accidents with less opportunity for staff surveillance. Therefore, studies of the costs, risks, and benefits of these interventions are needed. It is also argued that states should not succumb to the pressure to subsidize LTC services provided by the staffs of board and care homes. This view could be criticized on equity grounds. Some question the fairness of denying a care benefit to those living in board-and-care homes while providing such a benefit to those in assisted-living settings. However, it seems fair enough from the perspective of low-income consumers; once they are deemed to need a nursing level of services, they would be able to receive them in an enhanced environment. The main equity issue concerns providers seeking reimbursement. One cannot, however, expect the marketplace to change the paradigm of care if financing is provided in settings that meet neither minimal expectations as homes nor the staffing and health-related requirements of nursing homes. Ethicists might well turn their attention to these issues (Kane 1993b); in the meantime, obligations to consumers seem to trump any obligation to provide a market to providers. Analyses of the kinds of regulations and quality assurance provisions that would enhance the evolution of assisted living for older people with disabilities, such as recent work by Wilson (1995), are much needed.

Some advocates may object to any idea of relocating people with disabilities to assisted-living settings rather than leaving them in their own home. Here, however, we must distinguish between a person's own home and a person's original home. Many people experience multiple residential relocations over a lifetime. The value-laden question concerns what actually constitutes a home. A small group setting housing four individuals may be less of a "home" than is a small apartment for one person in an assisted-living complex that has sixty such apartments and a staff available to provide help and care in the unit.

Charting the future of the nursing home

What about nursing homes as we know them? There will still be people who cannot benefit at all from the privacy and autonomy inherent in an assisted-living model of care. For example, this service system makes no sense for people who are comatose or so severely demented that they are in vegetative states or do not interact with their environment in the slightest way. The model may not work for some medically unstable people who truly need around-the-clock high-tech care.

It is commonplace to note that the clientele of nursing homes has changed in the past decade. Residents are sicker than they used to be, and shorter stays, terminating in death or rapid discharge, are more common (Kodner 1993). Many proposals have been advanced for more effective nursing-home care in the future, some of which emphasize the need for the nursing home to be better integrated with care networks providing both acute care and LTC (Evashwick 1993). Recently, Burton (1994) has suggested that the nursing home could be at the hub of a service system for people with chronic disability, providing ambulatory care, home care for those living independently, and various types of group residential care for people with different needs. An alternative view (Kane 1993b, 1994) notes the heterogeneity of those now in nursing homes, and suggests that the nursing home as we know it (an institution that could never be mistaken for a home) should be reserved for people who cannot interact with their environment, who are so medically unstable that they need hospital-like medical attention, and who perhaps need intensive rehabilitation on an inpatient basis. (The jury is still out on the latter group, however, because physical environments and autonomy are important to the morale and outcomes of rehabilitation patients.)

Financing and payment

Financing of and reimbursement for home- and community-based care is beyond the scope of this chapter. Undoubtedly, however, both financing and reimbursement policies need rethinking in order to eliminate current barriers (Feder 1991) and to build on the developments I have described. The Health Care Financing Administration has initiated a process for examining the Medicare home health benefit, in part, to see if it could be more flexible and user friendly (Vladeck 1994). It will be important also to try to eliminate the differentials that make Medicare-covered services more expensive than those purchased privately or by other payers. Case managers for state programs will always be enjoined to find a federal payer when possible, and the general public is most concerned with the total public costs rather than which public payer gets the bill. Making flexible in-home and PAS services available to a wide range of users in a variety of settings possibly would work best with a disability allowance rather than a system of authorizing services, a stance that has its advocates (Batavia, DeJong, and McKnew 1991). Future studies should explore the advantages and disadvantages of various ways of making public dollars available to individuals with needs for service without inducing demand and increasing costs unduly.

Home-care and assisted-living providers could play pivotal roles in furthering a movement in LTC that would bring a home-care style of service to people who have established new homes in group residential settings so that their LTC needs are met. This will require flexibility and new paradigms for thinking, but the benefits for the lives of clientele are potentially enormous. One hopes that organized home care will be part of imaginative solutions to the care of functionally impaired older people rather than part of the problem that narrows and stultifies their lives.

Note

An earlier version of this chapter was commissioned by the Visiting Nurse Service of New York/Milbank Memorial Fund project on Home-based Care for a New Century, and discussed at a working conference held in Harriman, New York, on November 8th and 9th, 1993. Much of this material also appeared in the *Milbank Quarterly* (73: 2) (1995): 161–86, under the title, "Expanding the Home Care Concept: Blurring Distinctions Among Home Care, Institutional Care, and Other Long Term Care Services."

References

American Nurses Association. 1992. Position Statement on Registered Nurse Utilization of Unlicensed Assistive Personnel. Washington.

Applebaum, R.A., M. Harrigan, and P. Kemper. 1986. *Evaluation of the National Long-Term Care Demonstration: Tables Comparing Channeling to Other Community Care Demonstrations*. Princeton, NJ: Mathematica Policy Research.

Asch, A. 1993. Abused or Neglected Clients – Or Abusive or Neglectful Service Systems? In *Ethical Conflict in the Management of Home Care: The Case Manager's Dilemma*, ed. R.A. Kane and A.L. Caplan. 113–21. New York: Springer.

Batavia, A.I., G. DeJong, and L.B. McKnew. 1991. Toward a National Personal

Assistance Program: The Independent Living Model of Long-Term Care for Persons with Disabilities. *Journal of Health Politics, Policy, and Law* 16: 523–44.
Benjamin, A.E. 1992. In-Home Health and Supportive Services. In *In-Home Care for Older People: Health and Supportive Services*, ed. M.G. Ory and A.P. Duncker. 9–52. Newbury Park, CA: Sage.
Burton, J.R. 1994. The Evolution of Nursing Homes into Comprehensive Geriatric Centers: A Perspective. *Journal of the American Geriatrics Society* 42: 794–6.
Eckert, J.K., and S.M. Lyon. 1992. Board and Care Homes: From the Margin to the Mainstream in the 1990s. In *In-Home Care for Older People: Health and Supportive Services*, ed. M.G. Ory and A.P. Duncker. 97–114. Newbury Park, CA: Sage.
Evashwick, C.J. 1993. Strategic management of a continuum of care. *The Journal of Long-Term Care Administration* 21: 13–24.
Feder, J. 1991. Paying for Home Care: The Limits of Current Programs. In *Financing Home Care: Improving Protection for Disabled Elderly People*, ed. D. Rowland and B. Lyons. 27–47. Baltimore: Johns Hopkins University Press.
Friedlob, A. 1993. The Use of Physical Restraints in Nursing Homes and the Allocation of Nursing Resources. Unpublished doctoral dissertation, Health Services Research and Administration, University of Minnesota, Minneapolis, Minnesota.
Hawes, C., J.B. Wildfire, and L.J. Lux. 1993. *Regulation of Board and Care Homes: Results of a Survey in the 50 States and the District of Columbia: National Summary*. Washington D.C.: American Association of Retired Persons.
Jamieson, A. ed. 1991. *Home Care for Older People in Europe: A Comparison of Policies and Practices*. Oxford: Oxford University Press.
Kane, R.A. 1993a. Dangers Lurking in the "Continuum of Care." *Journal of Aging and Social Policy* 5: 1–7.
Kane, R.A. 1993b. Ethical and Legal Issues in Long-Term Care: Food for Futuristic Thought. *Journal of Long-Term Care Administration* 21: 65–73.
Kane, R.A. 1994. Transforming Care Institutions for the Frail Elderly: Trends in Group Residential Care. Paper delivered at an invitational meeting, "Caring for Frail Elderly People: Policies for the Future," sponsored by the Organization for Economic Co-operation and Development, Chateau de la Muette, Paris, July 5 and 6.
Kane, R.A., and A.L. Caplan. 1990. *Everyday Ethics: Resolving Dilemmas in Nursing Home Life*. New York: Springer.
Kane, R.A., L.H. Illston, N.N. Eustis, and R.L. Kane. 1991a. *Quality of Home Care: Concept and Measurement*. Minneapolis: Division of Health Services Research and Policy, School of Public Health.
Kane, R.A., R.L. Kane, L.H. Illston, J.A. Nyman, and M.D. Finch. 1991b. Adult Foster Care for the Elderly in Oregon: A Mainstream Alternative to Nursing Homes? *American Journal of Public Health* 81: 1113–20.
Kane, R.A., R.L. Kane, L.H. Illston, and N.N. Eustis. 1994. Perspectives on Home-Care Quality. *Health Care Financing Review* 16(1): 69–90.
Kane, R.A., C. O'Connor, and M.O. Baker. 1995. *Delegation of Nursing Activities: Implications for Patterns of Long-Term Care*. Minneapolis: University of Minnesota National Long-Term Care Resource Center.

Kane, R.A., and K.B. Wilson. 1993. *Assisted Living in the United States: A New Paradigm for Residential Care for the Frail Elderly.* Washington, D.C.: American Association of Retired Persons.

Kane, R.L., L.H. Illston, and N.A. Miller. 1992. Qualitative Analysis of the Program of All-Inclusive Care for the Elderly (PACE). *The Gerontologist* 32: 771–80.

Kane, R.L., and R.A. Kane. 1985. *A Will and a Way: What the United States Can Learn from Canada about Caring for the Elderly.* New York: Columbia University Press.

Kane, R.L., and R.A. Kane. 1994. Effects of the Clinton Health Reform on Older Persons and Their Families: A Health Systems Perspective. *The Gerontologist* 34: 598–605.

Kapp, M. 1993. Problems and Protocols for Dying at Home in a High Tech Environment. Paper presented at the Technological Tether Conference, sponsored by Montefiore Hospital, and held in New York City on February 18 and 19.

Kodner, D.L. 1993. Long-Term Care 2010: Speculations and Implications. *Journal of Long-Term Care Administration* 21: 80–5.

Lewis-Idema, D., M. Falik, and S. Ginsburg. 1991. Medicaid Personal Care Programs. In *Financing Home Care: Improving Protection for Disabled Elderly People,* ed. D. Rowland and B. Lyons. 146–77. Baltimore: Johns Hopkins University Press.

Litvak, S., H. Zukas, and J.E. Heumann. 1987. *Attending to America: Personal Assistance for Independent Living: A Survey of Attendant Service Programs in the United States for People of All Ages with Disabilities.* Berkeley, CA: World Institute on Disability.

Mollica, R.L., R.C. Ladd, S. Dietsche, K.B. Wilson, and B.S. Ryther. 1992. *Building Assisted Living for the Elderly into Public Long-Term Care Policy: A Guide for States.* Portland, Maine: Center for Vulnerable Populations, National Academy for State Health Policy.

National Council of State Boards of Nursing. 1990. Concept Paper on Delegation. Chicago.

Redfoot, D.L. 1993. Long-Term Care Reform and the Role of Housing Finance. *Housing Policy Debate* 4(4): 497–537.

Sabatino, C.P., and S. Litvak. 1992. Consumer-Directed Homecare: What Makes It Possible. *Generations* 16 (Winter): 53–8.

US General Accounting Office. 1994. *Medicaid Long-Term Care: Successful Efforts to Expand Home Services while Limiting Costs* (GAO/HEHS-94-167). Washington, D.C.

Vladeck, B. 1994. From the Health Care Financing Administration, Medicare Home Health Initiative. *Journal of the American Medical Association* 271(2): 1566.

Weissert, W.G., C.M. Cready, and J.E. Pawelak. 1988. The Past and Future of Home- and Community-Based Long-Term Care. *Milbank Quarterly* 66: 309–88.

Wilson, K.B. 1995. *Assisted Living: Reconceptualizing Regulations to Meet Consumers' Needs and Preferences.* Washington D.C.: Public Policy Institute, American Association of Retired Persons.

3

Home-Care Politics in the 1990s

A. E. Benjamin

Introduction

Home care seems to be on a roll politically. After decades of relative policy obscurity leavened with periodic controversy, home-care reform seems to have found a place on the federal policy agenda in the 1990s. The reasons for this are complex, but demographic trends, budget politics, and public opinion seem to have converged to make home care a centerpiece of recent reform discussions. As we learn more about the work of the Clinton Administration's health reform task force, home-care advocates can certainly find encouragement in the policy options developed by the long-term care work group. While strengthened income and resource protections for nursing-home residents have been included in all of the options proposed by the work group, the bulk of the proposed new funding is intended to expand home- and community-based services for people with severe disabilities. In the most generous, full social insurance model, home-care benefits would be phased in for several years before expanded nursing-home benefits are introduced.

These developments have taken many observers by surprise.

During the last decade, most policy scholars who examined the politics of long-term care reported little that made them sanguine about the prospects for reform. At least in part their pessimism was a product of the retreat from public solutions to social problems that characterized the Reagan–Bush years. But their conclusions were more than a mirror of the decade and were based upon analysis of what one author characterized as "the immobilism" of long-term care policy.

It is the argument of this chapter that the future of long-term care reform remains problematic and that the central obstacles involve both the general political environment and the character of home care. I will begin by briefly considering the relationships between home-care, long-term care and health-care reform within an historical context. Next, I will introduce alternative analytical perspectives for understanding the complexity of policy reform. Then using a series of interviews with policy actors and a review of literature in the field, I will review arguments that long-term care reform is close at hand and countervailing arguments that barriers to reform remain formidable. The chapter will conclude with an effort to synthesize these varied perspectives and to assess contemporary prospects for home-care policy within the context of long-term care reform.

Historical Context

If home care were a creation of the 1980s or, as is sometimes held, an invention of Medicare in 1965, it would be a relatively modest task to elaborate the historical context of home-care policy. In a very literal sense, however, home care is as old as the nation, and some of its political appeal comes from its deep historical roots. Not surprisingly, the ways that we think about home care have been transformed over time, yet some themes have persisted and continue to shape the debate about reform.

To simplify a much longer story (Benjamin 1993), three themes seem most significant. First, for much of this century, home care has been considered a residual set of services, at least somewhat apart from mainstream health care. At various times, home care has been what remained available for those too chronically ill to benefit from modern medicine, those too recovered to remain in the hospital, those too poor to pay for more expensive care, and too demanding or too uninteresting clinically to merit further medical attention.

Second, home care throughout its history has meant different things to different interests. With time and public funding, various service models have emerged, most notably postacute home health and social-supportive chronic-care variants, accompanied by suggestive but imprecise labels like "high technology" and "maintenance" services. Third, home care has long depended for its rationale upon its relationship to and impact on institutional care, first hospital and later nursing-home care.

It is the residual, varied and dependent character of home care that requires us to consider services at home in the more general contexts of long-term care and health-care reform, respectively. home care is considered part of the answer in both contexts, although the types of home care, the populations to be addressed, and the problems to be solved are likely to vary significantly with the context. A hierarchal dimension is added, moreover, when we consider the powerful argument that the occurrence and scope of long-term care reform will depend heavily upon the character of broader health-care (access) reform.

Two premises guide my initial focus on long-term care as the primary political context for a consideration of contemporary home-care reform. First, the primary focus of policy attention and resource allocation in home care historically, and especially since 1965, has been postacute, medical home care. Consequently, postacute home care has become an established component of public and private health-care coverage, while the most pressing and unresolved issues involve long-term, supportive care. Second, despite the persistent importance of this distinction, there are very significant interactions between acute and long-term care. Addressing this relationship will become an increasingly important part of reform efforts over time.

Analytical Context

Myriad factors shape the politics of long-term care. Any attempt to catalog or synthesize them implies a choice of conceptual lenses through which complex policy reality can be sorted. Three perspectives on public policy have contributed to my selection of analytical categories for trying to make sense of long-term care reform. Brown (1988, 1989) emphasizes the importance of the general policy context within which specific issues are considered, including prevailing economic and political conditions and agendas that shape what issues are considered salient and amenable to government response. Peterson (1993) suggests that the issue-specific political and structural contexts in which reform is debated shape the prospects for significant policy change. The political context includes the status of the conditions that underlie a given policy area (objective conditions) and the public attitudes and voting patterns related to a given policy arena (public values and attitudes). The structural context includes organized interests in a particular policy domain (demand structure) and patterns of governmental authority, access to which is critical in translating demand into policy consensus (governmental structure). Kingdon (1984) examines the federal agenda-setting process and, viewing government as an "organized anarchy," identifies three independent but related streams (or families of processes): problem recognition; the formation of policy proposals; and politics. Of immediate relevance to this discussion is his attention to the importance of technical issues and of the availability of viable policy alternatives (technology). More will be said later about the applicability of Kingdon's model to the politics of home care.

Opportunities and Barriers

Following the elections of 1992, optimism about the prospects for long-term care reform grew substantially. This renewed optimism derived from a conviction that profound changes have occurred in the political environment that have created new opportunities for long-term care to ascend the national policy agenda and to attract the support needed for comprehensive reform. Some political analysts have also identified a host of barriers likely to delay any significant long-term care reform in the foreseeable future. These analysts were writing in the mid- to late 1980s, following a period (the mid- to late 1970s) when reform optimism was high and a subsequent one (the 1980s) in which most hopes were dashed.

Borrowing from the analytical perspectives described earlier, opportunities for and barriers to reform can be grouped in terms of (1) the policy context, (2) objective conditions, (3) public attitudes and values, (4) the demand structure, (5) the governmental structure, and (6) technology. In the following discussion, I will use this framework to organize arguments that emphasize first opportunities then barriers. Within each category (e.g., policy context), the

Home-Care Politics in the 1990s 51

arguments will be presented with as much conviction as proponents might reasonably bring to them.

The Policy Context

Opportunities

After what might charitably be called a rough decade for government and the economy, some observers now argue that the context for reform has brightened considerably. This new sanguinity is based on anticipation of several things: renewed governmental activism following the 1992 elections; new public efforts to address the decline of the economy; fresh presidential leadership; and active efforts by the Clinton Administration to forge major health-care reform. Especially in the context of the latter, enthusiasts expect that long-term care reform can ride the coattails of broader change. Conviction that policy conditions are favorable goes beyond mere coattails, however, since many advocates (and some analysts) believe that important conditions affecting long-term care policy have improved notably in recent years (see below). Even if all the political groundwork has not been completed, a significant "window of opportunity" for reform has opened, and this is wide enough to accommodate long-term care.

Barriers

New public policy initiatives of all stripes have encountered a hostile fiscal environment since the late 1970s, and there is little convincing evidence that this will change appreciably or soon (Brown 1989). The economy has experienced a steady decline in real income and productivity over the past two decades (Pawlson 1990), and a modest upturn in the economy is unlikely to inspire new enthusiasm for taxation or governmental activism. Given expectations that any comprehensive long-term care initiative will be very costly, prospects for reform are heavily constrained by the anti-government, anti-tax attitudes that have limited domestic policy development since the late 1970s. Indeed, the report of the Pepper Commission (1990) soberly estimated that the cost of comprehensive long-term care reform would exceed that of providing basic health-care coverage to all uninsured Americans. To some in Washington, these cost data provided the "nail in the coffin" for reform; to the slightly less cynical, it meant banishment to the "back burner" for the foreseeable future. To those who cite the apparent enthusiasm of the new administration for tackling long-term care issues, skeptics point out that a crowded White House agenda that includes reviving the economy, reducing the deficit, and addressing health-care access and costs, probably means that long-term care will remain a third-order priority for the foreseeable future.

Objective Conditions

Opportunities

Marshalling data on conditions associated with chronic illness has been an essential and growing element of the contemporary policy process. At least four classes of conditions are important in characterizing the changing status of long-term care: (1) the demographics of chronic conditions, (2) the rising costs of the current system of care, (3) the inadequacy of coverage, and (4) inappropriate allocation of resources.

The number of persons over age 65 continues to grow steadily, the rate of increase in the population over 85 (on average, those most in need of care) is projected to be even higher, and we now understand much more about the large number and diversity of persons under 65 living with serious chronic conditions (LaPlante 1989). The sharply rising costs to federal and state governments of nursing-home services under Medicaid strain the ability of that program to finance home- and community-based services or health services to other low-income population. Because public benefits are so limited and eligibility so restrictive, while private insurance remains affordable only for relatively few, much of the burden of financing and care provision falls on needy individuals and their families. Even as the costs of care rise, public policy continues to support nursing-home stays far more readily than care at home, despite widespread popular preference for care in the community (Rivlin and Wiener 1988; Wiener and Harris 1990). At most, one-third of persons needing some assistance with daily activities receive formal (paid) home-care services (Families USA Foundation 1993).

While the prevalence of chronic conditions and illnesses is unlikely to change dramatically in the near term, what has changed is the quality and scope of the data we collect and report, our definitions of those with chronic care needs, and our understanding of the burden of caring for those with disabilities. Changes have occurred in both the numbers and types of persons with chronic care needs and the numbers of the citizenry who have direct experience with someone needing care. As the number of older persons grows steadily, so does (among others) the number with HIV infection, the number of children with special health needs, and the number of young adults living in the community with physical disabilities, many of whom need long-term care services. Objective conditions and public awareness of them are changing steadily over time, thus helping to create the political conditions necessary for reform.

Barriers

Politics is the process by which societal conditions are converted into problems meriting policy attention. Articulating objective conditions is a necessary but not sufficient step to policy reform (Peterson 1993). Although an abundance of research and data continue to highlight the steady growth in the population with chronic conditions, it is less clear in the short run that either the numbers or the severity of the circumstances under which people live have changed markedly. It is therefore unlikely that for political purposes a pressing problem, or crisis, has yet emerged, although with time it almost certainly will.

Current conditions thus may continue to be viewed through rather rosy lenses, although talking this way in public has its risks: All our data indicate that only a minority of the elderly have large long-term care expenses, and even fewer of those under 65 do. Most people with chronic care needs apparently manage to survive despite the many limitations of public programs. It is evident that families are not abandoning members in need in any large numbers and continue to provide significant, if not heroic, care outside the public purse. Despite the problems it creates, Medicaid has managed to fill some important service gaps (e.g., nursing-home care) and is addressing others (e.g., home care), however modestly (Vladeck, Miller, and Clauser 1993). Furthermore, important steps have been taken to humanize that program (e.g., protection of spousal assets). The real demographic crisis is still years away, so for long-term care, time is on our side politically.

Public Attitudes and Values

Opportunities

Since the federal election campaign in 1987–8 and with increasing regularity since, public opinion surveys have uncovered a growing interest among Americans of all ages in long-term care. What was once understood as relative public indifference has been replaced by more widespread experience with chronic illness and concern about the human and financial costs of chronic care. First, long-term care is no longer a hidden issue or one familiar to only a few. Roughly two-thirds of national samples report having experience with family members or friends with long-term care needs (R.L. Associates 1987; Daniel Yankelovich Group 1990). Nearly half of adults interviewed have had experience with their own or a family member's care needs (Daniel Yankelovich Group 1990), and those with direct experience are least confident and most concerned about their ability to deal adequately with this. Second, fewer Americans are content with prevailing approaches to paying for long-term care, namely out-of-pocket resources and Medicaid, with a very modest private insurance role.

Many citizens now support an expanded public effort to address the burdens of payment for needed chronic care. Nearly nine out of ten Americans believe that government must play a primary role in dealing with long-term care (ibid.). A similiar number indicate their support for a federal program of home care for the elderly, with about eight in ten also supporting a similar program for younger persons with disabilities (US Congress 1988). More than half report a willingness to pay higher taxes to support such a program (R.L. Associates 1987). Despite the persistence of anti-government and anti-taxation sentiment throughout the body politic, Americans in large numbers seem convinced that in the long-term care arena, individual and private-sector solutions have failed and a new role for government is required (Daniel Yankelovich Group 1990).

Finally, while concern about the cost of nursing-home care is widespread, public preference for care at home is strong. When asked to choose between the two care sites, two-thirds to three-quarters of respondents prefer care at home (R.L. Associates 1987; Long Term Care Management 1993b; US Congress 1988), with a majority opting for care by family members over paid care (Straw 1991). Disenchantment with nursing-home care is high, conviction that those with chronic conditions should be cared for at home is also pervasive, and many Americans are prepared to endorse governmental approaches consistent with these views.

Barriers
Certainly a bevy of surveys has documented growing public concern about a looming crisis in long-term care, as the baby boom generation begins to worry about the chronic-care needs in old age of their parents and themselves. The evidence may be more mixed than some advocates readily admit, however, given other attitudes that may act to soften public support for long-term care reform. First, while growing numbers of Americans have experience of chronic illness and its consequences, long-term care is almost always thought of as something that individuals must provide for someone else, and rarely do people acknowledge that they or their spouses might themselves someday require care (Daniel Yankelovich Group 1990). At first glance this may seem trivial in light of broader patterns, but to the extent that this suggests denial about the scope and impact of chronic illness, it may weaken political resolve to fashion new public solutions for chronic care.

Taken alone, this denial factor might not be consequential, but there is more. For example, although surprising numbers of those polled indicate support for a government program underwritten by modest tax increases, a minority is outspoken in its opposition. More conservative and prosperous than most citizens, this cohort challenges the need for a public program (since long-term care is perceived as a family responsibility), doubts the ability of government to run a program efficiently, and questions its affordability (ibid.). These attitudes are important because they are fundamentally American, have shaped welfare-state politics for decades if not centuries, and their persistence is a sober reminder of the difficulties associated with a significant expansion of public-sector authority and responsibility in long-term care.

Much has been made of widespread public preference for home care over nursing-home placement, but these attitudes are complicated by other, less touted findings. First, with the exception of (Medicare-style) home health care, many Americans are not well informed about home care (Straw 1991). Because this means that many are expressing approval for care options that sound sensible but are outside their range of experience, the support indicated may not be as stable or well-grounded as claimed. This conclusion is reinforced by a second observation, mentioned earlier, that much of the preference for home care may represent an endorsement of family care at home rather than paid, formal services. Care in a nursing home is a relatively well-specified and understood option as compared with home care, which for most persons is defined more by its familiar (as in, "of the family") setting than by the range of formal care provided there. While shifting public attitudes may provide a base for reform, a number of underlying issues seem unresolved and may continue to litter the path to significant public action.

Other public-survey results may also bear on prospects for long-term care reform. Foremost may be growing public awareness of 30–5 million (non-elderly) Americans with no health insurance at all, representing a salient, competing health-care issue for debate (Brown, 1989). Politically related is the persistent and troublesome sentiment that the elderly have benefited disproportionately from past public initiatives at the expense of other groups, and that their need (or "greed") for more governmental benefits seems boundless (Rosenbaum and Button 1993; Benjamin et al. 1991). The public tends also to equate long-term care with the elderly to the exclusion of younger adults and children with disabilities, thus magnifying the relevance of intergenerational issues in shaping a reform agenda. Finally, it remains less than clear that the public yet perceives a true public policy crisis in long-term care (Vladeck 1985). For all its shortcomings, Medicaid continues to provide nursing-home reimbursement, and private long-term care insurance is becoming a more visible option for some Americans.

The Demand Structure

Opportunities

In the past half decade, a sense of shifting public sentiment and emerging opportunity has activated aging interest groups and others to work for long-term care reform (and to commission still more surveys exploring and confirming public support for their efforts). The result has been, much more than previously, the forging of a broad common agenda and general agreement about the direction reform should take. One notable example of consensus-building has been the Long Term Care Campaign. In 1987 four organizations representing the elderly came together to work on a plan for long-term care in the context of the 1988 elections and in response to what was perceived as growing public sentiment for tackling the issue. These organizations (American Association of Retired Persons, Villers/Families USA, The Alzheimers Association, and The Older Womens League) targeted presidential and congressional candidates with an educational packet on long-term care, did polling in key primary states, and generated considerable publicity about chronic care issues within selected states and districts. Although the precise impact of the Campaign is difficult to measure, virtually all candidates in targeted primary states addressed the topic of long-term care, and electoral pollsters during the campaign for the first time incorporated the topic into their polling, and have continued to do so.

A related group of organizations (minus Families USA, plus several other aging interests, and with a more prominent role for AARP) mounted a different kind of effort during the 1992 election, focusing on educating voters in key states about candidate views on long-term care rather than targeting the candidates themselves. Again, results are difficult to assess, but the Campaign reports that 109 candidates for Congress in 1992 signed a pledge to support legislation ensuring comprehensive, universal and affordable care (half were elected), presidential candidate Clinton made a number of sympathetic statements on the subject, and Senator Dole stated that long-term care was one of the key issues facing the new President (Long Term Care Campaign 1992). In a related but less public way, these and other aging organizations are involved in continuing efforts to forge consensus on substance and strategy. The Leadership Council on Aging, an informal group of approximately 35 national organizations related to aging, has made long-term care a priority and provided a forum for educating diverse aging interests about long-term care policy and for developing a common focus on approaches to reform.

Not only are aging interests working more actively and coherently for reform, they have expanded the range of their collaborators. Specifically, they no longer define long-term care in terms of elderly issues alone and have begun to nurture relationships with non-aging interests around reform. Although pressures to seek collaboration have come from outside (i.e., from beleaguered friends in Congress following what everyone now terms "The Catastrophic Debacle" of 1988–9), aging interests seem to be coming to terms with the new "realpolitik" in long-term care. For example, in mid-1992 AARP invited the Consortium on Citizens with Disabilities (CCD) to review the long-term care component of a broader health-care reform proposal AARP was developing. As a result of a CCD critique, AARP redrafted the proposal, and the groups continued to collaborate during the Clinton task force process on a consensus approach to reform.

While substantive consensus has been elusive in areas like

functional eligibility criteria and case management, considerable agreement seems to have been achieved on basic principles like social insurance, eligibility based on disability not age, and the primacy of expanded home care. More fundamentally, interest groups representing the elderly and younger people with disabilities have discovered their common interests and confronted their differences on long-term care, and have taken significant steps toward crafting a common agenda. The result is likely to be more effective demand for reform.

Barriers

By many (informal and still unpublished) accounts, aging interest groups have lost influence at the federal level as a result of their role in the prologue to the repeal of The Medicare Catastrophic Coverage Act of 1988 (Binstock and Murray 1992). Primarily through a series of efforts at renewed coalition-building among aging groups, these organizations are currently laboring to dispel the mistrust and lingering perceptions of ineffectuality associated with that legislative debacle. Still, there is evidence that organizations representing the elderly have diverse interests of political consequence with respect to long-term care (Brown 1989; Torres-Gil 1989).

For example, despite widespread rhetoric calling for more home care, there is a perception that the middle-class elderly are much more concerned about impoverishment from nursing-home costs than about the availability or costs of home care (Binstock and Murray 1992). These and other differences get played out across groups with potentially competing priorities (e.g., AARP versus Families USA and OWL on the importance of Medicaid enhancement for low-income elderly and non-elderly). Although these differences are being addressed in the process of renewed coalition-building, the recent awakening of interest in long-term care has also made the stakes associated with different choices that much more apparent.

However the reform drama unfolds, the inevitable pressures toward political compromise can only make agreement on these choices more difficult. Further complicating the consensus calculus is persistent evidence that, despite public-opinion data suggesting the growing salience of long-term care, long-term care probably remains a third-order priority for many older persons and groups representing them, behind Social Security and Medicare. If (when) pressures mount to make cuts in either of the latter to support reform of the former, consensus among aging groups is likely to be strained further.

It is apparent that advocacy in long-term care is no longer the exclusive domain of the elderly; interest groups representing younger adults with disabilities, the mentally retarded and other consumers have become active and articulate players at the federal and state levels. This is a consequence of both successful advocacy for the Americans with Disabilities Act and a more general activation of interest in long-term care policy. While common needs and interests among disability populations have been articulated (Simon-Rusinowitz and Hofland 1993), there is considerable diversity in priorities and resources among these groups that makes consensus development and maintenance difficult (Torres-Gil and Pynoos 1986).

Although efforts to develop a common agenda between the elderly and younger disabled have yielded tangible results, there remains the sense that crucial differences and tradeoffs may not have been fully confronted within the relatively loose constraints of recent policy-development deliberations, especially since immediate legislation has not clearly been at hand (or at stake). This is complicated further by the fact that non-elderly disability interests are probably more diverse than elderly ones. There is at best a fragile unity among disability groups, with significant fissures apparent among those representing physical disability, mental retardation/developmental disability, and chronic mental illness. It is possible that agreement on reform substance and strategy can be forged and maintained, but it represents a politically daunting task.

Consumer groups are not the only interests that have been (or are likely to be) activated by new attention to matters of long-term care reform. In the context of a legislative system that generally gives an advantage to those seeking to obstruct reform (Kingdon 1984), the activation of various other interests seems likely to enhance political uncertainty and may generate additional barriers to reform. In fact, expert opinions differ about how certain powerful and well-heeled groups with stakes in long-term care will respond to reform proposals.

A priority for the private health-insurance industry has been development of private long-term care insurance, and in response to criticism it has tried to strengthen the home-care provisions of these policies (Rivlin and Wiener 1988; and US Congressional Budget Office 1991). Even more fervently, perhaps, the industry is fighting federal and state efforts to protect the assets of the frail elderly, since this threatens the pool of those buying private insurance policies. While the industry remains ambivalent about home care as an insurable risk and has shown few signs of lobbying hard against expanded publicly financed home care, its response to long-term care reform is likely to be determined by how nursing-home provisions are addressed. The nursing-home industry has joined the more powerful insurance lobby in fighting asset protection, and has publicly opposed home-care expansion in some states. Its role in reform involving home care remains ambiguous, particularly since the industry is diversifying into other venues (e.g., assisted living, board and care) where home-care services are expanding and into areas (e.g., subacute care) where home care is not an issue.

More surprisingly, perhaps, the role of the states in the reform debate also remains cloudy. As a group, on the one hand, state officials are the most rabid supporters of home care and continue to tout its role in reducing the costs of chronic care. Many states confront fiscal crisis, on the other hand, and feel squeezed by federal Medicaid mandates for women and children and the growing demand for long-term care. While the states would surely welcome expanded federal resources for home care, additional mandates without considerably more funds, discretion and flexibility are likely to be resisted.

The wildcard in building a coalition for expanded, federally funded home care may prove to be labor unions. Home care is a promising area for union expansion, and organizing efforts among home-care attendants in a few cities have led to tangibly improved wages and benefits. While varied interests can support improved working conditions for traditionally underpaid personnel, since these are expected to lead directly to enhanced service quality, such improvements also increase the cost of care. Moreover, the "individual provider" model favored by many in the independent living (disability) movement may collide with efforts to unionize workers and strengthen their working conditions (Feldman et al. 1990). Active participation by labor in long-term care reform may sharpen these issues and complicate the already complex process of building a coalition among advocates with diverse interests.

By most accounts, trade associations in home care will not be a major force in long-term care reform. This is true for at least two reasons. First, despite creation of the National Association of home care (NAHC) a decade ago, the field continues to be relatively fragmented, given four national associations with a mixed history of collaboration competing for political attention. (This alone would hardly support the argument, since it is true in most areas of the health and social services.) Second, the most influential home-care associations represent home health agencies that are oriented either to Medicare benefits or to private-pay patients. These organizations have been relatively uninvolved in past long-term-care debate and are unlikely to be central to current deliberations. While both NAHC and the Visiting Nurse Association of America have an interest in "unskilled" care, they have been most effective in monitoring Medicare home-care policy and the mechanics of program payment and eligibility. The historical preoccupation of home-care policy with Medicare postacute care is mirrored in the trade associations spawned by the program.

Governmental Structure

Opportunities

Demand for reform can only be effective if there is access to governmental decision structures and if those structures are able to respond in a coherent fashion to organized demands. Following the reform disappointments of the late 1970s and the reform despair of the late 1980s, there is good reason to believe that federal decision structures have become more responsive to the idea of long-term care as an agenda item for public action. Within both the executive and legislative arms of government, there is a growing perception that long-term care is a problem that will not go away and that whatever its (surely considerable) costs, it will have to be tackled in some meaningful way in the near future. Within government there are increasing numbers of decision makers who have personal experience of chronic care and of the limits of Medicare and public help generally, and this will surely alter the way they respond to organized demand for reform.

More concrete evidence supports the argument about more open governmental structures. However the outcomes of the Pepper Commission, for example, are judged, that body succeeded in converting what was at most an electoral issue in 1988 into a legislative one. As a result of its report, long-term care was converted from a rhetorical issue into one that could be broken down into a series of concrete decisions about policies and programs. Long-term care was "mainstreamed" into the broader context of health care, and arguments about a social insurance framework for home care and measures of functional status no longer seemed so exotic.

The Clinton task force took up where the Pepper Commission left off (and with some of the same staff leadership), and home care again became the centerpiece of the primary reform options under consideration. More generally, years of incremental reform under Medicaid and Medicare have produced a pool of Congressional members able to assume the role of legislative champions for long-term care along with a reservoir of Congressional staff and civil servants who understand the issues and are able to provide the needed expertise in forging a reform proposal and monitoring its implementation.

Barriers
While Congressional reorganization has probably increased the accessibility of that body to advocacy input (Peterson 1993), federal decision structures concerned with long-term care remain fragmented and weak and thus represent an unlikely vehicle for translating demand and forging political consensus. First, there is no focal agency with long-term care policy authority within the Executive Branch, and (as is true of health care generally) legislative authority within Congress is divided among several committees with varying commitments and agendas (Greenberg 1984). Second, although the presence of expert cadres within DHHS seems essential to the lengthy process of crafting and moving reform through government, those cadres have been depleted in recent years in the wake of conservative administrations bent on suppressing those who espoused active government and expanded public commitments (Brown 1989).

Third, there are few if any true champions of long-term care reform in Congress, especially since the death of Congressman Claude Pepper, and without them the prospects for Congressional action remain dim. This may be even truer in 1993 than in 1992, since the last election generated a significant turnover in Congress and diluted much of the educational impact of the 1988 Long-Term Care Campaign. There is also reason to believe that following the last election key allies of long-term care (e.g., Mitchell, Gebhart and Moynihan) may have been lost (in the eyes of advocates), not because they were defeated but because they must now be about doing the business of their President and the party occupying the White House.

Fourth, the absence in recent decades of Presidential interest in long-term care has critically undermined the prospects for reform (Vladeck 1985). By all appearances, this situation changed significantly following the 1992 election, because of the interest of the President and First Lady in long-term care issues and because their chief health-policy advisor (Magaziner) seems sold on the virtues of home care. Not all appearances have immediate consequences, however, for long-term care must now compete for attention with a host of other pressing (and costly) items on the current political agenda. With its complex access and cost issues, the health-policy-reform agenda may be sufficiently complex to consume the domestic "political capital" available to this (or any) administration.

Finally, an unhappy combination of circumstances makes this an unlikely time for displays of political courage with respect to long-term care. Persistent, nightmarish memories of the Catastrophic debacle, frightening estimates of the potential costs of comprehensive reform first from the Pepper Commission and more recently from the Clinton Task Force, and a White House agenda requiring both cost controls and new taxation, combine to make policymakers wary of significant reform in an area where demand seems pervasive but restrained and alternatives to comprehensive public solutions are available. Instead, for the foreseeable future political leaders will likely strive to maintain an appearance of interest and activism without endorsing any truly non-incremental initiatives or making any substantial new resource commitments.

Technology

Opportunities

With respect to long-term care, there is notable continuity between the work of the Pepper Commission and the Clinton Task Force, particularly in their priority on expanded home care, and their efforts reflect emerging agreement about the direction and content of long-term care reform (also see Harrington et al. 1991). While debate indeed continues regarding important issues like universality versus means-testing, allocating the burden of financing, and the balance between federal and state roles, such issues are hardly unique to this area and have accompanied all major social and health-policy choices. Strategic models have emerged to guide the reform debate, technical expertise has grown enormously in recent years, and lots of smart people in federal and state governments and in universities and think tanks are working on policy and program issues.

An example of new tools now available is the Brookings-ICF Long-Term Care Financing Model, a microsimulation model that makes possible systematic estimates of alternative financing options (Rivlin and Wiener 1988; Wiener et al. 1994) and is now widely utilized and respected. An example of new applications is the work of the task force/long-term care work group in which reform alternatives were specified and cost estimates were developed and released for discussion. While policy consensus does not yet exist, the technical base for achieving agreement has been developed.

Barriers
Analysts both inside and outside the field have suggested that long-term care reform founders not only on politics but also on technology. In a word, it is argued, experts disagree about what to do, how to do it, and how much it will cost. Long-term care represents a range of complex problems requiring diverse services in varied settings for a host of populations, and there seems to be little expert consensus about what the core issues are or how to solve them (Greenberg 1984; Brown 1989; Pawlson 1990). Uncertain knowledge is most apparent as we try to estimate the extent of the "woodwork effect" (i.e., the expectation that a new public benefit will attract users who previously relied on private, informal sources of care) and the projected costs of given options like the four developed by the Clinton task force.

Home care represents the starkest version of these problems. With medical and social models, a seemingly endless array of service and provider categories, and only the murkiest estimates about demand, home care seems like a muddle to many analysts and policymakers (Hudson 1990). At the heart of the confusion is the apparent absence of a broadly attractive strategic model around which experts can unite, and without such a viable alternative movement toward reform is extremely problematic (Kingdon 1984; Brown 1989). As was true in 1965 (Benjamin 1993), many in government continue to worry that expanded home care will mean (or seem to mean) "maid service" for the middle class at public expense.

Synthesis and Conclusions

Long-term care generally and home care most particularly have been bathing in the light from a new political window of opportunity. This may be a time of false hopes, however, since the character and length of the political agenda is highly constrained by the policy context in which it is developed. Most substantial social reform in our history has occurred in times of budget feast (e.g., the mid-1960s) or budget famine (e.g., the mid-1930s). In the latter context, reform was sold as part of a set of solutions to economic crisis. Although neither scenario accurately describes the current

Home-Care Politics in the 1990s   65

situation, the mood of the early to mid-90s clearly approximates the 1930s more than the 1960s. With considerable political skill, providing basic medical coverage for all Americans can be packaged as part of a solution to a troubled economy. In the political thaw of the immediate post-Reagan/Bush years, that is a much harder sell for long-term care, although advocates for younger adults with disabilities are more than willing to try. The national mood (Kingdon 1984) is hostile to expanded human service programs, and this is certain to narrow the window of opportunity for all social reform.

A narrow window might be adequate, if long-term care, and especially home-care expansion, were at the top of the domestic policy agenda; but it is certainly not. For political purposes, demographic conditions change glacially. Data on the number of chronically ill and disabled in the years 2020 and 2050 have relatively little significance for current politics. The case for a crisis in home care has not yet been made, despite abundant conviction that many Americans cannot arrange or afford services that are essential. While we know a great deal more about the numbers and circumstances of persons with chronic conditions, this has not yet translated into a marketable political message beyond one lamenting the financial burden of long-term stays in nursing homes.

Given this backdrop, how the public views the issue(s) may be critically important, since public opinion provides signals that help activate demand structures and alerts government structures to problems requiring immediate attention. Is home-care expansion an idea that has caught on? Will decision makers find it impossible to ignore a mandate for reform? The evidence on this remains ambiguous, despite an abundance of relevant polling data and related research (Stone and Kemper 1989). Public concern about caring for the chronically ill and disabled clearly has grown, as has general awareness about alternatives to nursing-home placement. Yet support for publicly financed expansion of non-medical, home-based services seems less firm than advocates would wish. The presence of vocal opponents creates further problems, since politicians characteristically distance themselves from initiatives that are zealously challenged by even a few; for an example, witness the Catastrophic stampede (Binstock and Murray 1992). Public opinion can be an important starting place for public action (Kingdon 1984) but in the case of expanded home care probably falls well short of a solid mandate for reform.

The activation and diversification of interests working for reform is perhaps the single most important development of the last half decade in long-term care. This has helped to lift reform above categorization as an issue of intergenerational conflict (Benjamin et al. 1991) and to widen the base of real and prospective support. In part this has been possible because "home care" is broad in scope, means different things to different interests, and thus can attract diverse supporters. But this also means that important differences in priorities among supporters remain submerged or at least manageable only as long as policy language is broad and imprecise, and policy options are budgeted at levels sufficient to provide something adequate for everyone. In the current (and foreseeable) budget environment, this coalitional equilibrium will be difficult to sustain as concrete legislative proposals are framed, modified and debated.

Growing numbers of public officials and other policy influentials have direct, family experience with someone who is chronically impaired. This brings an immediacy and familiarity to long-term care that until recently was missing in policy circles. In a different way, familiarity was strengthened by the Pepper Commission and, more immediately, the health-reform task force, as a common policy language and set of issue labels was integrated into the policy debate and a set of experts was acknowledged and mobilized. At the same time, familiar issues of administrative fragmentation, elusive Congressional championing, and uncertain Presidential leadership have not disappeared and continue to cloud prospects for reform. The weight of other domestic agenda items remains heavy, as do comparative estimates of the costs of competing initiatives, in which significantly expanded home care fares poorly. In 1993–4 government has been more open to reform than at any time since the late 1970s, but a steamroller of demand is necessary to translate openness into action.

As more details have become available about task force options and about the substance of the Administration's reform agenda (prior to the 1994 election), and as professional and public debate ensues, the claim that relative consensus exists about a strategic model for reform will be sternly tested. The policy problem seems far less that no expert consensus exists than that no effective way has been found to convey the content of that consensus to a broader policy or public audience. As long as the boundaries of home care remain obscure to many serious observers, faced with services as diverse as intravenous therapy, personal care, and homemaker services, building broader political agreement about the content and scope of reform will remain difficult.

Medical, postacute home care was incorporated into the basic benefit package recommended by the Clinton task force. Long-term, supportive home care was left outside the core reform proposal, awaiting political judgments about how to deal with long-term care. Many observers have argued that the demands of the elderly can be assuaged by a prescription drug benefit, which while not irrelevant, is a long way from comprehensive long-term care reform. Laying out a timetable for reform is politically valuable, but taken alone it also permits policymakers to avoid the hard decisions about how to pay for new benefits.

The safe course in any assessment of the prospects for reform is to emphasize the barriers and be wary of easy optimism. This is so both because policy reform is an extremely complex and interactive series of processes that defy our best predictive powers and because most scholars try to avoid looking completely foolish. Most of the important, non-incremental policy events in our recent history have been described coherently only with hindsight (Marmor 1973). A common feature of these events, even in retrospection, is the political surprise, usually a convergence of events that propels an issue to the top of the policy agenda and makes a policy solution politically necessary and feasible. Such surprises rarely occur in a vacuum but instead follow decades of political groundwork that establishes the contextual possibility for policy reform. Much of the groundwork in long-term care has been laid in recent years, and the process continues apace.

References

Benjamin, A.E. 1993. An Historical Perspective on Home Care. *The Milbank Quarterly* 71(1): 129–66.

Benjamin, A.E., Paul W. Newacheck, and Hannah Wolfe. 1991. Intergenerational Equity and Public Spending. *Pediatrics* 88(1): 75–83.

Binstock, R.H. 1983. The Aged as Scapegoat. *The Gerontologist* 23(2): 136–43.

Binstock, R.H. 1990. The Politics and Economics of Aging and Diversity. In *Diversity in Aging*, ed. S.A. Bass, E.A. Kutza, and F.M. Torres-Gil. 73–99. Glenview, IL: Scott, Foresman and Company.

Binstock, R.H., and T.H. Murray. 1992. The Politics of Developing Appropriate Care for Dementia. In *Dementia and Aging: Ethics, Values, and Policy Choices*, ed. R.H. Binstock, S.G. Post, and P.J. Whitehouse. 153–70. Baltimore: Johns Hopkins University Press.

Brown, L.D. September 1988. Health Policy in the United States (occasional paper no. 4, Ford Foundation Project on Social Welfare and the American Future), Ford Foundation.

Brown, L. 1989. The Static Politics of Long-Term Care. In *The Economics and Politics of Long-Term Care*. Conference proceedings, October 11–13. Irvine/Long Beach: University of California, Irvine and the FHP Foundation.

Daniel Yankelovich Group, Inc. 1990. *Long Term Care in America: Public Attitudes and Possible Solutions.* Prepared for the American Association of Retired Persons, Washington, D.C.

Families USA Foundation. 1993. *The Heavy Burden of Home Care.* Washington, D.C.: Families USA Foundation.

Feldman, P.H., A.M. Sapienza, and N.M. Kane. 1990. *Who Cares for Them?: Workers in the Home-Care Industry.* New York: Greenwood Press.

Greenberg, G.D. 1984. Health Policy Debate in the Executive Branch: The Case of Long-Term Care. In *Health Politics and Policy,* ed. T.J. Litman and L.S. Robins. 114–25. New York: Wiley.

Harrington, C., S.Wollhandler, and the Working Group on Long-Term Care Program Design, Physicians for a National Health Program. 1991. A National Long-Term Care Program for the United States: A Caring Vision. *Journal of the American Medical Association* 266(21): 3023–9.

Hudson, R. 1990. Home Care Policy: Loved by All, Feared by Many. In *Home Health Care Options, A Guide for Older Persons and Concerned Families,* ed. C. Zuckerman, N.N. Dubler, and B. Collopy. 271–301. New York: Plenum Press.

Kingdon, J.W. 1984. *Agendas, Alternatives, and Public Policies.* Glenview, IL: Scott, Foresman and Company.

LaPlante, M.P. 1989. Disability in Basic Life Activities Across the Life Span. *Disability Statistics Report* 1(1): 1–42.

The Long-Term Care Campaign. 1992. *Insiders' Update.* November/December. Washington, D.C.: The Long-Term Care Campaign.

Long Term Care Management. 1993a. Task Force Debates LTC Options, April 21, Special Report.

Long Term Care Management. 1993b. Conflicting Polls Indicate Varied Views on LTC Reform, May 5, pp. 3–4.

Marmor, T.R. 1973. *The Politics of Medicare.* Chicago: Aldine-Atherton.

Pawlson, L.G. 1990. Health Policy and Health Politics: The Ever-Growing Dilemma of Long-Term Care. *Journal of the American Geriatrics Society* 38(9): 1053–4.

Pepper Commission (US Bipartisan Commission on Comprehensive Health Care). 1990. *A Call for Action.* Washington, D.C.: US Government Printing Office.

Peterson, M.A. 1993. Political Influences in the 1990s: From Iron Triangle to Policy Networks. *Journal of Health Politics, Policy and Law* 18(2): 395–438.

R.L. Associates. 1987. *The American Public Views Long-Term Care.* Princeton, New Jersey: R.L. Associates.

Rivlin, A.M., and J.M. Wiener. 1988. *Caring for the Disabled Elderly: Who Will Pay?* Washington, D.C.: The Brookings Institution.

Rosenbaum, W.A., and J.W. Button. 1993. The Unquiet Future of Intergenerational Politics. *The Gerontologist* 33(4): 481–90.

Simon-Rusinowitz, L., and B.F. Hofland. 1993. Adopting a Disability Approach to Home Care Services for Older Adults. *The Gerontologist* 33(2): 159–67.

Stone, R.I., and P. Kemper. 1989. Spouses and Children of Disabled Elders: How Large a Constituency for Long-Term Care Reform? *The Milbank Quarterly* 67(3/4): 485–507.

Straw, M.K. 1991. *Home Care: Attitudes and Knowledge of Middle-Aged and Older Americans*. Washington, D.C.: AARP.

Torres-Gil, F. 1989. The Politics of Catastrophic and Long Term Care Coverage. *Journal of Aging and Social Policy* 1(1/2): 61–86.

Torres-Gil, F., and J. Pynoos. 1986. Long-Term Care Policy and Interest Group Struggles. *The Gerontologist* 26(5): 488–95.

US CBO (US Congress, Congressional Budget Office). 1991. *Policy Choices for Long-Term Care*. Washington, D.C.: Congressional Budget Office.

US Congress (House of Representatives Select Committee on Aging). 1988. *Hearings on the Need for Long-Term Care: A Survey of Public Opinion*. 100th Congress, 29 March. Washington, D.C.: US Government Printing Office.

Vladeck, B.C. 1985. The Static Dynamics of Long-Term Care Policy. In *The Health Policy Agenda: Some Critical Questions*, ed. M.E. Lewin. 116–26. Washington, D.C.: American Enterprise Institute for Public Policy Research.

Vladeck, B.C., N.A. Miller, and S.B. Clauser. 1993. The Changing Face of Long-Term Care. *Health Care Financing Review* 14(4): 5–23.

Wiener, J.M., and K.M. Harris. 1990. Myths and Realities: Why Most of What Everybody Knows about Long Term Care is Wrong. *The Brookings Review* 8(4): 29–34.

Wiener, J.M., L.H. Illston, and R.J. Hanley. 1994. *Sharing the Burden: Strategies for Public and Private Long-Term Care Insurance*. Washington, D.C.: Brookings Institution.

4

Integration of Home- and Community-Based Services: Issues for the 1990s

Robyn I. Stone

As the expansion of coverage for and access to home- and community-based care (HCBC) has become a priority long-term care policy concern for the 1990s, policymakers are exploring ways to efficiently and effectively achieve these dual goals by integrating these services along several dimensions. The purpose of this chapter is to examine the following four areas of integration of HCBC:

1   acute and long-term care services;
2   the administration of and/or funding for state HCBC programs;
3   programs for diverse long-term care populations; and
4   formal and informal services.

The first section describes the state of the art in the integration of HCBC within each of these areas, drawing on the literature and consultation with experts from the policy, program, and academic arenas. This is followed by a discussion of the policy implications of current integration initiatives, including possible areas for future policy development. The chapter also highlights areas for further research to assist policymakers in making important decisions about the scope and direction of their integration efforts.

What We Know about Integration of HCBC

There is a prevailing notion among many policymakers that the integration of HCBC on the four dimensions noted above will lead to more rational long-term care policy, and ultimately to the more efficient and effective financing and delivery of services. At the same time, it is important to note at the outset that there is little extant research to support the success of integration on these various dimensions. Policymakers have proceeded more on the basis of faith in the concept of integration as an efficient and effective strategy for improving access to HCBC than on empirical evidence supporting this contention. The following section provides a discussion of current efforts to integrate HCBC, and presents the limited information currently available on the success or failure of these initiatives.

Integration of Acute and Long-Term Care Services

Over the past decade, there has been increasing recognition of the need to integrate the financing and/or delivery of acute and long-term care services. Federal and state policymakers, as well as the private sector, have focused most of their efforts on developing integrated models that serve a disabled elderly population. With the increasing emphasis on managed competition as a framework for achieving health-care reform, the question of whether and how to integrate a broad continuum of services for the *elderly and nonelderly* disabled has received closer scrutiny by researchers (see for example, Schlesinger and Mechanic 1993) and policymakers. President Clinton's comprehensive health-care reform proposal, the Health Security Act of 1994, included a large-scale demonstration project to test models of integrated care for a variety of populations including the elderly, younger physically disabled, and mentally retarded/developmentally disabled. A range of approaches to integrating the financing of acute and long-term care services are currently being tested or are in the early, exploratory phases in both the public and private sectors. These include: (1) capitating the financing for a comprehensive set of services for the disabled (primarily the elderly); (2) capitating the financing for dually eligible Medicare/Medicaid enrollees; (3) bundling the financing of acute and long-term care services (e.g., using an expanded DRG (Diagnosis Related Group) episode approach); and (4) developing corporate retiree programs that combine Medicare with supplemental acute and long-term care coverage. Most of the information on existing integrated models is descriptive; there has been little evaluative research examining the success and failures of efforts to integrate *financing and delivery* of a broad range of services. Some of the key models of integration currently being explored at the federal, state, and private-sector levels are described below.

Social health maintenance organizations (SHMO). Since 1985, the Health Care Financing Administration (HCFA) has been experimenting with the SHMO concept, which combines Medicare HMO coverage for the elderly with chronic-care benefits (e.g., short-term nursing-home care, personal care, homemaker chore services) and other expanded benefits (e.g., prescription drugs and eyeglasses). There is a single, capitated monthly payment for all services, and participants are charged a monthly premium. The SHMO was designed to provide a broad range of benefits with no expected increases in total per member cost. This outcome is to be achieved through a gain in caregiver efficiency and more control over the level and intensity of care (Newcomer et al. 1993).

The SHMO model has been tested in four sites – two HMOs (Kaiser Permanente in Portland, Oregon, and Seniors Plus in Minneapolis) and two community-based organizations (Elderplan in New York and SCAN in Long Beach, California). Monthly premiums range from $25 to $57; between $6,500 and $12,000 in expanded long-term care (primarily HCBC services) are available to nursing-home certifiable enrollees. While there was slow enrollment at the start of the experiment, all four sites have reached break-even membership levels (Leutz et al. 1991). At a recent conference on integrated models sponsored by the American Association of Retired Persons, staff from the SHMO sites noted that the promise to keep disabled elderly at home through coverage of a range of HCBC services and prescription drug coverage were the two major reasons for enrollment in the program.

All four sites assumed full financial risk in 1987. Until 1988, three of the four sites experienced significant losses due to high administrative and marketing costs. These losses were greatest for the two non-HMOs because of the inability to take advantage of economies of scale (Leutz et al. 1991). One important lesson learned from this experiment is that starting from an existing HMO base is easier and less expensive than attempting to build a SHMO around a long-term care, community-based organization.

Researchers at the University of California San Francisco recently completed a HCFA-sponsored evaluation of the SHMO demonstration project. While there are some concerns about the methodology and quality of the data, preliminary findings suggest that the SHMOs have not achieved the goal of integrating the delivery of acute and long-term care services (Newcomer et al. 1993; Harrington 1993). Although these organizations were successful at creating a prepaid financing system covering a wide range of services, they were not able to effectively coordinate the efforts of the primary-care providers, case managers and community-based long-term care providers. Capitation alone does not provide the incentive to integrate the medical and non-medical, socially-oriented chronic-care services. In fact, this evaluation found that the primary-care physicians and the long-term-care case managers operated in isolation. Consequently, the coordination required to integrate a comprehensive set of benefits was not achieved. The evaluators argued that the primary function of the case manager in a SHMO model should be to link medical and social interventions rather than making allocation decisions. They also noted that few practitioners were trained in geriatrics and that insufficient attention was paid to identifying and treating medically at-risk members.

A second generation of SHMO demonstration sites was required by OBRA '91. Newcomer et al. (1993) in their evaluation of the first generation of SHMO models made several observations which have implications for the design of these projects. First, long-term care organizations and state Medicaid programs need to understand the considerable staff and financial resources and prepaid-health-care managerial expertise that is necessary for the SHMO startup. Second, researchers and policymakers must examine the tradeoffs associated with expanding case management and home- and community-based services as substitutes for hospital, physician and nursing-home services. Unless hospital, nursing-home, and/or physician use can be reduced, budget-neutral expansion of nonskilled care will not be achieved. Third, the SHMO package was limited compared to other long-term care products. The evaluators suggested that integrated models need to provide more home- and community-based care options targeted to people with moderate as well as severe disabilities. Fourth, SHMOs and other integrated models need to make more use of geriatricians, geriatric-nurse practitioners, and gerontological clinical nurse specialists. Finally, in the design of the next generation of SHMOs, special attention should be paid to refining how these organizations select "high risk" cases, focusing not just on nursing-home certifiable enrollees but also on persons with high medical risk.

Six sites have been selected to participate in the project, which will focus on refining the targeting and financing methodologies and benefit design, emphasizing geriatric care and the expansion of the model to special populations (e.g., dual eligibles or rural beneficiaries). The sites will receive technical assistance for one year from the University of Minnesota and the University of California San Francisco; enrollment will begin in January 1996 with approximately 85,000 beneficiaries.

Program of all-inclusive care for the elderly (PACE). PACE is a HCFA-sponsored evaluation designed to test the replication of the San Francisco-based OnLok model of acute and long-term care service integration. OnLok serves a very frail, nursing-home certifiable, elderly population, with service delivery built around an adult day health model. Core services include adult day health care and case management using a multidisciplinary team approach. Physician, therapeutic, ancillary, and social support services are provided on site, whenever possible. The vast majority of participants are dually eligible for Medicare and Medicaid, with financing achieved through prospective capitation.

Ten geographically diverse sites are currently participating in the PACE replication and evaluation, with over 1,700 frail elderly served. Legal authority exists for up to 15 sites. A preliminary, qualitative assessment (Kane et al. 1992), however, reports that enrollment has been less than expected due to the potential clients' resistance to change physicians as well as resistance to the day-care model that is central to the PACE approach to health-care delivery. Some sites have had difficulty in developing a stable care-management team, delaying implementation of the PACE services under full capitation in at least one site. These evaluators also noted that PACE sites have experienced considerable turnover of physician staff; their analysis suggests that the demands for practice in a very different model of care have made recruitment and retention of physicians in PACE difficult.

Gruenberg et al. (1993) examined the cost effectiveness of the PACE program, comparing 1990 PACE data to 1984 National Long-Term Care Survey data. They found that in comparison to a fee-for-service setting, the PACE program provides Medicare with a 9 to 34 percent saving depending upon the analytical assumptions and the sites selected. Data compiled by On Lok Inc. (Shen 1993) has shown that inpatient hospital utilization rates for frail elderly PACE enrollees are much lower than those for a comparable frail population, and hospital days per thousand PACE enrollees have been shown to be fewer than of the general elderly population. Nursing-facility use is also lower than expected for such a frail group of elderly.

In comparing the SHMO and PACE models, it is important to highlight the major differences. The SHMO is an insurance model where all those who enroll do not need long-term care at entry. The long-term care benefits (available to enrollees who are nursing-home certifiable) are primarily home- and community-based with very little, if any, nursing-home care provided through the extant models. In contrast, Onlok and the PACE replication sites enroll only nursing-home certifiable elderly persons; the majority are dually eligible for Medicare and Medicaid. The PACE models rely heavily on a multidisciplinary assessment team to develop the care plan and to provide a range of acute and long-term care services for which they are financially at risk; furthermore, the case managers are also the service providers. The SHMO sites separate the case-management and service-provision functions, and do not, for the most part, use a team approach.

State initiatives. A number of states are exploring the integration of acute and long-term care services. Arizona's Long Term Care System (ALTCS) incorporates long-term care for the elderly and physically disabled and individuals with MR/DD (Mental Retardation/Developmental Delays) into the state's basic managed-care system, the Arizona Health Care Cost Containment System (AHCCCS). Individuals are eligible for the program if their income is up to 300 percent of the SSI eligibility level and if they are at risk for institutionalization. As of January 1994, about 12,000 elderly and nonelderly physically disabled individuals were served by one program and 6,500 individuals were served through the MR/DD program. For the first program, the state contracts with either the county government or a private entity in each county to provide services. For the MR/DD program, the state contracts with the Arizona Department of Economic Security to provide services. Program contractors receive a monthly capitation from the state and are responsible for providing (either directly or through subcontract) both acute and long-term care services. Once enrolled, a case manager employed by the program contractor formulates a care plan for each enrollee.

One important area of concern is the phenomenon that some ALTCS members' health status improves to the point that they are no longer at risk for institutional care, therefore making them ineligible for the program (Irvin et al. 1993). Another area for concern is the ALTCS risk pool, which is smaller and sicker, by definition, than the pool for the general AHCCCS program. This may be a consideration for HMOs at risk for providing cost-effective services for these individuals when bidding for ALTCS contracts.

Integration of Home- and Community-Based Services

An evaluation of the overall AHCCCS program conducted by Laguna Research Associates (McCall and Korb 1994) compared the long-term care program costs of ALTCS with a traditional Medicaid program. The results indicate that ALTCS costs were 6 percent less in FY 1990, and 13 percent less in FY 1991 than the costs of a traditional program. However, the per capita costs of caring for the elderly and younger physically disabled individuals in ALTCS were higher than those for the traditional program. The researchers attribute the overall savings of the program to those incurred in serving people with developmental disabilities.

The Florida Medicaid Prepaid Health Plan/HMO Frail Elderly Option is designed to provide care to the state's elderly Medicaid population through integrating medical and social services so as to delay or avoid institutionalization (Irvin et al. 1993). Frail elderly are eligible for this program if they

1. are eligible for SSI/Medicaid;
2. are enrolled in a health plan that receives a capitated rate from the state to care for Medicaid recipients; and
3. qualify for the Frail Elderly Option Program (must be nursing-home certifiable and able to be cared for in the community).

As of 1993, the Frail Elderly Option was operational in two Medicaid contract plans. Capitation rates are calculated by the state for health plans contracting to serve Medicaid members. Community and institutional experience data are used to calculate an enhanced capitation rate for the Frail Elderly Option. The health plan receives this enhanced rate for as long as members utilizing the Frail Elderly Option continue to meet the eligibility requirements. If the individual is no longer able to remain in the community, the health plan is responsible for covering nursing-facility care for the remainder of the contract year. There is intense case management which provides access to the support services necessary for each enrollee to remain at home. It is similar to the goals of the SHMO and PACE projects, but does not pool Medicare and Medicaid funds into one capitated rate.

Minnesota recently received waivers from HCFA under Section 1115 of the Social Security Act (Medicaid) and under Title 42, Section 1395b-1 of the United States Code (Medicare) to conduct the Long Term Care Option Project (LTCOP), a demonstration that will pool Medicare and Medicaid funding for primary, acute and long-term care services for the state's dually eligible elderly population. (Other populations would be phased in over time.) LTCOP builds on the state's current managed-care system, recognizing that many elderly residents are already enrolled in prepaid health plans. This is the first effort in which a state is taking the initiative to design a new financing and delivery system for both the institutional and noninstitutional elderly population.

In developing this project, the state was motivated by several interactive factors. First, separate Medicare/Medicaid administration, rate structures and provider groups have led to inefficiencies and duplication as well as cost shifting between providers and funding sources. Second, physicians have little incentive to manage care across settings. Third, there is little incentive to provide care in alternative settings or care at the lowest level of appropriate service (i.e., home- and community-based care). By combining state and federal funding sources, Minnesota hopes to eliminate cost-shifting incentives that lead to less effective and more costly care. The state also seeks to promote prevention, early intervention and provision of services in the least restrictive setting by emphasizing managed-care systems in which the service providers share financial risk with the state and federal governments (Saucier and Riley 1994).

It is important to note that the negotiation process for these waivers was long and difficult (National Academy for State Health Policy 1995). There was no clear authority for the state to have HCFA make capitated Medicare payments to the state Medicaid agency, which would, in turn, enter into risk-based contracts with plans to provide the entire range of Medicaid and Medicare services for dually eligible persons. The final agreement between HCFA and Minnesota treats the state like a health plan, which is responsible for purchasing both Medicare and Medicaid services for dually eligible beneficiaries through a contracting procedure. Plans will receive the Medicare portion of their payments directly from HCFA, but for the LTCOP members, the state will manage both Medicaid and Medicare through a single contract. HCFA and the state also agreed on single enrollment, grievance and quality-assurance procedures for dually eligible persons.

LTCOP differs from the PACE models in that it will not be restricted to community-based frail elderly persons; individuals are eligible regardless of level of need or residence, including institutions. This model differs from the SHMO concept in that it focuses on the Medicaid as well as Medicare-enrolled population and offers a more expansive long-term care package. The design of this new program involves an intensive geriatric clinical-management system. The plan also calls for the provision of some acute medical

Integration of Home- and Community-Based Services

services in assisted-living settings and in the home, where appropriate.

Oregon is considering incremental steps toward integration as it moves to implement its health-care reform. Although the plan clearly distinguishes between medical and long-term care services (covering the former only), the state and prepaid health plans are exploring strategies for integrating services for dually eligible enrollees.

Other initiatives. The Community Medical Alliance (CMA) is an integrated system of care in Boston for people with severe disabilities and AIDS (Master et al. 1995). To date, very few Medicaid recipients with disabilities have been enrolled in managed care because of clinical, financial and regulatory concerns. CMA represents one of the first attempts in the US to adapt managed-care contracting widely used for employed and AFDC populations to address problems in the care and cost for people with disabilities. CMA offers two programs – one serves severely physically disabled individuals and the other serves people with AIDS. In both programs, CMA uses teams of nurse practitioners and physicians to provide primary care and case management across a full range of settings, including the home, medical clinics and hospitals.

The National Chronic Care Consortium (NCCC) is a consortium of providers in 14 states that are dedicated to the integration of acute and long-term care services through various models. Most of the NCCC sponsors include a comprehensive hospital system and a comprehensive long-term care network either under the same auspice or strategically aligned. The NCCC considers its members as natural laboratories for the examination of how organizations can achieve successful integration of a comprehensive package of services for chronically disabled persons of all ages. NCCC has established a task force to develop a tool to measure the degree of integration that exists in managed-care systems serving persons with chronic-care needs. This tool is intended to be used for evaluation purposes as well as for a report card to inform consumers and advocates.

Integration/coordination of state long-term care programs

Programs that fund long-term care services have historically been administered by separate state agencies. This has created a fragmented system that prevents the disabled and their families from identifying programs and services that will meet their needs. A number of states, however, have begun to address this problem by establishing case-management programs to guide clients through the maze and by streamlining the administration of the financing and delivery systems (IHPP 1988).

There have been several descriptive reports of integration/coordination efforts by states to consolidate administrative structures and/or financing streams to better meet the long-term care needs of the elderly and, to a lesser extent, other disabled populations. Success stories, however, are based frequently on anecdotal accounts from program directors. There have been no rigorous evaluations of these efforts to examine the effects of this integration on the allocation of resources, the delivery of services, the health and well-being of clients and their families, and cost savings. The following discussion highlights initiatives at two levels of integration: overall integration of the administration of state HCBC programs and the linkages of HCBC programs with nursing-home care and other providers.

Integration of state HCBC programs. In 1988, 12 states had statewide home- and community-based care systems for the elderly with multiple funding sources devoted to HCBC, and state-level organizational structures for consolidating long-term care management responsibilities. Justice (1988) conducted a six-state case study of state long-term care integration, identifying three basic models of integrating multiple financing and delivery systems primarily serving the elderly.

The first model consolidates all long-term care responsibilities covering both institutional and HCBC into a single, sole-purpose agency – a "one-stop shopping" approach. Such consolidation requires a major reorganization of state government. Oregon's Senior Services Division, which exemplifies this model, manages the Medicaid nursing-home and HCBC waiver programs (including the 1915D waiver), Older Americans Act funds, and state general revenues. All long-term care expenditures are consolidated into one budget so that resource allocation between HCBC and institutional care is a direct and visible tradeoff.

The second model creates a human-services umbrella structure with some internal shifting of responsibilities and increased interdivisional coordination. The Wisconsin Community Options Program (COP) is an example of this approach, coordinating all federal, state and local resources for HCBC. The state establishes guidelines for counties to develop plans for coordinating existing service programs. County governments handle the local implementation of the programs. The flexibility and control given to the counties allows COP case managers to tailor care plans without regard for traditional restrictions on the types of services provided.

Integration of Home- and Community-Based Services 81

The third model of integration retains independent, cabinet-level agencies, but establishes an official interagency long-term care committee to keep agencies informed of each other's activities and to coordinate the development of interagency policies. Illinois and Maryland exemplify this approach. Under this arrangement, the state office on aging or the state Medicaid agency usually is assigned primary responsibility for long-term-care program management.

In examining the motivation for program integration, Justice (1988) distinguished between incremental and structural models of change. Arkansas, Maryland, and Illinois began funding HCBC gradually in the late 1970s without a conscious attempt to achieve reform in the overall long-term care system or to reduce the growth of Medicaid nursing-home expenditures. In contrast, Maine, Oregon, and Wisconsin deliberately set out to control long-term care expenditures through statewide changes. The first three incremental states began their integration initiatives before state budget crises. The structural-change states, in contrast, faced fiscal crises, and nursing-home capacity controls became an integral component of strategies to expand HCBC.

In all cases, coordinating committees were established involving participants from inside and outside the government. These policy work groups tended to have higher-level officials as members, and all were part of an official research or planning effort. Where collaboration was most successful, substantial time was devoted to discussing philosophy and goals, and people at the highest levels were involved.

It is important to note that even though structural integration may be achieved, it is very difficult to integrate funding. Although Oregon funnels dollars through one agency, the case manager still must allocate resources to each client according to the program in which that person is enrolled. Illinois appears to operate the most seamless HCBC program; case managers working for the state Community Care Program and Medicaid-waiver program through the Department on Aging allocate resources to each client regardless of the program in which s/he is enrolled. Claims from the respective programs are reconciled at the end of each month; the client, however, is not aware of the funding source.

Delaware has streamlined the administration of programs for the elderly and physically disabled. The Long-Term Care Oversight Committee in the state's Office of Community-based Long-Term Care recommended the creation of a single division that has merged the Social Services Long-term Care Unit, Public Health Day Care Programs, and the Office on Aging. The Division for the Visually

Impaired has remained separate and has expanded its responsibilities to serve the needs of the deaf and hearing impaired. A single case-management system has been developed to help create a more seamless system and to realize savings in administrative overhead.

Vermont is developing a Community Assisted Independent Living (CAIL) program for disabled adults aged 18 and over. The Department on Aging and Disabilities is currently conducting hearings on three models. The *Access* model expands information and referral and benefit counseling services as well as creating a resource development function to stimulate new ways to pay for services; the *Coordination* model adds to the previous model by including a function that will assist consumers in gaining access to the system; the *Integrated* model consolidates funding streams, simplifies access to the delivery system, broadens the array of services available and promotes consumer choice. There would be "one-stop shopping" with the entry-point agency in each region responsible for the assessment and allocation of resources and for developing other resources to augment public funds. For each of these models, linkages would be established with the proposed universal health-care system in Vermont.

Linking HCBC programs with nursing homes and other providers. Most statewide HCBC programs designate a single local agency in selected parts of the state to serve as the access point for receipt of HCBC. This centralized entry helps to reduce the fragmentation; locating nursing-home screening programs in the same agency that serves as the single entry point for HCBC increases the potential for successful coordination of care. A 50-state study of state infrastructure for long-term care (Pendleton et al. 1989) found that 15 states had a statewide pre-admission screening program (PAS); seven other states had a PAS program that excluded non-Medicaid persons likely to spend down in a nursing home. The PAS and the Comprehensive Assessment, Care Planning and Care Management (CAPM) programs, however, were coordinated through state- or local-level agencies in only 12 states.

In five of the six states participating in a recent study of case management in community-care programs (Justice 1991), the same staff that conducts assessments of clients seeking HCBC was responsible for assessing people seeking nursing-home care. In three of the states, case managers maintained in their case loads some clients who had been admitted to nursing homes if they had the potential to move back to the community.

With respect to linkages with other types of providers, all six states participating in the case-management study indicated that the case managers attempted to maintain cooperative relationships with hospitals. The 50-state infrastructure survey (Pendleton et al. 1989), however, found that in only four states did local CAPM programs have explicit agreements with area health-care providers such as physicians; only one of these agreements was statewide.

Integration of HCBC programs for diverse long-term care populations

Long-term care programs tend to be categorical, serving distinct populations. Programs that serve more than one population usually target the elderly and the younger physically disabled. There has been increasing interest over the past few years in integrating HCBC programs for people with disabilities across the age span. A number of consumer groups have been seeking common ground as exemplified by efforts of aging and disabilities' advocates to establish the Consortium of Citizens with Disabilities and a spate of articles in gerontological and disability journals focusing on the similarities and differences in needs and service interventions for various populations.

Researchers have identified a number of barriers to the integration of programs serving different populations (Ansello and Eustis 1992; Simon-Rusinowitz and Hofland 1993). Two major impediments are differences in philosophy and language. For example, day-care programs for the developmentally disabled tend to focus on habilitation and vocational training while programs for the elderly tend to provide recreational activities and custodial care for the more disabled. Younger physically disabled people prefer the term "services" rather than "care" (e.g., personal assistance services vs. personal care), and are more likely than disabled elderly people to demand consumer-driven services with heavy reliance on independent providers. There are also differences in the use of unpaid caregivers with the elderly more likely to be receiving and accepting informal care from family and friends. Significant turf problems, particularly in times of scarce resources, create barriers to integration, with some groups (the mentally retarded/developmentally disabled in particular) fearing the loss of benefits if programs are consolidated. In addition, there is a shortage of cross-trained personnel to serve diverse populations, although there is little research indicating the degree to which HCBC providers require generic versus specialized skills to address the needs of people with different disabilities.

A number of factors affect a state's decision to develop generic versus categorical HCBC programs. The decision is driven, in large part, by the type and level of advocacy group activity in the state. The existence of coalitions of consumer organizations is associated with a more generic approach to program development. Historical considerations also play a role. If, for example, a HCBC program for one group is already firmly in place in a state or local community, separate programs for other populations are likely to develop. The existence of a human-services umbrella agency at the state level also is more likely to encourage the development of a HCBC serving diverse populations.

The Wisconsin Community Options Program (COP) is one of the few statewide HCBC programs designed to serve all populations in need of long-term care including the elderly, physically disabled, developmentally disabled, chronically mentally ill, and chemically dependent. COP was developed and implemented in a state with a long history of program integration, a strong focus on client choice, and a desire to create a very flexible program that would tailor services to the needs of each client. Although the program is integrated at the administrative level, it is important to point out that eligibility criteria for the program and the assessment tools used to determine eligibility differ according to the needs of the particular population.

While COP is frequently cited as *the success story* in the development of a generic HCBC program, state officials are currently considering a return to a categorical approach after a decade of struggling to administer a comprehensive program designed to meet the diverse needs of a range of disabled populations (D. McDowell, personal communication, Washington D.C., April 1993). The state's romance with a generic approach has faced the realities of providing widely divergent services to people with very different philosophies, needs, and preferences. At the same time, state officials have also acknowledged that a return to categorical programs may be difficult to achieve, as there is now strong political support from coalitions of consumers for continuing an integrated program. One option may be to maintain an umbrella organization that would oversee separately administered categorical programs.

Integration of formal and informal care
Research over the past two decades has underscored the finding that informal care provided by relatives, friends and other unpaid helpers is the mainstay of the long-term care system. Approximately 81 percent of the noninstitutionalized elderly and 85 percent of the nonelderly disabled living in the community rely primarily on informal care (US Department of Commerce, SIPP 1990). While

there has been some increase in the use of formal care among disabled elderly persons between 1982 and 1989 (from 9 percent to 13 percent), the bulk of the care is still provided informally (Doty et al. 1995). Policymakers involved in the development of more effective and efficient HCBC programs are concerned about how the informal care system links with the formal care system, and the extent to which the two systems are, or should be, integrated.

Theories of formal/informal care linkages. Noelker and Bass (1989) identified four theoretical models of linkages between the formal and informal care systems. The *complementary* model (Litwak 1985) posits that each system manages the kinds of tasks for which it is best suited. Informal care is more appropriate for unpredictable, nontechnical tasks; formal providers are better equipped to handle specialized and predictable tasks. These complementary roles have been termed "dual specialization." According to the *supplementation* model (Edelman 1986), the formal system supplements the care provided by the formal sector, rather than being specialized in particular tasks. In contrast to these two models, the *substitution* theory argues that formal care substitutes for or replaces informal care, particularly when publicly subsidized services are available. This is of special concern to policymakers, who fear that families will reduce the amount or level of care they provide if formal care is available. A fourth model of the linkage between formal and informal care indicates essentially *no relationship*; according to this theory, kin independently meet the needs of disabled relatives, regardless of the availability of formal care. In fact, informal providers may even obstruct or preclude the disabled person's access to formal care.

Substitution of formal for informal care. Driven primarily by cost concerns, but also by a philosophy that recognizes the importance of familial obligation, much of the policy research in the area of the link between the formal and informal sectors has focused on the extent to which paid care substitutes for unpaid care. Most of the findings do not support the substitution hypothesis; while the availability of paid care may increase the overall amount of care provided, it does not tend to replace informal care. Weiner and Hanley's (1992) critical review of a meta-analysis conducted by Weissert et al. (1988) found that the majority of the 53 evaluation studies on the relationship between formal and informal care cited by this meta-analysis reported results that were not statistically significant. Seven studies suggested a statistically significant increase in unpaid care, and only one noted a decrease in unpaid care. None of the studies demonstrated a reduction in the total amount of unpaid care; several studies indicated a trend toward changes in certain types of informal care, suggesting a complementary rather than a substitutive role for formal care.

One early study testing the substitution hypothesis among participants in the California Multipurpose Senior Services Project (Smith-Barusch and Miller 1985) found a 10 percent increase in formal care use, but only a 1.2 percent decrease in informal care used by people living with others. Christianson (1988) observed only a small reduction in the percentage of disabled elderly persons receiving unpaid assistance in the National Channeling Demonstration. There was a nonsignificant decrease in the amount of visits per week provided by informal caregivers and a nonsignificant increase in the number of hours per day provided by the primary caregiver. The only statistically significant reductions in unpaid care were by nonfamily caregivers.

Three other major studies (Moscovice et al. 1988; Edelman and Hughes 1990; Hanley 1991) found no evidence of reductions of informal care. In particular, researchers examining the relationship between paid and unpaid assistance in the Five-Hospital Program Community Care Project (Edelman and Hughes 1990) observed no significant decreases in either the total number or volume of services provided by informal caregivers between baseline and a 9-month and 18-month follow-up, despite significant increases in formal care use.

Integration of informal care in the assessment and resource-allocation process. As policymakers explore options for expanding access to HCBC, one critical issue that has received increasing attention has been the extent to which the availability of informal care should be considered in making assessment and resource-allocation decisions. Doty (1990) differentiates between implicit and explicit policies. The implicit policy takes the informal caregiver for granted and assumes that care will be provided, to the extent possible, by family, friends and other unpaid helpers. In determining eligibility for Medicare home health benefits, for example, professional judgments are made about whether informal supports are available to facilitate the safe and effective delivery of services in the home.

Explicit policies involve an active effort to integrate publicly-funded services with informal supports. The majority of state HCBC programs build individual care plans around the informal support system; a few states (e.g., Oregon, Illinois, Wisconsin) use availability of informal care in determining eligibility for the program. A recent study of case-management standards (Justice et al. 1993) found that most of the documents include language requiring the case managers to consider family supports in the resource-allocation

Integration of Home- and Community-Based Services

process and in the development of the individual plans. These requirements include communicating with the families about their role in the provision of HCBC, and actively soliciting a caregiver's opinion on types and level of services needed. The standards state, furthermore, that a change in the family caregiver support system would immediately trigger a reassessment.

The inclusion of family supports in the eligibility determination, resource allocation, and/or care planning processes raises an important equity issue. To the extent that the availability of family members is explicitly built into eligibility criteria for benefits or unofficially through inclusion in a care plan, an elderly or nonelderly disabled person with the same level of disability as another without family supports would perhaps not qualify for the program or would receive fewer benefits (Kemper 1990; Stone 1991). On the other hand, some have argued that if disability level is the only criterion used, individuals with substantial informal support may receive more formal care than they need, while those with weak or no supports may receive less than adequate formal help (Doty 1990). A related concern is how the case manager actually measures the availability of informal support. Programs that incorporate informal care may or may not take into consideration the fragility of that system. Consequently, reduced access of disabled people with families to public-program benefits may place additional burdens on informal caregivers, perhaps leading to an erosion of the very system of informal care many policymakers pledge to support.

Paying informal caregivers. The ultimate form of integration of the formal and informal care systems is making the unpaid helper a paid helper through direct payment to the caregiver. Payments to informal caregivers can be categorized by those providing compensation for work done and those compensating only for out-of-pocket expenses incurred by caregivers (Keigher and Stone 1992). *Wage programs* provide compensation directly to the caregiver, with pay related to the work either needed or actually performed. Relatives or neighbors may be hired like other home-care workers, except that most programs provide neither full-time employment nor fringe benefits to persons caring for one or two recipients. *Allowance programs* provide a flat grant geared to family or caregiver need and the care recipient's condition. Caregivers may be eligible because of categorical eligibility for income assistance, shared household status, or simply being related to the disabled person.

Caregivers may also receive *compensation for out-of-pocket expenses* for supplies or for paying privately for home care, respite care and day care. Finally, a number of programs (e.g., Senior Companion Program) also *reimburse volunteers* who provide long-term care.

Payments to informal caregivers have been very controversial. While most of the industrialized countries provide financial assistance to informal caregivers through such mechanisms as care allowances and wage compensation (Glendenning and McLaughlin 1993; Keigher 1992), policymakers in the US have been reluctant to monetize services that they believe should be the responsibility of family members and others in the informal network. To many, family payments are morally reprehensible as well as an additional drain on already constrained budgets. Despite federal regulations restricting personal care benefits to medical or medically-related care provided by a qualified medical professional "who is not a relative", some states have used a significant amount of Medicaid financing to pay informal caregivers. A 1990 survey of state long-term care provisions for the elderly (Linsk et al. 1992) identified 35 of the 50 states that made some form of financial payment to relatives and other informal caregivers for provision of homemaker, chore, personal care and attendant care. States that allow payment to relatives typically have restrictions. Some pay only certain relatives (four exclude adult children and three exclude grandchildren/grandparents). One state would pay only a co-residing relative; six states prohibited co-residence. Nine states require that the caregiver also be eligible for public assistance or be impoverished, and nine require that the caregiver relinquish outside employment.

A 50-state study in 1989 of publicly subsidized programs supporting families caring for developmentally disabled relatives found 25 states providing some type of financial assistance (Bradley et al. 1990). In seven states, the programs were pilot projects; nine served less than 100 families. Financial assistance, furthermore, was frequently viewed as a supplement to services available, rather than a stand-alone benefit. Five distinct forms of assistance include:

1 discretionary cash subsidy;
2 vouchers;
3 cash reimbursement;
4 cash allowances; and
5 line of credit.

The eligibility criteria for these financial assistance programs vary across states, as do maximum dollar amounts. In Minnesota, for example, a family with a mentally retarded child at risk of institu-

Integration of Home- and Community-Based Services 89

tionalization is eligible for $3,000 per year to purchase a wide range of services including homemaker services, therapies, respite care, special equipment, and transportation. In Georgia, families with incomes under $30,000 are entitled to up to $5,000 per year to cover a broad range of needs from clothing and nutrition to nurse training and respite care.

There has been very little rigorous evaluation of programs that pay informal caregivers. One evaluation of four pilot family-support projects in Pennsylvania (Ellison et al. 1991) concluded that financial assistance is a useful way to help families cope with raising a disabled child. Families demonstrated that if allowed to spend the cash on whatever they choose, they can be trusted to use the money appropriately.

Policy Implications and Future Directions

Integration of HCBC on a number of dimensions will undoubtedly receive increasing attention from policymakers at both the federal and state levels as both entities examine ways to reform long-term care policy in this country. States are struggling to find more cost-effective strategies for financing and delivering care to the disabled population under severe budget constraints, and are experimenting with waiver authority to develop more integrated systems of care. The Clinton administration's health-care reform proposal would have expanded access to a comprehensive array of acute and long-term care services while at the same time containing costs. The integration of HCBC services at the financing, administrative and service-delivery levels will, therefore, be an issue for the 1990s. The following section discusses some of the major policy implications of current efforts to integrate HCBC, including possible directions for future policy and research.

Integration of Acute and Long-Term Care Services
The development of models that integrate acute and long-term care services for a range of disabled populations is still in the embryonic stage. Aside from Arizona's integrated system of care for the Medicaid population and the new Minnesota waiver to experiment with integrated services for the dually eligible population, states have been reluctant to address the administrative and financial barriers to integration. The SHMO and PACE demonstration projects reflect the "state of the art" in the integration of services through

provider networks, and both are limited to the elderly. In sum, the integration of acute and long-term care services is more rhetoric than reality.

At the same time, the graying of the population, the passage of the Americans with Disabilities Act, recent legislative proposals to drastically reduce the rate of growth in the Medicare and Medicaid programs, and the rapid movement of the health-care industry into managed care portend a greater emphasis on the development of integrated systems of care in the next few years. In their desire to contain costs while ensuring quality of care, however, policymakers and providers will undoubtedly proceed with extreme caution. To achieve their dual goals through the integration of acute and long-term care, they must address a number of important issues recently outlined in a background paper prepared by staff at the Department of Health and Human Services (ASPE 1995).

The first critical design decision in the development of integrated systems for people with disabilities is whether to enroll a population of healthy and disabled individuals or just an already disabled population. Identifying the target population is essential because decisions regarding the capitation rate, reimbursement method, scope of benefits, and risk arrangement depend on the selection of the risk pool. Even within plans that carve out a particular population with disabilities, there is considerable concern regarding the level of severity that can be accommodated. For example, the Community Medical Alliance enrolls a mix of already disabled persons such as individuals with cerebral palsy who have a relatively flat clinical course, individuals with AIDS who have a progressive course requiring more long-term care services later, and individuals with spinal cord injury who require more front-loading of acute and rehabilitative services (Master et al. 1995). Unfortunately, few data are available from traditional managed-care providers in the private sector to facilitate an examination of the tradeoffs between inclusive models versus specialized plans. From the viewpoint of the prospective consumer, considerable skepticism has been expressed about equal access to care in a "separate but equal" health-care system; many people with disabilities, particularly younger physically disabled individuals, fear that care in a "disabled only" system will be severely constrained and of inferior quality.

A second key design issue is the extent to which and how long-term care services should be integrated with acute care. A number of administrative, financial and clinical barriers impede the integration of services including:

1 lack of financial incentives;
2 difficulty in establishing capitation rates;
3 the predominance of organizational and care-delivery structures that bifurcate around acute medical and long-term care service lines;
4 lack of clinical pathways for various disabilities;
5 an inability to predict potential expenditures and risks associated with integration; and
6 resistance from state bureaucracies to pool funding streams.

A third issue – and one that has received relatively little attention – is the need to develop a workforce that is trained in how to address the full range of care needs of the consumer (and family) and how to coordinate efforts to achieve this goal. Graduate medical education, nursing, social work, pharmacy, and therapy programs have not tended to focus on the interdisciplinary needs of people with disabilities, and few training models have adopted such an approach. While the field of geriatrics provides a framework that may be useful in designing educational curricula and practice guidelines for serving the under 65s as well as the elderly population, this concentration is currently physician dominated and tends to ignore the nonmedical aspects of long-term care.

The final issue relates to the absence of financial incentives to encourage providers to develop integrated systems of care for people with disabilities. Managed-care plans, in particular, attempt to select the "good risks" while avoiding bad ones. There is little guidance from past experience about how to set rates in such a way as to reflect potential costs. If higher premium rates are charged, more healthy participants are likely to opt for lower-cost plans, leaving the plan financially vulnerable. Two types of financial incentives are being explored to try to address the special problems of incorporating disabled populations into integrated care systems: risk sharing and risk adjustment. One major question that needs resolution relates to how risk can be shared between payers and providers, especially in the context of integrated funding streams. Progress in risk adjustment for people with disabilities is in its infancy. There is a lack of actuarial information to facilitate the modeling of service use and costs. The tremendous variation in the characteristics, service needs and utilization patterns of the disabled impede the development of risk adjustment methodologies. A National Chronic Care Consortium task force is developing a risk contracting model to help providers interested in integrating acute and long-term care services. The Community Medical Alliance is experimenting with new severity-of-impairment measures and functional-status measures to improve the ability to accurately predict future service use and cost. While these models are specific to particular disabilities such as spinal cord injury and AIDS, the lessons learned from these activities may help in the development of more general risk-adjustment methodologies.

Integration of state HCBC programs

As HCBC programs proliferate across the country, more states are exploring mechanisms for integration at the program and service-delivery levels. States have consolidated programs through single agencies, or have developed coordination of programs through umbrella organizations. Even if a state has been successful at achieving this integration, however, questions still remain as to the ultimate effects of this integration. First, and most important, is the extent to which this integration has produced positive outcomes in terms of improving access to HCBC services, enhancing the quality of care and reducing or at least controlling costs. A second question is whether integration at the administrative and/or service-delivery levels is sufficient if funding streams remain fragmented and targeted to different populations. Third, policymakers must assess whether the outcomes outweigh the costs of reorganization, including major turf battles, that were required to achieve administrative integration. Fourth is the extent to which these integration efforts are replicable in other states and communities. Many policymakers, for example, have looked to Oregon, Wisconsin and other administratively integrated states as models for their respective states. However, several state officials (R. Ladd, D. McDowell, personal communication, Washington, D.C., April 1993) have emphasized the fact that integration depends largely on the unique sociopolitical and economic environments as well as the client characteristics and service needs of the particular state and community. What works in one state will not necessarily be successful in another state.

The variation in state approaches to HCBC program integration is of particular concern to a small group of analysts in the US Department of Health and Human Services that has been charged with devising a plan for integrating "residual Medicaid programs" (e.g., 2176 waiver, personal care program) that would remain if Medicaid acute care services are folded into a national guaranteed benefits package. Options have ranged from maintaining separate programs but requiring formal administrative linkages to creating HCBC block grant programs to capping all long-term care services in a state, including institutional care. Given the difficulties that

Integration of Home- and Community-Based Services

states have encountered in integrating programs and the idiosyncratic nature of state initiatives, there is some question as to whether the federal government can, or should, mandate a particular option.

An increasing number of states have developed single points of entry and are attempting to integrate, or at least coordinate, care across settings through preadmission screening and case management. The few descriptive studies that have been conducted, however, have failed to examine empirically the extent to which these efforts have succeeded in achieving the goals of improving access to and delivery of care as well as controlling costs. There is a great need for more information on how various models work in different environments, and a detailed analysis of the factors that allow or impede successful integration of services. These include the auspice of the case management and/or pre-admission screening organizations, the entities responsible for these functions, and the degree to which actual (not just paper) linkages have been created across the full range of providers (i.e., hospital, physician, nursing home, home care). Finally, researchers need to examine the outcomes of these efforts, focusing not only on the process but also on the effects of single points of entry, pre-admission screening, case management and other mechanisms for the health and well-being of disabled consumers and their families.

Integration of HCBC Programs for diverse populations

The debate over the appropriateness of a generic versus a categorical approach to the financing and delivery of HCBC will continue and probably intensify as policymakers at the federal and state levels struggle with how to achieve long-term care reform. As advocates for the elderly and younger people with disabilities forge coalitions to lobby for universal health and long-term care coverage, there is pressure to develop HCBC programs that serve people of all ages and a range of disabilities. The Consortium for Citizens with Disabilities, a coalition of consumer groups representing the elderly and younger people with disabilities, has been working on draft language for a set of eligibility criteria that would be applicable to diverse populations. At the same time, Wisconsin's COP program, frequently cited as the premier example of a generic system, is now seriously contemplating a return to categorical programs with loose administrative integration.

These conflicting trends create confusion for policymakers involved in long-term care reform. The White House Task Force on Health Care Reform's Long-term Care Workgroup, for example, proposed a generic plan that would have required states to use a series of eligibility triggers to target services to severely disabled persons of all ages. The exact nature and design of the program, however, was left to each state. While the Health Security Act was defeated in Congress, the debate over the long-term care provisions raised the question of a generic versus specialized service system to a new level of priority.

As is true in the other areas of integration, there is a critical need for more evaluative research that examines the advantages and disadvantages of a generic approach to developing a HCBC program. Researchers should use the natural laboratories that exist in states serving multiple populations, including close scrutiny of the policy decisions made in Wisconsin. Currently, most of the programs that serve more than one population tend to target the elderly and younger physically disabled. To what extent is this "marriage" working? Are the service needs of other groups, particularly the MR/DD population, so different that separate programs are necessary?

Integration of formal and informal care
It is clear that relatives, friends and other informal helpers will remain the backbone of the HCBC delivery system in the US. Policymakers at the federal and state levels are focusing on how best to integrate the informal and formal care systems. While the findings from a variety of demonstration projects and state experiences in building care plans around informal networks provide little evidence of substitution, policymakers are still concerned that formal care will replace informal care if a large-scale, publicly subsidized program were implemented. This question may be more salient for the future as the elderly and nonelderly disabled become more comfortable with the use of formal services.

Descriptive studies and anecdotes documenting the care planning and resource-allocation process indicate that programs can successfully work with families to tailor services to the needs of the disabled person and existing informal supports. What is less clear is the extent to which the availability of families can, or should, be explicitly considered in determining eligibility for benefits. While several states have indicated no problems with this approach, there may be significant ethical, and perhaps even legal, consequences of developing a more comprehensive, federal program that denies benefits to people with informal networks.

The future of programs that pay informal caregivers is uncertain. As some states move aggressively in this direction, others have cut back on the discretion afforded to disabled persons and their families. There is an increasing trend toward more consumer choice and autonomy in long-term care policy, fueled in large part by the efforts of younger people with disabilities and the development of the independent living movement. Consistent with the consumer-choice orientation of the Clinton administration's health-care reform initiative, the White House Task Force's Long-Term Care Work Group recommended that cash payments, including the ability to hire family caregivers, be included in the plan. This issue will remain the subject of debate as the federal and state governments continue to explore long-term care reform alternatives. In order to make informed decisions, policymakers need better information on the relative advantages and disadvantages of paying informal caregivers. How do families use the funds? Are the payments adequate? Does paying informal caregivers increase the costs of HCBC programs? How is quality ensured?

To this end, DHHS has sponsored a study of independent providers in California that will, in part, examine the effects of paying family caregivers on quality of care. In addition, DHHS is collaborating with the Robert Wood Johnson Foundation to fund a large-scale demonstration and evaluation of state programs that offer cash instead of services to individuals who need personal care and long-term support in the community. The results of these two studies will provide new insights into the relative advantages and disadvantages of paying family caregivers and providing more choice and autonomy to consumers.

In conclusion, it is clear that integration has become a buzzword for long-term care reform, and that policymakers will continue to explore strategies for integrating HCBC on the four dimensions examined in this chapter. It is time, however, to go beyond the rhetoric of success. Rigorous evaluations are required to assess the degree of success with these initiatives and to identify the factors determining success or failure.

References

Ansello, E., and N. Eustis 1992. A Common Stake? Investigating the Emerging Intersection of Aging and Disabilities *Generations* 16(1): 5–8.
Office of the Assistant Secretary for Planning and Evaluation (ASPE). 1995. Managed Care for People with Disabilities: Developing a Research Agenda. Unpublished paper presented at an expert meeting sponsored by the US Department of Health and Human Services, Washington, D.C., January.
Bradley, V.J., J. Knoll, S. Covert, et al. 1990. *Family Support Services in the United States: An End of Decade Status Report*. Final report prepared by the

Human Services Research Institute for the Administration on Developmental Disabilities, US Department of Health and Human Services, Cambridge, MA.

Christianson, J.B. 1988. The Evaluation of the National Long-Term Care Demonstration, 6. The Effect of Channeling on Informal Caregiving. *Health Services Research* 23(1): 99–117.

Delaware Long-Term Care Oversight Committee, Office of Community-Based Long-Term Care. 1993. *Report on the Community-based Long-Term Care Needs of Delaware's Elderly and Physically Disabled.* Delaware Health and Human Services, Wilmington, DE.

Doty, P. 1990. Family Caregiving and Access to Publicly Funded Home Care: Implicit and Explicit Influences on Decisionmaking. Paper presented at the conference on Family Caregiving in Long-Term Care – Next Steps for Public Policy. Morgantown, WV, December.

Doty, P., R. Stone, B. Jackson, and M. Adler. 1995. Informal Caregiving. In *The Continuation of Long-Term Care: An Integrated System Approach*, ed. C. Evashwick and W. Evashwick. Albany: Delmar Publishers.

Edelman, P. 1986. The Impact of Community Care to the Homebound Elderly on Provision of Informal Care. *The Gerontologist* 26: 213.

Edelman, P., and S. Hughes. 1990. The Impact of Community Care on Provision of Informal Care to Homebound Elderly Persons. *Journal of Gerontology Social Sciences* 45(2): S74–84.

Ellison, M., et al. 1991. *Testing Family Support and Family Empowerment: Key Findings across Four Pilots.* Final report prepared by the Human Services Research Institute for the DHHS Administration on Developmental Disabilities. Cambridge, MA.

Glendenning, C., and E. McLaughlin. 1993. *Paying for Care: Lessons from Europe.* Social Security Advisory Committee Research Paper No. 5. London: Her Majesty's Stationery Office.

Gruenberg, L., A. Rumshiskaya, and J. Kaganova. 1993. An analysis of expected Medicare costs for participants in the PACE demonstration. Presented before the PACE annual demonstration meeting, May.

Hanley, R. 1991. Will Paid Home Care Erode Informal Support? *Journal of Health Policy, Politics and Law* 16: 507–21.

Harrington, C. 1993. Managed Competition for the Frail Elderly: Case Study of the SHMOs. Unpublished paper prepared at the Institute on Health and Aging, University of California San Francisco.

Intergovernmental Health Policy Project (IHPP). 1988. *State Financing of Long-Term Care Services for the Elderly, Volume I: Executive Report.* Washington, D.C.

Irvin, K., T. Riley, M. Booth, and Fuller. E. 1993. *Managed Care for the Elderly: A Profile of Current Initiatives.* Portland, ME: National Academy for State Health Policy.

Justice, D. 1988. *State Long-Term Care Reform: Development of Community Care Systems in Six States.* National Governors' Association, Center for Policy Research, Washington, D.C.

Justice, D. 1992. *Case Management in Community Care Programs: Selected State Approaches.* Report prepared by the National Association of State Units on Aging, Washington, D.C.

Justice, D. 1993. Case Management *Standards in State and Community Based Long Term Care Programs for Older Persons with Disabilities.* Report prepared by the National Association of State Units on Aging. Washington, D.C.

Kane, R.L., L.H. Illston, and N. Miller. 1992. Qualitative Analysis of the Program of All-Inclusive Care for the Elderly (PACE). *The Gerontologist* 32(6): 771–80.

Keigher, S. 1992. Family Compensation for Care of the Elderly in Other Nations: Options, Lessons, and Evolving Concerns. In *Wages for Caring: Compensation Family Care of the Elderly,* ed. N. Linsk, S. Keighter, L.G. Simon-Rusinowitz, et al. 39–62. New York: Praeger Press.

Keigher, S., and R. Stone. 1992. Payment for Care in the US: A Very Mixed Policy Bag. Paper presented at the International Meeting on Payment for Dependent Care. Vienna, Austria, July.

Kemper, P. 1990. Case Management Agency Systems of Administering Long-Term Care: Evidence from the Channeling Demonstration. *The Gerontologist* 30(6): 817–24.

Leutz, W., et al. 1991. Adding Long-Term Care to Medicare: The Social HMO Experience. *Journal of Aging and Social Policy* 3(4): 69–87.

Linsk, N., S. Keigher, L.G. Simon-Rusinowitz, et al. 1992. *Wages for Caring: Compensating Family Care of the Elderly.* New York: Praeger Press.

Litwak, E. 1985. *Helping the Elderly: The Complementary Roles of Informal Networks and Formal Systems.* New York: Guilford Press.

Master, R., T. Dreyfus, S. Connors, et al. 1995. The Community Medical Alliance: An Integrated System of Care in Greater Boston for People with Severe Disability and AIDS. Paper presented at a conference on Chronic Care Initiatives in HMOs. Washington, D.C., April.

McCall, N., and J. Korb. 1994. *Combining Acute and Long-Term Care in a Capitated Medicaid Program: The Arizona Long-Term Care System.* San Francisco: Laguna Research Associates.

Moscovice, I., et al. 1988. Substitution of Formal and Informal Care for the Community-Based Elderly. *Medical Care* 26(10): 971–81.

National Academy for State Health Policy. 1995. Preliminary Report of the Subcommittee on Dual Eligibility. Unpublished report presented May 22, 1995 to the National Steering Committee on Managed Care for Older Persons and Persons with Disabilities, Washington, D.C.

Newcomer, R. J., C. Harrington, K. Manton, et al. 1993. Case-Mix Adjusted Service Use and Expenditures in the Social HMO Demonstration. Unpublished report prepared at the Institute on Health and Aging, University of California, San Francisco.

Noelker, S.L., and D.M. Bass. 1989. Home Care for Elderly Persons: Linkages between Formal and Informal Caregivers, *Journal of Gerontology Social Sciences* 44(2): S63–70.

Pendleton S., et al. 1989. *State Infrastructure for Long-Term Care: A National*

Study of State Systems. National Aging Resource Center: Brandeis University, Waltham, MA.

Saucier, P., and T. Riley. 1994. *Managing Care for Older Beneficiaries of Medicaid and Medicare: Prospects and Pitfalls.* Portland, ME: National Academy for State Health Policy.

Schlesinger, M., and D. Mechanic. 1993. Challenges for Managed Competition from Chronic Illness. *Health Affairs* 12 (Supplement): 123–37.

Shen, J.K. 1993. Program of All-Inclusive Care for the Elderly (PACE). From Session 9 of "Long-Term Care: A Workshop for Senior State and Local Health Officials," Miami, December.

Simon-Rusinowitz, L., and B.F. Hofland. 1993. Adopting a Disability Approach to Home Care Services for Older Adults, *The Gerontologist* 33(2): 159–67.

Smith-Barusch, A., and I.S. Miller. 1985. The Effects of Services on Family Assistance to the Frail Elderly, *Journal of Social Services Research* 9(1): 31–46.

Stone, R. 1991. Defining Family Caregivers of the Elderley: Implications for Research and Public Policy. *The Gerontologist* 31(6).

US Department of Commerce, Bureau of Census. 1991. Survey of Income and Program Participation. Washington, D.C.

Weiner, J.M., and R.J. Hanley. 1992. Caring for the Disabled Elderly: There's No Place like Home. In *Improving Health Policy and Management: Nine Critical Research Issues for the 1990s,* ed. S. Shortell and U.E. Reinhardt, 75–110. Ann Arbor: Health Administration Press.

Weissert, W.G., C.M. Cready, and J.E. Pawelak. 1988. The Past and Future of Home- and Community-Based Long-Term Care, *Milbank Quarterly* 66(2): 356.

5

Home Health Services in a Managed-Care System: Policy Recommendations from a Program of Research

Merwyn R. Greenlick and Kathleen K. Brody

Introduction

The policy recommendations of this chapter are particularly timely because, in our assessment, the delivery of home-care services to managed-care populations in its current form is very similar to service delivery for other populations. This is true because organization of care within HMOs has been driven by imperatives from the fee-for-service world. But it appears that state and national health policy changes are going to force the development of a set of new population-based clinical practice models for care generally – that is, models that balance the needs of individual patients with the needs of the population at large – and the organization and delivery of home health services should follow those models. But, generally speaking, the experience of managed-care systems with home care is being ignored when the history of the field is reviewed. (See, for example, Benjamin (1993) for an otherwise excellent review that totally overlooks this aspect of the field.) In this chapter, we review the program of home health research at the Center for Health Research – from our pioneering skilled home-care research in the 1960s through the current Social HMO demonstration – and offer some policy recommendations for adapting to new models of care and health-care reform on the horizon.

Early HMO Research in Home Care

Agencies were providing organized home health services decades before HMOs made their way onto the medical care stage. But the early HMO models, primarily staff and group-model prepaid group practices, did not include these services within their scope of benefits or within their delivery models prior to the implementation of Medicare in 1966. The Medicare legislation provided organized financing for post-hospital skilled services available in extended-care facilities and by home health agencies for the elderly population of the United States. That meant that for the first time a large number of people in this country would present themselves to service-providing agencies with a need for services and with a card that represented a blank check that could be filled in by providers to pay for their services. This situation motivated researchers to seriously inquire into the dynamics of providing skilled home health services to the elderly population.

One of the first questions to be addressed in this research was what would be the effective demand for these newly entitled services. The legislative reports, produced as a part of the policy-development process, seemed seriously flawed to some observers because no population-based data on the demand for these services were available in the early 1960s when the legislation was being developed. Moreover, in order to keep the revenue required for the new legislation at a minimum, the framers of the legislation underestimated, rather than overestimated, the potential demand for these services. A group of investigators at the Kaiser Permanente Center for Health Research (CHR) began, in 1964, a project to develop a more precise national estimate of the demand for skilled nursing-care services.

The study design for this project involved three stages. The first was to develop simple, objective criteria that would allow measurement of physical condition and functional capacity, and were related to the need for post-hospital skilled nursing care. The second stage was to evaluate a probability sample of selected discharges on the

Home Health Services in a Managed-Care System

basis of these criteria and on questionnaire data gathered from the patients. The third stage included analyzing these evaluations and formulating estimates of need in the population. Work in the assessment of functional capacity had only just begun in the United States at that time and there was not much science to guide the effort, but the dimensions of patient disability that were posited to be most important would now seem very familiar to professionals in the field. These dimensions were mobility, continence, need for rehabilitative services, mental state (especially agitation, confusion, and coma) and, finally, the need for special procedures.

After the selected medical records were reviewed using standardized instruments, the relative probability of having a high need for post-hospital skilled services was assessed for the population. (Patients were included in this category if they had two or more areas of disability or if they had only one area of disability but had no one in the home to constantly care for them.) The study concluded that the estimates included in the planning for Medicare were dramatically understated. The study found that approximately 18 percent of the nearly 3.5 million projected discharges each year for people 65 years or older would be prime candidates for some form of post-hospital skilled nursing care. The authors noted that "perhaps 600,000 people will have both the high probability of need for post-hospital skilled nursing care and the financial capacity to demand it" (Greenlick, Hurtado, and Saward 1966).

This project provided a very accurate estimate of demand for post-hospital skilled nursing services in the United States. The Social Security Administration's report for the fiscal year 1967 indicated that under the Medicare program 448,500 persons were admitted to extended-care facilities and that 260,000 persons received a "start of care" notice for home-care services (US Congress 1969). Since many beneficiaries are in both counts, it is likely that about 600,000 people actually received services.

The project's estimate was that as many as 14,000,000 persons under 65 years of age could benefit from the same skilled nursing services, stimulating the Public Health Service to fund, in 1967, a demonstration study by the same investigative group at Kaiser Permanente in Portland. This second study was designed to provide the home-care and extended-care facility services available under Medicare to those over 65 years of age to a population of more than 100,000 people under 65 receiving care in Kaiser Permanente in Portland. (Greenlick, Burke, and Hurtado 1967; Hurtado et al. 1972; Hurtado, Greenlick, and Saward 1972).

The specific objectives of this project were:

1. To determine the feasibility of integrating home-care and ECF services into an ongoing, comprehensive, prepaid group practice plan;
2. To evaluate the impact of these new services on hospital utilization patterns;
3. To determine the utilization and costs associated with providing such services to a large population;
4. To train new personnel to provide professional services commonly undertaken by nurses, social workers, physical therapists, and occupational therapists.

To carry out the project a home health program was created within the prepaid group practice plan, with all services to be provided by the staff of that program. Also, an extended-care facility (what would more recently have been called an SNF) was developed that was physically connected to the HMO hospital. All artificial organizational barriers to the use of both services were eliminated.

The project used an objective algorithm to guide the decision on when a patient should be treated in the hospital, in the ECF, under the home health service, or in ambulatory care, or should be simply discharged to home (see figure 1). The then current Medicare definition of an appropriate ECF case was strictly applied; only patients with specific needs for skilled nursing or rehabilitation services qualified for admission. When ECF patients needed only custodial care, they were rapidly transferred to their homes, with or without home-care agency services, or to a nursing home.

All patients in the hospital were reviewed daily to determine if they should be moved to the ECF or discharged to the home-care program. It was an experiment to determine the outer limits of skilled home health and skilled care-facility use within an integrated medical-care system for both aged and younger members of the system.

Since the Medicare legislation had created the position "home health aide," a job title that was virtually unknown at that time, the project decided to create a very special kind of home health aide, one specially trained to demonstrate the outer limits of service potential for this new kind of health personnel. The training program for home health aides involved six weeks of didactic training, as well as continued supervision and training throughout the project. Each aide was trained to provide, as prescribed by a professional, member-specific physical therapy, nursing, social work, and occupational therapy in the home. As a result, one-half of the visits made by agency personnel were made by the home

Home Health Services in a Managed-Care System

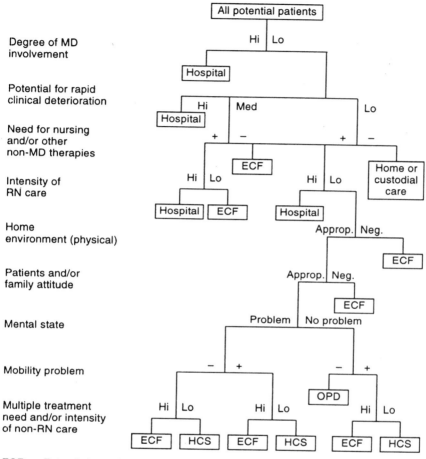

ECF — Extended care facility
HCS — Home care service
OPD — Outpatient department

Source: M. R. Greenlick, A. Hurtado, and E Saward. "The Objective Measurement of the Post-hospital Needs of a Known Population," *American Journal of Public Health* 56, no. 8 (1966): 1193-98.

health aide, who provided a majority of physical therapy procedures as well as a substantial portion of nursing services. Many social work visits in the home were provided by home health aides.[8] The more highly trained professionals devoted a large portion of their time in the home-care service to supervising and training these aides.

The aides were not specialized; each provided patient care from all disciplines, according to a care plan and under the supervision of the appropriate professionals. Consequently, supervision of a single aide by more than one professional was fairly common. This required greater communication among professionals. But the result of this experiment was that the full range of services provided under this program to a total population of nearly 100,000 people was delivered by four registered nurses, one physical therapist, one licensed practical nurse, a half-time social worker, and eight home health aides.

Patients accepted the services of this special aide with great ease, and the supervising professionals reported that the aides provided effective service in the field. There were no reports of services detrimental to the patient; the aides were able to recognize developing problems and changes in patient status very quickly, and to obtain appropriate supervisory help.

Overall, the project findings were dramatic and led to the eventual institutionalization of both home health and skilled care-facility services within the benefit package and, in the case of skilled home health, within the service-providing capacity of Kaiser Permanente and other group- and staff-model HMOs. In fact, in the situation of the ECF physically integrated with the acute hospital, the addition of ECF and home-care services did not increase the overall per capita cost of medical care for the younger population, because every two days of ECF care appeared to be associated with a one-day reduction of much more expensive hospital care. And although the home health services in the younger population did not produce significant cost-offsets, the per capita costs were relatively low (a few cents per member month in those days), encouraging the HMO to add the home health benefit at the conclusion of the project.

The ability of Kaiser Permanente to provide home health services to its entire population was at its zenith when the project concluded in 1970. Two sets of factors led to the eventual regression of the home health program within this HMO to the mean of the field. First was the increasing formalization of Medicare rules that were imposed on home health services, even services organized within risk-based HMOs. And perhaps more important were the growing legal, regulatory, and normative restrictions of the freedom of home health aides to provide services that, to the investigators and professionals of the project, seemed perfectly safe and appropriate for them to perform. Consequently, by the time one of the first-round Medicare risk demonstration sites was implemented at the Center for Health Research in Portland (Greenlick et al. 1983), the home health program at KP was virtually indistinguishable from a competent home health agency serving fee-for-service patients in a

Home Health Services in a Managed-Care System

medium-sized American city anywhere. The reason we review this research is to remind ourselves of what is possible, to compare this with what has actually emerged, and to see what we can learn from that comparison.

Current Delivery of Home-Care Services in Managed Care

The provision of home health care through health maintenance organizations was reviewed by Parker and Polich (1988) in an InterStudy project in 1988 and a review of their findings provides the basis for much of the material in this section of the chapter. The focus of their investigation was the provision of home health services for Medicare beneficiaries, partly because of their funding source (HCFA), and partly because a major portion of the home health activity of most HMOs is in the Medicare arena. There were 648 HMOs operating in the United States in 1988 and only 159 of them were serving Medicare beneficiaries. Seventy percent of the HMOs serving Medicare beneficiaries were operating under TEFRA (1982 Tax Equity and Responsibility Act) risk contracts, 18 percent had Medicare cost contracts and 12 percent operated under Health Care Prepayment Plans. Only two HMOs reported more than one type of Medicare contract in 1988, Kaiser Permanente Northwest Region being one of these.

Table 5.1 Home health services provided by Medicare HMOs*

Service	Percentage of HMOs that cover service
Skilled nursing	100
Physical therapy	97
Speech pathology	92
Home health aide	81
Occupational therapy	74
Medical social worker	66

*Source: M. Parker and C. Polich, *The Provision of Home Health Care Services Through Health Maintenance Organizations* (Excelsior, Minnesota: InterStudy, 1988) p. 26.

HMO Medicare federal contracts require that beneficiaries receive, at a minimum, the mandated Medicare benefits of skilled nursing, physical therapy, and speech pathology. According to

InterStudy, the services provided by HMOs fell largely into these main categories (see table 1). Conditional services include occupational therapy, medical social work, and home health aid. Sixty-six percent of the HMOs surveyed did not offer any type of supplemental services such as meal preparation, housekeeping, hospice, transportation, telephone reassurance, or respite care.

Four percent of the HMOs provided internally all home health care service, 70 percent contracted with an outside agency to provide home health care, and the remainder used a combination of internal and external provision. Various service payment methods, capitation, fee-for-service, and discount rates are employed by the HMOs, each with its own set of unique problems. Nearly half of the HMOs without internal home health care services expressed an interest in developing an agency (Louden 1986).

The Medicare home health benefit has clearly emerged within an acute-care context, providing professional care at home to serve post-hospital acute needs and shortening the length of hospital stay. Needs for acute-care home health services are generally episodic in nature and the services are targeted to reduce or eliminate the highest end of medical service trajectory – inpatient stays (Louden 1986). After examining the data from Medicare HMOs, Parker and Polich conclude that "HMO home health care services mirror the inadequacies of Medicare Home health care in that they are acute care-focused and not intended to fill the supportive and maintenance care needs of chronically ill elderly (Parker and Polich 1988, 33).

The goal noted as primary by 93 percent of the HMOs in the InterStudy project was to provide short-term skilled home health care to shorten or substitute for inpatient or skilled nursing-home care rather than maintaining the independence of chronically ill elderly. The main difference to the beneficiaries of receiving care in an HMO is that the HMO determination of eligibility for home health care is a bit more flexible than the guidelines and limitations imposed by Medicare retrospective determinations. Utilization still appears to be controlled by traditional gate keeping, prior authorization, determining visit length, or by requiring additional member copayments or deductibles (although none of the group models required copayments). On the other hand, 90 percent of the HMOs stated that they had no specific visit cap connected to the home health benefit. InterStudy found that 41 percent of the HMOs serving Medicare beneficiaries developed their own discharge plan from hospitals. Geriatric case-management programs had been instituted in 24 percent of the risk-contract HMOs and another 10

Home Health Services in a Managed-Care System

percent were in the process of developing the program. Ninety-four percent of the Medicare HMOs used prior authorization for home health, some with time limits.

Outside HMOs, home health services represent the fastest growing segment of Medicare expenditures. It is predicted that the home will be the primary site of clinical care in the 21st century (Griff and Lerman 1987). Reasons for the surge in home health generally, beyond the aftermath of instituting Diagnostic Related Groupings for inpatient stays, are: legislative changes, new technology suited to the home, consumer preference, and the unique needs of a population which is growing older. Because of what is happening in the field, many believe that HMOs will become even more dependent on home-care providers to supply a cost-effective alternative to hospital care (Roeder 1986).

There is some evidence that HMOs are beginning to expand the scope of services available under the home-health rubric. In an earlier study of 41 risk-contract HMOs surveyed, all reported that home health services were based on medical need. However, one-fourth indicated they were beginning to provide limited supportive home care, not mentioned in their marketing literature, but available on a case-by-case basis as a cost-effective alternative to institutional care (Iversen and Polich 1986, 1987). On the one hand, Kramer, Fox, and Morgenstern (1992) report that HMO home health agencies appear to serve members with higher activity than fee-for-service home health agencies. On the other hand, Parker and Polich (1988) reported that over 70 percent of the HMOs felt that home health care should be expanded to provide a smooth, safe transition from hospital to home and to provide terminal care. The study clearly reported that these unmet needs are in the area of supportive care and social service. The study also reported that there was consideration for a new set of services to be provided in members' homes, although those on the list of players discussed do not sound like supportive care providers. HMOs gave some consideration to expanding the variety of home health professionals, to include laboratory technicians, intravenous therapists, nutritionists, respiratory therapists, dialysis nurses, and other nursing specialists.

Recommendations

The policy recommendations following this analysis fall into three areas, each of which is offered in the context of improving home health services within managed-care systems.

The first set of recommendations proposes ways to integrate population-based models for delivering care within capitated managed-care systems. The weight of these recommendations would move regulatory and management practices away from those developed in a fee-for-service world to a new approach to home health, based on fitting it into the world of managed care.

The second set of recommendations relates to integrating community-based long-term care and skilled acute-care-based home health services. These recommendations derive from data from the Social HMO models being tested in the United States today.

The third set of recommendations suggests finding ways to change the current approach to home health personnel policy. These recommendations speak of enhancing the role of the home health aide and to creating new models for nurse–family interaction, including significant expansion in the role of the home health nurse.

Area 1: Integrating population-based models within managed-care systems

Context. While one could argue that the delivery of home health services within HMOs is, by definition, population-based, the delivery models that have emerged do not seem to be based on meeting members' overall needs and aspirations. Nor do they seem to be designed to fully meet the needs of the health-care systems within which they reside. In our early research, and particularly in our demonstrations, we developed the population-based model, with the only a priori constraints being the nature of the population at risk and the specific needs of those people. While needs were assessed patient by patient, the assessment methodologies were designed with simultaneous consideration of not only patient satisfaction but also program effectiveness and health-care services efficiency.

What stimulated that original design work was the inclusion of skilled home-care services under Medicare when it began in 1966. Because Medicare became the major funding source for skilled home-care services in managed-care systems, Medicare rules and regulations eventually overwhelmed the traditional HMO perspective. This was true even when the HMOs began to include coverage for services for the younger population. Because the critical decision makers in operationalizing Medicare rules are the directors of the home health services, or the directors of the agencies with which managed-care systems contract, the HMO home-care programs are skewed under Medicare rules.

Because Medicare has been oriented to controlling costs in the fee-for-service environment, it should come as no surprise that the Medicare regulations focused in three areas – ensuring that people receiving services are really *home bound*, that they really need *skilled* home health services, and that the *proper* personnel deliver *professionally* appropriate services.

These concerns are not necessarily the wrong basis for criteria development. But they are not the dimensions that would emerge normally from an analysis of how home health services "ought" to be designed to fit within a rational package of services and benefits for members of an HMO. A systems approach to specifying the criteria for serving HMO members in their home includes a requirement to balance the needs of the population at large (through a broader efficiency definition) with the service needs of individual patients. That balancing process should allow a full set of trade-off decisions, especially concerning the definition of the proper place for the delivery of the full range of services needed by members of the population. In the ideal situation any artificial barriers between the hospital, the nursing facilities, the office, and the home should be eliminated, especially barriers that are developed to avoid inappropriate behavior in the fee-for-service world. That does not seem possible in the current situation. At least we did not identify any current models that looked properly seamless.

It was not that way in the beginning of Medicare. In the discussion of the KP home-care project above, the addition of home health and extended-care-facility services was hailed as the final implementation of what was referred to as "progressive patient care" (Somers and Somers 1961). Home care and ECF services were provided to patients according to their needs, without regard to their physical location at the time of assessment. The project demonstrated that the addition of these services within an HMO allowed the patients to flow to the appropriate medical-care setting according to the intensity and nature of their need. And since the patient's single medical record was the vehicle for sharing the care plan approved for a patient and for documenting the services provided, it was possible in that project to create a situation where neither the structure of the payment mechanism nor the organization of care encouraged unnecessary utilization of more expensive services. The level of care received was determined by need alone, unrestricted by financial or other administrative barriers. Unfortunately, that is not the case 25 years later.

There is a pressing policy need to redefine home health services within a broader context. (As it happens, there is also a need to redefine hospital and ambulatory care, but we will save that for another day.) In a capitated managed-care system all of the available dollars are put into a single pot at some level of the organization. (All of the population's needs are put into a single pot as well.) It is then the job of the strategic planners of the program to develop a model that properly allocates resources, usually dollars in the first instance, for meeting the needs of the membership in the most effective way possible. In the decisions for any single year (tactical decisions) there are always many constraints, including primarily the inertia of how things have been done in past years. But the more relevant factors are the defined long-term constraints, such as the medical care market in an area or how hospital and physician services are to be purchased or delivered.

In the home-care field one of the most important strategic constraints is defined by the set of Medicare regulations (and customs) about the delivery of skilled home-care services. This constraint has narrowly defined the field. Consequently, the delivery of home health services within HMOs and other managed-care organizations has not emerged as a major area of innovation.

The InterStudy conclusions discussed above pointed out the traditional nature of HMO home health services, as did a recent study of innovations in geriatric care within HMOs (Kramer, Fox, and Morgenstern 1992). The latter reiterated that HMOs are not precisely bound by traditional Medicare home health restrictions to only provide care to homebound patients who need skilled home health services on an intermittent and generally short-term basis. HMOs could, at least in concept, ignore the relatively stringent eligibility criteria and could provide the home health services that they regard as cost effective. And the investigators observed that some HMOs used home health care more aggressively. But, other than the Social HMO demonstration in place in KP in Portland and Group Health in Minneapolis, they could point to no major innovation in the use of home health services in the HMOs they visited. It is definitely time to change that situation.

Recommendations in Area 1

- HCFA's approach to ACR and AAPCC methodology should be revised to reward risk-contract HMOs that use home health services more aggressively.
- HCFA should support research to validate ways to expand home health use within managed care and aggressively disseminate findings from this research.

First, HCFA should revise ACR and AAPCC methodology to specifically reward HMOs serving Medicare beneficiaries for using home health services more aggressively. HCFA should support work to create research models that demonstrate cost-effective ways of expanding home health services. And they should work to disseminate these findings in a set of consensus conferences designed to create a new standard for HMO use of home care and related modalities.

Secondly, work should proceed to help home health agency directors and staff to understand the issues relevant to HMO managers, such as service integration models and capitation and risk-adjustment issues. They need to understand the issues involved in operating managed-care systems. As health reform bases the financing for most health care on population-based, capitation models, home health agencies will have to integrate their activities within new health-care systems whose incentives and problems will mirror those of current HMOs. When home health services are provided within these systems they become cost rather than revenue centers and the objectives of the agencies will, perforce, change. It is important that these changes are understood. Currently even the home health directors working within HMOs are so influenced by their peers in the home health field that they continue to view the world through fee-for-service glasses, rather than managed-care contact lenses.

Area 2: Integrating community-based long-term care and home health services

Context. In addition to dealing with the isolation between skilled home health services and the rest of the medical-care world, there is the problem of appropriately defining the patient's situation as one that calls for "skilled" services. The traditional Medicare definition of services, invented and refined during the 1960s as a part of institutionalizing the new Medicare program, clearly created a gulf between skilled home care and other care services that were needed to care for the patient in the home (chronic care or community-based long-term care). This skilled-care restriction has gone beyond Medicare-covered services, at least in HMOs, and sets the limit for covered home health services across populations. The legislation that created Medicare permitted post-hospital coverage in extended-care facilities and services by home health agencies only if either is "primarily engaged in providing skilled nursing care or related services" (US Social Security Administration 1965).

The problem is that a patient's need for care is a composite of physical, functional, emotional, social, and medical levels. Unfortunately, the skilled services directed to demonstrable acute needs are frequently not sufficient to care for the aggregate needs of patients.

Therefore, the next policy issue we address is the desirable link between skilled home-care services and community-based long-term care services that fosters stability, especially for chronic-care patients. Community-based long-term care (LTC) services include those supportive personal-care services that are needed to enhance or maintain normal body function, to address emotional comfort, and to assist the patient in independent living. (This definition of services was what guided the work of the home health aide in the original home health demonstration project of the CHR. It was assumed to be what Medicare originally intended to cover. These services become necessary in a variety of medical care situations, including situations of convalescence from a specific acute episode, for a medical flare-up of a relatively stable chronic condition, during an end-stage illness episode, for respite for informal caregivers, or to care for a very frail and declining patient (Greenlick et al. 1988).

During the two decades from the end of the original home health projects, CHR investigators were involved in several demonstrations that are relevant to these recommendations, but two are particularly apposite. We were involved in the first round of Medicare HMO risk demonstrations and the Social HMO national demonstration project (Greenberg et al. 1985). These demonstrations honed our concern for and our knowledge about the provision of services to Medicare beneficiaries within an HMO. In the first we demonstrated the feasibility of integrating the organization and financing of care for elderly people within a group-practice HMO. And with the Social HMO demonstration we learned about the feasibility and importance of integrating community-based long-term care services into the spectrum of services available within any managed-care program, but especially within a managed-care system caring for elderly participants.

The Social HMO demonstration was conceived by scholars at the Heller School of Brandeis University and includes four service sites throughout the United States: Elderplan, Brooklyn, NY; Senior Care Action Network (SCAN Health Plan), Long Beach, CA; Seniors Plus, within Group Health, Inc. of Minneapolis, MN; and the Medicare Plus II program in Kaiser Permanente in Portland, OR. The National Social HMO Research Consortium's Data Center is housed at the CHR in Portland. The demonstration currently enrolls, in integrated

Home Health Services in a Managed-Care System 113

managed-care programs, about 25,000 Medicare beneficiaries across the sites. Each of the beneficiaries receives the full range of medical care benefits, including coverage for community-based long-term care services. These benefits are funded through member premiums valued at around $40 per member per month. The total revenue for the program comes from a combination of funds from Medicare and Medicaid as well as, in some plans, from member premiums. The HMO savings at two of the sites offset some or all of the member premium.

Members are regularly assessed at the sites for need for services, and integrated referral networks have been developed to ensure that eligible members who need LTC services gain access to those services. Each site has developed an integrated approach for delivering community-based long-term care services that is integrated within the managed-care system's delivery approach.

Data from the Social HMO national demonstration project are very useful for assessing the need for linking skilled and community-based LTC services. Because the Social HMO includes the resources for providing community-based long-term care services to large HMO Medicare populations, it is possible to assess the extent that there exists a concurrent need for skilled and LTC services. While it is clear that there is bound to be overlap between utilization of Medicare skilled care services and community-based LTC services, Social HMO data show that this overlap is indeed substantial.

Among Social HMO patients receiving Medicare skilled care, 37 percent were found to concurrently qualify for and receive care from the Social HMO's LTC benefit during their first month on skilled care. On the other hand, new community LTC patients often need and qualify for Medicare skilled services. Fully 37 percent of the community LTC plans for Social HMO members made during their first month of community LTC eligibility contained concurrent authorizations for Medicare-covered skilled services. That is, more than one-third of newly identified "long-term care" patients were eligible for and receiving Medicare-covered skilled services during that same month (Abrahams et al. 1992; Leutz, Greenlick, and Capitman 1994).

In both these situations the overlap was managed by community LTC case managers. These case managers work closely with post-acute and skilled care staff to ensure that each understands the targeting criteria and services covered by the other and to maintain close contact regarding shared patients and transfers. This coordination is particularly important in cases that are medically or socially complex, or that involve transitions across settings. In the current HMO system, where only Medicare-covered skilled services are available, these patients are left without access to particularly important services and the health-care system struggles, dealing with the consequences of fragmented care.

Recommendation in Area 2

- Congress should create a new entitlement for a modest amount of community-based long-term care services under Medicare or under Medicare supplemental insurance programs.

It is clear that the debate on health reform in the United States is going to have to address these issues of long-term care generally, but certainly one lesson has been learned from the Social HMO experience in the United States. That lesson is that it is both desirable and feasible to add community-based long-term care services to the benefits and to the available service package of any managed-care system providing care to the elderly (Leutz, Greenlick, and Capitman 1994).

If we are going to deal with reforming home health care in the United States it is particularly important to begin to expand the current limited definition of what is a Medicare-covered home health service. While we probably will not be able to create an entitlement to provide access to total community- and institutional-based long-term care services, we certainly can take the first step. That first step is to create entitlement, under Medicare or under Medicare supplemental insurance programs of various kinds, to a modest amount of community-based long-term care services. The pressing need for these services and the evidence, from the Social HMO demonstration and from other demonstrations, that it is reasonable and feasible to include them in an entitlement system, make this area an extremely high priority.

Area 3: Re-examining home health personnel policy

Context. The final recommendation relates to the scope of allowable or appropriate practice of home health workers. There has been a major change in health manpower policy in the field of home health care since the implementation of Medicare in 1966. When we began the home health study discussed above, the field was relatively primitive and straightforward. While home health services had been available for decades, to a large extent they were available from visiting nursing service agencies. These agencies, in most communities, really focused on the delivery of nursing services, although included in the definition of what a visiting nurse did in those days were a great many of the "caring" as well as "curing" services. To be sure, there had been experiments in the delivery of home nursing services and the service definition had begun to grow. As hospitals began to expand their sphere of influence in the Hill-Burton era, several began integrated, hospital-based, home health agencies, delivering a range of services, including nursing, physical therapy, and social-work services (Ryder and Stitt 1967; Mather and Hobaugh 1967).

The introduction of Medicare coverage for home health aide services into this rather unstable situation created an environment that fostered change, both positive and negative. As the demand for skilled home health services grew, many agencies began to grow to meet the demand. A variety of approaches were put forward for defining the proper role of the players in the field, with the result that the role of each of the professionals in home care began to crystallize and to move toward a more and more narrow definition. The nurse remained dominant. The narrowly defined role of the physical and occupational therapists, the social worker, and the speech pathologist still left each profession with significant responsibilities in the field.

At the same time the professionals began to narrow the scope of responsibility of the home health aide. And because of the resultant narrow definition of the home health aide, a variety of other kinds of aide-level professionals began to be introduced into the field: personal care aide, physical therapy aide, certified nursing assistant, homemaker and a variety of others across the states. Currently, the job definition of each is quite narrow. We do not even allow trained aides to do things in the home that we are quite willing to train a totally unskilled family member to do.

This situation creates problems in the organization and delivery of care within an integrated system, or perhaps in any system. In fact, enlightened industrial practice world-wide is reversing earlier management engineering practices that created over-specialized industrial workers. In the health-care field it is especially difficult to organize services efficiently when personnel are so specialized. Data from the original home health study indicate that the dramatically less specialized personnel of that day produced more than twice as many visits per year as do current personnel. And since a single aide was primarily responsible for most direct-care services to a single patient, the patient and the aide were able to develop a closer relationship. Further, the aide was able to use the flexibility of the role to provide whatever services were needed on any particular day. The job was a more interesting one, and since agencies made such an investment in the training of the aides, they were much more interested in creating a service career for each aide. The turnover, therefore, was relatively low.

Recommendation in Area 3

- Programs should be created at the state and national level to stimulate the creation and deployment of nonprofessional-level service personnel who have a much greater scope of responsibility than do current nonprofessonal home health workers.

The first recommendation in this area is to explore what can be done to create and deploy nonprofessional-level health-service personnel with a much greater scope of responsibility. Certainly, professionals need to be involved in training, mentoring, and supervising the aide-level personnel. But it is urgent that we develop the resources for a set of research and demonstration projects investigating how to recreate a category of home health worker with a job description that is greatly expanded in breadth and depth. Having such workers available would allow us to organize services in an efficient manner, would reduce the number of workers that need to be in the home of a patient, and would develop an enhanced occupational role for a potentially large number of talented workers in the health-care field. This change in policy could go a long way toward eliminating a potential shortage of home-care workers as the population ages.

Even if we can demonstrate the cost effectiveness and the quality of such personnel models, we will still need to find a way to overcome the barriers in state laws and regulations, and in Medicare and Medicaid regulations, that make it difficult to deploy such personnel. Indeed we must find ways to motivate agencies to hire, train, and deploy such personnel to the greatest extent possible. And we must make certain that there are no financial disincentives to expanding the role of aide-level personnel within federal, state, or private health-care programs. If the legal, regulatory, and financial barriers to this expansion are removed, it seems inevitable that we can succeed in changing the way care is given in the home.

Finally, we should find ways to expand the role definition of all existing home health professionals to ensure that they are doing all that is possible to enhance the informal system that currently provides most of the home health services in the United States. We need personnel who have a greater understanding of how they can train, supervise, support, empower, delegate, and develop ongoing relationships with family members, caregivers, and other health attendants.

The Institute of Medicine Committee on a National Agenda for the Prevention of Disabilities took this issue head-on, noting: "There are few incentives for practicing the types of longitudinal care this committee advocates, and health professionals who follow these careers historically have had little recognition and prestige within their professional groups" (Pope and Tarlov 1991). One of the recommendations made by the committee was to provide more training opportunities for family members and personal attendants of people with disabling conditions and to develop new health-care service delivery strategies for caring for these people.

A recently completed research pilot, conducted jointly by CHR and Oregon Health Sciences University investigators, focused on training caregivers in an effort to increase the stability of the care-giving situation. The pilot study tested a home health nursing intervention aimed at expanding the role of home health nursing. (Archbold et al. 1995). This intervention was designed to increase the preparedness and competence of family members providing long-term care for frail older people, to make unpredictable care-giving situations more predictable, and to enrich care-giving processes.

One of the main goals of the pilot was to enhance the nurses' assessment skills of the healing arts and to tone down the ingrained nursing education patterned on physiology and treatment. The intervention required home health nurses to change their practice in substantial ways, and to shift from an individually oriented, skilled-care model to a long-term care, family-driven model focused on care-giving preparedness, predictability, and enrichment. The patient was defined as a dyad — that is, as a care receiver and a caregiver existing in an environment of established strengths and weaknesses and being jointly affected by disease processes, aging, financial issues, time constraints, worry, relationships, and other relevant problems.

Pilot results indicate that it is possible not only to expand the perspective of the nurse, but, more importantly, to redefine the role of the family and to create a new environment where the family caregiver can safely take on an entirely different role relative to the professional.

Research resources should be provided to test this kind of expanded role for the health professional and we should search for and encourage existing models that move toward enhanced independence for family members as they care for a member of their family. As the new models become available, we need to find ways to facilitate their introduction into the field.

The above recommendations for change come from demonstration projects, which tried the various approaches and found them both feasible and effective when used within the context of a managed-care system. Most of the innovations (except the very newest ones – those from the Social HMO demonstration) guided the development of services within the HMO, only to be eliminated by the pressure of meeting the regulations imposed upon home health agencies by external regulators. Since changes in health policy are likely to continue the movement toward managed care, the recommendations go beyond suggestions for HMOs as we know them.

Combined, these recommendations could shift the paradigm for current home health service delivery. With dramatic proposals for changing the overall organization and delivery of health care on the way, it is time to find ways to revolutionize home health care as well.

References

Abrahams, R., T. Von Sternberg, D. Zeps, S. Dunn, and P. Macko. 1992. Integrating Care for the Geriatric Patient. *HMO Practice* 6(4): 12–19.

Archbold, P.G., B.J. Stewart, L.L. Miller, et al. 1995. The PREP System of Nursing Intervention: A Pilot Test with Families Caring for Older Members. *Research in Nursing and Health* 18: 3–16.

Benjamin, A.E. 1993. An Historical Perspective on Home-Care Policy. *Milbank Quarterly* 71(1): 129–66.

Coate S. and E.A. Nordstrom, Jr. 1969. Experiment in Upgrading the Nonprofessional Worker. *Social Casework* 50: 401–6.

Greenberg, J.N., W. Leutz, S. Ervin, M. Greenlick, D. Kodner, and J. Selstad. 1985. S/HMO: The Social Health Maintenance Organization and Long Term Care. *Generations* 9(4): 51–5.

Greenlick, M.R., D. Burke, and A. Hurtado. 1967. The Development of a Home Health Program within a Comprehensive Prepaid Group Practice Plan. *Inquiry* 4(3): 31–9.

Greenlick, M.R., A. Hurtado, and E. Saward. 1996. The Objective Measurement of the Post-Hospital Needs of a Known Population. *American Journal of Public Health* 56(8): 1193–8.

Greenlick, M.R., S.J. Lamb, T.M. Carpenter, Jr, T.S. Fischer, S.D. Marks, and W.J. Cooper. 1983. Kaiser Permanente's Medicare Plus Project: A Successful Prospective Payment Demonstration. *Health Care Financing Review* 4(4): 85–97.

Greenlick, M.R., L.L. Nonnenkamp, L. Gruenberg, W. Leutz, and S. Lamb. The S/HMO Demonstration: Policy Implications for Long-Term Care in HMOs. 1988. *Journal of Long-Term Home Health Care* September: 15–24.

Griff, S.L. and D. Lerman. *The Future of Home Care: Positioning the Hospital for the Future.* Chicago: American Hospital Publishing Inc.

Hurtado, A., M.R. Greenlick, B.A. McCabe, and E. Saward. 1972. The Utilization and Cost of Home-Care and Extended Care Facility Services in a Comprehensive Prepaid Group Practice Program. *Medical Care* 10(1): 8–16.

Hurtado, A., M.R. Greenlick, and E. Saward. 1972. *Home-Care and Extended Care in a Comprehensive Prepayment Plan.* Chicago: Hospital Research and Educational Trust.

Iversen, L.H., and C. Polich. 1986, 1987. *December Update on Medicare Enrollment in HMO.* Excelsior, Minnesota: InterStudy.

Kramer, A.M., P.D. Fox, and N. Morgenstern. 1992. Geriatric Care Approaches in Health Maintenance Organizations. *Journal of the American Geriatric Society* 40(10): 1055–67.

Leutz, W.N., M.R. Greenlick, and J.A. Capitman. 1994. Integrating Acute and Long-Term Care. *Health Affairs* 13(4): 58–75.

Louden, T.L. 1986. *Home Care-HMO/PPO Perspectives.* Chicago: Louden and Company.

Mather W.G., and R.J. Hobaugh. 1967. Physician and Patient Attitudes toward a Hospital Home Care Program. *Inquiry* 4(3): 47.

Parker M., and C. Polich. 1988. *The Provision of Home Health Care Services through Health Maintenance Organizations.* Excelsior, Minnesota: InterStudy.

Pope A.M., and A.R. Tarlov (eds), for the Committee on a National Agenda for the Prevention of Disabilities. 1991. *Disability in America: Toward a National Agenda for Prevention.* Washington, D.C.: National Academy Press.

Roeder, B. 1986. Positioning for the Future: HMO Contracting. *Caring* 5:12–15.

Ryder C.F., and P.G. Stitt. 1967. Physician Involvement in Home Care. *Inquiry* 4(3): 41.

Somers H.M., and A.R. Somers. 1961. *Doctors, Patients and Health Insurance: The Organization and Financing of Medical Care.* Washington, D.C.: Brookings Institution.

US Congress, House. 1969. *Second Annual Report, Operations of Medicare Program.* H. Doc. 9157, 91st Congress 1st session, January 20, 1969, appendix C. Washington, D.C.

US Social Security Administration. 1965. *Health Insurance for the Aged: Information for Providers of Service.* Washington, D.C.: Government Printing Office.

6

Home-Care Dollars and Sense: A Prescription for Policy

William G. Weissert

Home care that is too expensive is home care that will almost certainly remain unavailable. Fear of runaway budgets has kept coverage restricted for three decades and will probably continue to restrain its growth. Home-care demonstration projects have produced almost exclusively disappointments, higher costs and few patient benefits.

The reasons appear to be two-fold: inappropriate policy goals, and faulty implementation.

Inappropriate Goals

The goal most policymakers have ascribed for home care is to reduce nursing-home use to justify itself. But the tools available to case-managers are not effective instruments for selecting a population of clients who are exclusively at risk of nursing-home entry. Green (1987) has shown that even designing highly accurate instruments is probably impossible. The results: three out of four clients admitted to home care were not at much risk of nursing-home entry. This makes the nursing-home-use-reduction goal irrelevant for three out of four patients. Yet the Clinton Health Care Reform proposal which called for substantial expansion of home-care benefits, again predicated coverage on the notion that home care will substitute for nursing-home care (The White House Domestic Policy Council 1993).

Pursuing irrelevant or inappropriate goals directs energies away from more appropriate goals which might actually have produced some desirable benefits.

An example may illustrate the point. The National Channeling Demonstration project, an expensive and highly visible project reflecting the collected wisdom of two dozen earlier home-care demonstrations, sought to reduce hospital use. Yet despite this goal, and though 62 percent of its home-care patients were hospitalized, it had no effect on those hospitalizations (Kemper 1988). Why not? A potential answer: Its intervention lacked the kind of patient-care management needed to help patients prevent the specific types of hospitalizations over which home care might have had some control. Since home care is for most of its patients not a medical or invasive intervention, it is unlikely to affect physiological change. It must therefore affect knowledge, attitudes, and behavior. Two types of hospitalization in which knowledge and attitudes might affect behavior are those resulting in death and those resulting in nursing-home placement. While neither may be avoidable in any given case, it seems quite reasonable to assume that some might be avoidable in some cases. Yet the Channeling intervention included no special program targeted at these types of hospitalization. Their occurrence was not defined or their prevalence counted, patients' risks of experiencing them were not evaluated, and results of the project were not judged against the criteria of avoiding this specific subgroup's success in avoiding hospitalization despite the fact that they constituted nearly a fourth of all patients (Weissert et al. in review).

This is not a failing of the Channeling Demonstration project, per se. It is a failing of our whole approach to home care. Assuming that it would reduce hospitalization and nursing-home use, we failed to do our homework, defining just what it can do and for whom, before we began trying to prove our hunches.

Implementation Problems and Agency Theory

Thinking of the home-care policy and implementation problem as an example of what economists and political scientists call "agency theory" is instructive (Prottas 1979; Lipsky 1980; Moe 1984; Arrow 1985). It conceptualizes the relationship between a principal and an agent as one in which the agent will act perfectly in the interest of the principal only if the task is well defined, training and technologies are adequate, sufficient monitoring is performed, and the right incentives are in place to induce the desired behavior.

Home-care case managers are agents with two masters: the payer source, which wants efficient and effective care, and the patient, who wants effective care but doesn't much care about efficiency. Furthermore, their training and the tools they use for screening and care planning are inadequate, the goals they are given are inappropriate, and the budgeting assumptions under which they operate doom them to failure in their quest to save money. These factors make the policymaker and payers ineffective principals. Not surprisingly, their goals for home care are rarely met.

Patients and their families, on the other hand, and rightly or wrongly, often know what they want. Unlike acute-care patients cowed by technology and expertise, in a long-term care setting, Nyman, Levey, and Rohrer (1987) and others have argued that patients and their families can be very knowledgeable consumers. Patients do not have the same goals for home care as do policymakers and payers. Most patients are likely to have little regard for efficiency or overall costs. Indeed, some are in the program because they want their costs shifted from private to public funds – a perfectly reasonable patient goal, but not one which helps the policymaker achieve the public goal of lower public costs. Other patients want merely caregiver relief, again, a worthwhile goal, but not one which will save money. And if the care is free, patients and families have little incentive to worry about how expensively it is achieved. Still others may want improvements in physical functioning despite the fact that an enormous body of research shows that home care simply does not produce improved physical functioning – though much continues to be spent trying to prove otherwise.

Worse, despite delivery of expensive services, some of which appear to be in pursuit of futile or inappropriate goals, some patients fail to get care which might have served both their interests and those of policymakers. An example is the potentially avoidable hospital use mentioned above. Some of these admissions may be avoidable, but with no effort directed at identification and reduction of this risk, in this case, the case manager failed to act as effective agent of either the payer or the patient. Poor task definition, poor training, inadequate monitoring and feedback of results, and an incentive structure which makes the case manager and his or her employer in no way liable for the costs of hospitalization may have been contributing causes of this failure of implementation. To the extent that the two principals conflict, the case manager will move in the direction of the one which provides the clearest task definition, the most monitoring, and the strongest incentives for conformity. Often that is the family. When it is not, it may be nobody, if the payer has not articulated relevant, clear, and well-defined goals. In the face of vague, irrelevant, or unachievable goals, agents are likely to respond to situational exigencies and circumstances rather than weighing options against policy objectives. They are likely to fall back on standard operating procedures and professional norms – not necessarily producing behavior in the payer's interests (Wilson 1989).

Exceptions to the rule prove the rule. In South Carolina, a determined program manager intent on meeting a nursing-home avoidance goal actually went into nursing homes and took clients out (Brown et al. 1985). She rigorously applied the same standards of admission to home-care clients as to nursing-home applicants. In New York, the Access program focused on avoiding hospital use, identifying high users and going even to the lengths of increasing nursing-home use if it would substitute for hospital care (Berkeley Planning Associates 1987). On Lok, another promising effort, focuses on avoiding hospital use, keeping costs down, and managing both acute and long-term care services (Zawadski et al. 1984).

Home-care programs, if they are to be effective, must assess patients' risks, design protocols which will mitigate those risks at the lowest possible cost, train case managers in implementing the protocols, monitor their activities, provide them with feedback on their success, and create incentives such as global budgets which force providers to allocate resources efficiently, making tradeoffs among patients so that marginal costs maximize marginal benefits. Modest copayments and deductibles can encourage patients and families to honor efficiency both in the home care provided and in the acute care avoided. Integrating long-term and acute care payment and service delivery can further enhance efficiencies and incentives to substitute the cheaper for the more expensive.

To that end, some practical principles for affordable home care are presented, based upon the notion that home care suffers two kinds of problems which must be addressed in future efforts: Policy must more clearly state appropriate goals for home care, and implementation must include effective task definition, training, risk-assessment methodologies, monitoring, feedback, and appropriate incentives for case managers and their employing firms. The principles represent a preliminary effort at gleaning lessons which can help set home care on an affordable path. The effort is preliminary because while the research on home care has been extensive, it has failed to focus adequate attention on the questions of for whom benefits can be produced, the mix and amount of care needed to produce them, and the incentive structure, task definition, risk factors, and training which must be put into place to encourage appropriate behavior by providers and patients.

Some Practical Principles

Principle Number 1: Policymakers must adopt more realistic goals and expectations for home-care. Goals must fit the needs of the client population and capabilities of the program.

Most home-care patients are not at risk of nursing-home entry or long stays, so it makes no sense to make avoiding nursing-home use the primary goal of home care. For a few patients, it is the appropriate goal; for most, it is not.

Several other outcomes may also be unreasonable policy expectations for home care. Three dozen studies show that home care does not slow the rate of physiological decline toward death, it does not improve physical functioning, or even slow its rate of decline (Weissert, Cready, and Pawelak 1988; Hedrick, Koepsell, and Inui 1989). Indeed, there is some evidence that home care makes physical functioning decline (Hughes, Cordray, and Spiker 1984; Weissert, Cready, and Pawelak 1988).

For most patients, care plans should not be designed to produce these outcomes and the success of home care should not be judged against them.

Carefully designed to do so, for some very carefully selected patients, home care might be able to alter attitudes toward hospitalization and responses to health-status changes over which itself it has no control. Why has it not done this? The explanation may be that lacking a precise set of expectations, the intervention was not effectively designed to produce this benefit for the subgroup of home-care patients for whom it might have been effective (Granneman, Grossman, and Dunstand 1986).

For most patients the benefit produced is improved well-being of the patient, the caregiver or both. Some patients seem to receive no measurable benefits at all.

Principle Number 2: Implementation of home care must work within a realistic budget constraint.

The reality that few dollars will be saved by substitutions for inpatient or institutional care means there must be a limited budget for home care. It should be what would have been spent without home care, plus the value of added benefits. Most patients would have spent nothing or very little on nursing-home care. And their most likely benefit is improved well-being. While the benefit to society of this outcome has not yet been fixed and may never be, physicians routinely work with this level of ambiguity, making decisions that potential benefits justify only limited expenditures of caring resources. These same judgments must be applied to home care. Though demand can be controlled and cost-saving potential can be enhanced by striving to serve a case mix which approximates nursing-home patients' disability level, this is not enough to produce efficient operation (Weissert and Cready 1989).Many patients will be admitted who are not "at risk." It follows that the budget for their care should not be predicated on the assumption that they would otherwise have been in a nursing home. Doing so guarantees that home care will raise overall costs. Instead, for patients not at risk – which is most home-care patients – some other home-care budget target must be set. One that makes sense, and is the guiding principle in the rest of medical care, is adjusting services to patients' benefit potential. Priorities have to be set so that resources are spent where they will do the most good. If the goal is improved well-being, care planners must ask themselves what minimal level of support will produce these benefits. More expensive interventions must be saved for patients who are likely to benefit from higher levels of treatment. While past studies have included spending caps, because they were based on nursing-home care costs, they were a binding constraint on only the most expensive patients. That is, the caps were so high that most patients used significantly less care than the caps provided. This left the way open to spending levels which may have been higher than they needed to be to produce the modest benefits found.

A related issue is the widespread belief that home care is currently unavailable. In reality, most individuals who seek expanded home-care benefits turn out to be already receiving them from a variety of existing sources (Kemper 1988). For them, the expanded benefits merely increase frequency and range of services consumed. In light of diminishing returns, this may in part explain the poor showing of expanded home-care benefits – they may be delivering what has been called "flat of the curve medicine." In an era of constrained resources, initial services to a previously unserved client should take precedence over extra increments of care to someone already being served.

Principle Number 3: Home care needs greater physician involvement and they need to be trained in its effective use.

Typical physician involvement in home care is often limited to signatures on authorization to commence services and telephone reauthorizations of continued service use. Payment methods do not reward them for making careful assessments of patient risk factors, care needs, expected outcomes, and progress toward achieving those outcomes. Under current policy, the physician has little incentive to learn how to use home care as a support mechanism to avoid more expensive forms of care which are more directly under the physician's control (e.g., hospitalization). Systems of care such as capitated payment are needed as well as training physicians in using home care to manage chronically ill ambulatory-care patients.

Principle Number 4: Performance must be monitored and feedback on success and failure provided.

Quality assurance in home care must be redefined to emphasize risk assessment, tailoring care to mitigation of risks, comparison of outcomes to expected population-based norms for patients who faced similar risks, training of case managers in these tasks, monitoring outcomes and costs, and feeding back results. Appropriate incentives in the payment system to produce desired efficiencies and effectiveness should also be part of quality assurance.

Home-care quality assurance now is substantially a paper review of documentation: eligibility determination, care-plan documentation, service-delivery confirmation, reassessment, and agency organizational and staffing capabilities (Schlenker et al. 1989). Shifting the focus of review to an assessment of the clinical basis for care plans, expected benefits of the treatment, the face validity of the linkage between the patient's problem and the services being delivered, efficiency of the care plan, and overall program costs in relation to benefits would change the criterion variable for care planning from meeting "needs" to producing outcomes. Home-care programs should be able to demonstrate the risks faced by a patient, the relationship of the care plan to amelioration of those risks, and assurance that the choice of services is the least costly for the result sought for that specific patient.

Principle Number 5: The incentive structure of home care must be improved.

Moral hazard and induced demand – both consequences of the insurance effect on patient and provider behavior – are problems at least as serious in home care as in other types of health-care use. They produce incentives which make both the provider and the patient act in ways not in the interests of the payer.

Fee-for-service home care with budgets set in relation to nursing-home care annual costs and ineffective patient or provider incentives to conserve resources are prescriptions for waste, inefficiency, and high cost. Potentially effective incentives include: per capita payments and global budgets, responsibility for both acute and long-term care payment, copays and deductibles, effective risk assessment and care-planning protocols, training, monitoring, and performance feedback.

Past studies have generally ignored the provider in trying to improve home-care effectiveness and efficiency. They have not recognized the theoretically useful principal–agent relationship between the home-care payer and the care manager. In general, studies have not even reported data on care-manager characteristics, variation in services prescribed by them for controlling for patient characteristics, or the type of intensity of training, monitoring, and feedback which they received.

Nor can home care alone achieve health-system economies. It must be delivered within a system of care in which incentives favor efficient use of all types of services to produce the best overall outcomes at the lowest cost.

Principle Number 6: Research is needed to help redesign home care to make it more effective and efficient.

Research demonstrating that poorly designed interventions produce disappointing outcomes has been done in more than sufficient quantity. Needed instead are panel designs guided by principles such as those suggested by agency theory: evaluating the clients' risks and transition rates to various outcomes so that appropriate goals can be set; assessment of effects of varying mixes and intensity of services for specific subgroups so practice guidelines can be developed (Weissert and Hedrick 1994); estimation of substitution rates among types of care and dose–response relationships to improve efficiency; and elasticities of demand under varying copayments and deductibles to encourage appropriate use rates. Training, monitoring, feedback, and incentive structures of the principal–agent relationship should be described and manipulated to produce greater effectiveness and efficiencies.

Until research efforts are focused at the same rigorous level of subgroups and their outcomes that is common for other forms of health care, home care will continue to be ineffective.

Implications for Health Reform

The Clinton health reform package (38) was responsive to some of these concerns but not others.

Home care will be available for people of all ages suffering severe dependency, defined as needing at least standby assistance in at least three activities of daily living. Leaving aside the issues of costs and benefits for this generous package, at least two issues were disturbing:

- The policy objective set for home care was once again the avoidance of nursing-home care – a goal irrelevant for most patients and therefore leaving care managers without policy guidance for most of the patients they serve.
- Far from acknowledging the need to improve implementation by putting more responsibility into the hands of care planners to allocate scarce resources where they will do the most good, the package required a minimum expenditure of $2,000 for each client.

On the other hand, because it was offered as part of a larger package which sought cost control through global budgets and integrating acute and long-term care, the proposal offered the promise that appropriate incentives would be in place to encourage health plans to focus on efficient implementation and cost-limited interventions.

In addition, the Clinton plan called for a demonstration to integrate acute and long-term care services, and for evaluation of performance of home-care programs against criteria which (if carefully constructed in regulations) could address issues of training, risk assessment, appropriateness of care in relation to patient outcome goals, and incentives for appropriate physician involvement.

Should home-care expansion pass Congress in some future reform plan without these kinds of incentive, costs will surely rise, benefits will be minimal, and opportunities to make home care do a better job are likely to be lost.

Conclusion

Home care is expensive and largely ineffective. It has not been well designed. Past efforts were directed more or less unthinkingly at proving that it will substitute for nursing homes. That it does not do much of that should long ago have led not to more efforts to prove that it does, but rather to efforts to document just what it can do, for whom, and at what cost, and to implement training, monitoring, and appropriate incentives to make it do it better and cheaper than it has in the past.

References

1. Bergner, M., L. Hudson, D. Conrad, et al. 1988. The Cost and Efficacy of Home Care for Patients with Chronic Lung Disease. *Medical Care* 26(6): 566–79.
2. Katz, S., A.B. Ford, T.D. Downs, et al. 1972. *Effects of Continued Care: A Study of Chronic Illness in the Home.* DHEW Pub. No. (HSM) 73–3010. Cleveland: Case Western Reserve University School of Medicine.
3. Posman, H., L.S. Kogan, A. LeMat, et al. 1964. *Continuity in Care for Impaired Older Persons: Public Health Nursing in a Geriatric Rehabilitation Maintenance Program.* New York: Department of Public Affairs and Institute of Welfare Research, Community Service Society of New York.
4. Hanchett, E., and P.R. Torrens. 1967. A Public Health Home Nursing Program for Outpatients with Heart Disease. *Public Health Reports* 82(8): 683–8.
5. Hughes, S.L., D.S. Cordray, and V.A. Spiker. 1984. Evaluation of a Long-Term Home-Care Program. *Medical Care* 22(4): 640.
6. Hughes, S.L., J. Cummings, F. Weaver, et al. 1990. A Randomized Trial of Veteran's Administration Home Care for Severely Disabled Veterans. *Medical Care* 28(2): 135–45.
7. Hughes, S.L., J. Cummings, F. Weaver, et al. 1992. A Randomized Trial of the Cost Effectiveness of VA Hospital-Based Home Care for the Terminally Ill. *Health Services Research* 26(6): 801–17.
8. Papsidero, J.A., S. Katz, M.H. Kroger, and C.A. Akpom, eds. 1979. *Chance for Change: Implications of a Chronic Disease Module.* East Lansing, MI: Michigan State University Press.
9. Selmanoff, E.D., R.U. Mitchell, F.W. Widlock, et al. 1979. Home Care

of Geriatric Patients by a Health Maintenance Team. Paper Presented at the Annual Meeting of the American Public Health Association, New York, November.
10. Wade, D.T., R. Langton-Hewer, C.E. Skilbeck, et al. 1985. Controlled Trial of a Home-Care Service for Acute Stroke Patients. *Lancet* 9 (February): 323–6.
11. Zimmer, J.G., A. Groth-Junker, and J. McCusker. 1985. A Randomized Controlled Study of a Home Health Care Team. *American Journal of Public Health* 75: 134–41.
12. Weissert, W.G., T.T.H. Wan, B. Livieratos, et al. 1980. Cost-Effectiveness of Homemaker Services for the Chronically Ill. *Inquiry* 17 (Fall): 230–43.
13. Blenkner, M., M. Bloom, M. Nielsen, et al. 1970. Home Aide Service and the Aged: A Controlled Study. Part I: Design and Findings. Part II. The Service Program. Cleveland: The Benjamin Rose Institute.
14. Nielsen, M., M. Blenkner, M. Bloom, et al. 1972. Older Persons after Hospitalization: A Controlled Study of Home Aide Service. *American Journal of Public Health* 62(8): 1094–101.
15. Hedrick, S.C., M.L. Rothman, M. Chapko, et al. Summary and Discussion of Methods and Results of the Adult Day Health Care Evaluation. *Medical Care*. In press.
16. Eagle, D.J., G.H. Guyatt, C. Patterson, et al. 1991. Effectiveness of a Geriatric Day Hospital. *Canadian Medical Association Journal* 144(6): 699–704.
17. Weissert, W.G., T. Wan, B. Livieratos, et al. 1980. Effects and Costs of Day-Care Services for the Chronically Ill: A Randomized Experiment. *Medical Care* 28(6): 567–84.
18. Mor, V., D.S. Greer, and R. Kastenbaum, eds. 1988. *The Hospice Experiment*. Baltimore: The Johns Hopkins Press.
19. Kane, R.L., J. Wales, L. Bernstein, et al. 1984. A Randomized Controlled Trial of Hospice Care. *Lancet* 1: 890–94.
20. Lawton, M.P., E.M. Brody, and A.R. Saperstein. A Controlled Study of Respite Service for Caregivers of Alzheimer's Patients. *The Gerontologist* 29(1): 8–16.
21. Berkeley Planning Associates. 1987. *Evaluation of the ACCESS: Medicare Long-Term Care Demonstration Projects: Final Report*. Berkeley, CA.
22. Birnbaum, H., G. Gaumer, F. Pratter, et al. 1984. Nursing Home Without Walls: Evaluation of the New York State Long-Term Home Health Care Program. Cambridge, MA: Abt Associates.
23. Blenkner, M., M. Bloom, and M. Nielsen. 1971. A Research and Demonstration Project of Protective Services. *Social Casework* 52: 483–99.
24. Brown, T.E. Jr, D.K. Blackman, R.M. Learner, et al. 1985. South Carolina Long-Term Care Project: Report of Findings. Spartanburg, SC: South Carolina State Health and Human Services Finance Commission.
25. Commonwealth of Massachusetts. 1975. *Home Care: An Alternative*

to Institutionalization: Final Report. Boston: Commonwealth of Massachusetts, Department of Elder Affairs.
26 Gaumer, G.L., H. Birnbaum, F. Pratter, et al. 1986. Impact of the New York Long-Term Home Health Care Program. *Medical Care* 24(7) 641–53.
27 Kemper, P. 1988. The Evaluation of the National Long-Term Care Demonstration: 10. Overview of the Findings. *Health Services Research* 23(1): 161–74.
28 Maurer, J.M., N.L. Ross, Y.M. Bigos, et al. 1987. Final report and Evaluation of the Florida Pentastar Project. Tallahassee: Florida Department of Health and Rehabilitative Services.
29 Oktay, J.S., and P.J. Volland. 1986. Evaluating a Support Program for Families of the Frail Elderly. Paper presented at the annual meeting of The Gerontological Society of America. Chicago.
30 O'Rourke, B., H. Raisz, and J. Segal. 1982. *Triage II: Coordinated Delivery of Services to the Elderly: Final Report.* Vol. 1–2. Plainville, CT: Triage, Inc.
31 Pinkerton, A., and D. Hill. *Long-Term Care Demonstration Project of North San Diego County: Final Report.* 1984. NTIS no. PB85 – 10391. San Diego: Allied Home Health Association.
32 Sainer, J.S., R.S. Brill, A. Horowitz, et al. 1984. *Delivery of Medical and Social Services to the Homebound Elderly: A Demonstration of InterSystem Coordination: Final Report.* New York: New York City Department for the Aging.
33 Seidl, F.W., R. Applebaum, C. Austin, et al. 1983. *Delivering In-home Services to the Aged and Disabled: The Wisconsin Experiment.* Lexington MA: Lexington Books.
34 Skellie, A., F. Favor, C. Tudor, et al. 1982. *Alternative Health Services Project: Final Report.* Atlanta: Georgia Department of Medical Assistance.
35 Sklar, B.W., and L.J. Weiss. 1983. *Project OPEN (Organization Providing for Elderly Needs): Final Report.* San Francisco: Mount Zion Hospital and Medical Center.
36 Zawadski, R.T., J. Shen, C. Yordi, et al. 1984. *On Lok's Community Care Organization for Dependent Adults: A Research and Development Project (1978–83): Final Report.* San Francisco: On Lok Senior Health Services.
37 Greene, V.L. 1987. Nursing Home Admission Risk and the Cost-Effectiveness of Community-Based Long-Term Care: A Framework for Analysis. *Health Services Research* 22(5): 664–9.
38 The White House Domestic Policy Council. 1993. *The President's Health Security Plan.* New York: Times Books.
39 Weissert, W., J. Lafata, B. Williams, and C. Weissert. Potentially Avoidable hospital Stays Among Home Care Patients: Predictors and Treatment Effects. In review.
40 Arrow, K.J. 1985. The Economics of Agency. In *Principals and Agents: The Structure of Business,* ed. John W. Pratt and Richard J. Zeckhauser, 37–51. Boston: Harvard Business School Press.
41 Lipsky, M. 1980. *Street-Level Bureaucracy: Dilemmas of the Individual in*

Public Services. New York: Russel Sage.
42. Moe, T.M. 1984. The New Economics of Organization. *American Journal of Political Science* 20: 739–77.
43. Prottas, J.M. 1979. *People Processing: The Street Level Bureaucrat in Public Service Bureaucracies.* Lexington, MA: Lexington Books.
44. Nyman, J., S. Levey, and J. Rohrer. 1987. RUG: Equity of Access to Nursing Home Care. *Medical Care* 25: 361–72.
45. Wilson, J.Q. 1989. *Bureaucracy.* New York: Basic Books.
46. Weissert, W.G., C.M. Cready, and J.E. Pawelak. 1988. The Past and Future of Home-and-Community-Based Long-Term Care. *Milbank Quarterly* 66(2): 309–88.
47. Hedrick, S.C., T.D. Koepsell, and T.S. Inui. 1989. Meta-Analysis of Home-Care Effects on Mortality and Nursing Home Placement. *Medical Care* 27(11): 1015–26.
48. Grannemann, T.W., J.B. Grossman, S.M. Dunstand. 1986. Differential Impacts among Subgroups of Channeling Enrollees. Princeton, NJ: Mathematica Policy Research, Inc., Enterprise Business Center.
49. Weissert, W. and C. Cready. 1989. A Prospective Budgeting Model for Home-and-Community-Based Long-Term care. *Inquiry* 26: 116–29.
50. Schlenker, R., J. Miller, Berg, K. Bischoff, and P. Butler. 1989. *Future Research on the Quality of Long-Term Care Services in Community Based and Custodial Settings.* Denver, CO: Center for Health Services Research, University of Colorado.
51. Weissert, W.G., and S.C. Hedrick. 1994. Lessons Learned from Research on Effects of Community-Based Long-Term Care. *Journal of American Geriatrics Society* 42: 348–53.

7

Financing Long-Term Care
Robert B. Friedland

Introduction

This chapter is about the organization of financial obligations for care at home and care in an institution. It is intended to be an overview of what we know and do not know about financing long-term care and what that may mean for the political debate that is likely to ensue about reforming the current financing of long-term care. The chapter will proceed with a brief definition of terms and issues. This will be followed by an overview of how long-term care is currently financed and the consequences of this arrangement. Broad options for reform will be outlined with a discussion of both the political and practical considerations.

Defining Terms

Long-term care is the medical, nursing, and social services needed by people who are dependent on other people to function from day to day over an extended period. These are people whose illnesses, impairments, or social problems have become disabling, and this has limited their ability to carry out independently the customary activities of daily life. Those who are chronically ill, disabled, frail, or cognitively impaired and in need of long-term care are people who, without assistance, are most likely to become acutely ill.

It is, however, one thing to state a definition that conveys the target and the goal. It is quite another to put such a definition into practice in a public or private program that finances this care. Carving out acute care from long-term care can be difficult. Sorting out services that should be provided, as opposed to those that might be nice to receive is tricky. Determining the appropriate site of care – a home, community-based institutions such as an adult day-care center, or an institution, such as a nursing home – only complicates the array of service choices. This is only confounded more by the fact that long-term care needs generally might not serve the needs of the mentally ill, mentally retarded, or developmentally disabled.

Despite our inadequacies in defining long-term care precisely, we do know that every day, millions of Americans of all ages struggle to obtain assistance with basic human functions. While estimates vary, the number is not insignificant. There may be about 12 million people, approximately 5 percent of the population, who are now chronically dependent on hands-on assistance from others. About 40 percent are under the age of 65. But what is more important, while most of the population is not now in need of long-term care or consumed by providing or making arrangements for such care to a loved-one, almost everyone will eventually either worry about the long-term needs for family or friends or need care themselves.

Primarily because of the growth in the proportion and number of elderly, the number of people who need assistance is expected to grow. By 2030, the number of elderly likely to need long-term care will almost double. The number of elderly living in the community who need long-term care is expected to increase from about 7 million in 1990 to nearly 14 million by 2030, and the number requiring nursing-home care will triple from 1.5 million to 5.3 million (Pepper Commission, 1990).

Most long-term care is provided by family and friends. But the availability of family and friends to provide assistance is likely to diminish over time (Stone and Kemper, 1989). Changes in birth rates already portend fewer adult children and more elderly persons without any children. Between 1990 and 2030, the number of elderly women without children is projected to increase by more than 47 percent (Zedlewski, Rafferty, and McBride 1992). The incidence of divorce is more likely to leave many elderly alone, and as second marriages become more common, some adult children may find themselves conflicted with the long-term care needs of extended family. Geographic mobility can result in isolation as fewer elderly have children nearby. The number of elderly living alone has been projected to more than double from 10.4 million in 1990 to 25.5 million in 2030.

All of these factors point toward increased demand for paid assistance, particularly in the home. In some sense this pressure may have already begun. The evidence, of expenditures, facilities, encounters, or visits is sketchy, but indicates tremendous growth in the demand for services and the supply of services, as well as the unit cost of care. Expenditure for home health care, for example, is the fastest growing among all the national health-care accounts. From 1980 to 1991, while all personal health care, other than home health care, increased 198 percent, home health care increased 654 percent.

The Costs of Long-Term Care

The cost of long-term care varies considerably. Care in a nursing facility can easily exceed $80 a day and certainly can approach $140 a day. Care at home through a licensed agency with certified caregivers can cost $15.00 to $20.00 an hour, and unskilled and often unlicensed care from an independent attendant may cost $5.00 an hour. Since the care needed can last for years, the total cost of care can easily exceed the financial means of most people. An episode of long-term care can put the economic well-being of spouses and children at serious risk. Most people have not incorporated the prospect of paying for long-term care into their retirement planning. In part, this may be due to the relatively high cost, but it is more likely to be because the prospects of needing long-term care are denied or incorrectly presumed to be covered by health insurance.

Studies have shown that the elderly with high overall health-care costs also had high out-of-pocket costs for nursing-home care and prescription drugs (Rice and Gabel 1986). Furthermore, among elderly in the community, 10 percent had out-of-pocket acute care costs that exceeded 10 percent of their income (Feder, Moon, and Scanlon, 1987). Among chronically disabled elderly, 41 percent had out-of-pocket costs from acute health care, prescription drugs, home care, and nursing-home care that exceeded 15 percent of their income (Liu, Perozek, and Manton 1993).

More fundamental is the question of whether people should, or even could, include the cost of long-term care as a part of their saving goals. These are two different questions. On the question of could people include long-term care as a part of their savings, one need only look to our experience with tax-encouraged, but individual-directed, retirement planning. Despite current tax incentives people, generally, are not saving according to their expectations for income during retirement.[1] Concern about people withdrawing their retirement savings before retirement has led Congress to impose and repeatedly increase the tax penalty of using the money before age 60.

It has taken effort and additional tax incentives such as Simplified Employee Pensions, to encourage employers to establish tax-favored retirement plans, for individuals to participate or save on their own, and then to keep their savings for retirement. Yet, there are concerns that personal savings are inadequate. Views about retirement are not subject to the same level of denial and misunderstanding as long-term care. The calculation of needed savings relative to a retirement-income goal is relatively straightforward. People speak positively about retirement and in fact the propensity towards earlier retirement has been one of the most pervasive labor-force trends. If the desire to retire cannot yield higher savings' rates, it seems unrealistic to expect the fear of possibly needing long-term care to be an even stronger source of encouragement for savings.

Differentiating Saving from Insurance

Even if people would or could save for long-term care, there is still the question of whether they should. Although the lifetime risk is not insignificant, long-term care is not a certain event. Moreover, the cost of care varies by the amount of care that is needed, the duration of that need, and the extent to which family and friends are participating in providing care and assistance. Given the variations in unit cost, duration of need, and the extent of care needed, this makes for a very high variation around a relatively high average cost. As a result, it is quite likely that one will either save too much or too little. While saving for its own sake may be desirable, and perhaps because of its fundability, ought to be encouraged, insuring for the possibility of needing long-term care is more efficient than saving for this contingency.

Saving for an event is efficient when the occurrence of that event is fairly likely and the costs are predictable. But in the case of long-term care, sharing the financial consequences of the risk through either public or private insurance is much more efficient. Grouping individuals together for the purpose of spreading the financial risk enables everyone in the group to pay a portion of the average cost without worrying if they are saving too much or too little. The portion paid would be a fraction of the average cost of care, based on the probability that any one individual would need care. Insurance reduces both the risk of having to pay the full average cost of care and the variation in the cost of care.

Private long-term care insurance has been around, in one form or another, since the mid-1970s. Most of the early policies were just for nursing-home care, often in distinct areas. National insurers only began to market insurance, for both care at home and nursing-home care, nationally in the late 1980s. Private long-term care insurance is now widely available. Continuing Care Retirement Communities, in which housing, home care, and nursing-home care is integrated and financed by the community have been around since the 1930s.

But why is it that this market has not grown so that private insurance is a significant portion of the financing of long-term care? Perhaps long-term care really is not an insurable event. For most of this century, most insurers did not think so. There was little noticeable market demand. There are also data and measurement problems. Little was known about the average cost of care, or the probability of needing such care. Moreover, it was even less clear how to define when long-term care was needed, never mind define what long-term care is. On all of these fronts, and only in the past decade, have researchers begun to develop answers. But there are still serious limitations in existing data and critical differences in definitions that make comparisons of fundamental descriptive statistics difficult.

Insurers worry about how and where to draw the lines that would define long-term care. Their inability to define the risks makes it impossible to define the insurance. In response, the products that have emerged do not cover long-term care. Instead they are a fixed dollar amount for a specific duration for those who are certified as needing specific long-term care services. The purchase of a $100 a day, nursing-home benefit, for example, will provide $100 a day, regardless of the cost of the nursing-home stay. If the difference between the cost and the policy is out of the reach of the policy holder, then a situation may emerge where one is too rich to qualify for Medicaid, but still too poor to obtain access to care.

To keep these policies affordable, their price is based on the age at initial purchase and the price incorporates the risks of needing care that year and prefunds the expected risk in the future. This enables the funds to accumulate reserves so that premiums remain level over the course of one's lifetime. This is similar to the comparison between whole life insurance and term life insurance. At younger ages term life insurance will be much less expensive than whole life, but at older ages term insurance will be substantially greater than the whole life premium. This may be appropriate for life insurance since the need for life insurance – which for most people is intended to insure against the risk of a premature death during working years – is of less importance after the children have grown and one is retired. The relative importance of long-term care insurance, however, only increases with age. For this reason, long-term care policies have been priced and sold as "whole life" policies rather than on a "term" basis.

While the market for private long-term care insurance has expanded dramatically, it has not yet become a significant form of financing long-term care. In fact, despite the increase in health-insurance coverage of nursing-home care and home health care as a substitute for hospital care, the proportion of privately insured nursing-home care and home health care has stayed essentially the same.[2] Perhaps 300,000 elderly persons live in Continuing Care Retirement Communities and 2.4 million persons of all ages have private long-term care insurance (Somers 1993; HIAA 1993).[3] Altogether it would be generous to say that more than 1 percent of the elderly had any form of long-term care insurance. The proportion of the non-elderly population with such protection is virtually nonexistent.

Insurance companies have put many resources into the marketing and selling of long-term care insurance. It is a new product and has required a great deal of effort to sell. It has required the training of sales agents and then the education of the consumer. Repeated telephone conversations and multiple face-to-face discussions with prospective purchasers are usually necessary. Despite the hard sell and the financial consequences of needing long-term care, people are aware of long-term care needs and many say they are willing to purchase long-term care insurance. But opinions and action are inconsistent. In a Gallup poll conducted May 1993 for the Employee Benefit Research Institute, 21 percent indicated that someone in their family had received long-term care in the past five years, 22 percent indicated that they personally expected to need long-term care assistance during their life, and 42 percent indicated that if they needed to pay for long-term care it would be financed by a long-term care insurance policy. Also, in this survey, 51 percent knew that Medicare did not cover long-term care and 69 percent said they would support a government-funded program to provide long-term care assistance for the elderly, even if it meant an increase in their income taxes.

Long-term care insurance is also not inexpensive. It is somewhat of an academic debate to argue what proportion of income or assets people will be willing to spend for long-term care insurance.[4] It should be sufficient to point out that 40 percent of the current elderly have incomes of less than 200 percent of poverty, and therefore coverage for most of the elderly will take time. If people with $10,000 in assets who are not now in need of long-term care would be willing to spend 10 percent of their income on a long-term care insurance policy, then one-half of all people age 45 to 64 and 7 percent of all elderly could afford a long-term care insurance policy.[5] If one-half of all people age 45 to 64 and 7 percent of all people age 65 or older purchased insurance today, and continued to hold that policy over the rest of their lives, then in 20 years, 43 percent of the elderly might have private long-term care insurance. More of the non-elderly would have insurance and private long-term care insurance would be a substantial part of the long-term care economy.

How is Long-Term Care Currently Financed?

In 1991, approximately $73 billion was spent on nursing-home care and home health care. Most of this expenditure (82 percent) went toward the cost of care in a nursing facility. The most significant cost missing from this estimate is the direct value and forgone opportunities associated with the care provided by family and friends. Most people (81 percent) who need long-term care live in the community and most (84 percent) of this care is provided by family and friends.

Of the nearly $60 billion spent on nursing-home care, half was publicly financed. Most of the public financing (88 percent) was through Medicaid, not Medicare. Virtually all the private financing was directly out of pocket and not through insurance. Slightly more than 47 percent of nursing-home expenditure was financed by Medicaid and 43 percent was financed directly from those in nursing homes or their families. Medicare covers short stays in skilled nursing facilities, but this only financed 4.4 percent of nursing-home care. Private insurance, including acute health-care insurance, financed 1 percent of nursing-home expenditure.

Almost three-quarters of all home *health* expenditures, as distinct from home-care expenditures, were publicly financed. In this case, however, 62 percent of the public funding was from Medicare, not Medicaid. In 1991, expenditures on home health care reached $9.8 billion. Almost 45 percent of this was financed by Medicare. Medicaid financed nearly 27 percent, and individuals paid 12 percent directly out of pocket. Private insurance, including acute health care and Medigap policies, financed 7.1 percent. In fact, private health insurance paid more in home health-care claims than in nursing-home claims.

Using the 1987 National Expenditure Survey, Lewin-VHI used population growth and expenditure per user from Medicare and Medicaid trend data to estimate home care for 1992. Their estimate for 1992 was $22.9 billion. To the extent that this also includes home health care, then this estimate might suggest that half of this nearly $23 billion is home- and community-based care and the other half is for skilled home health care. They estimated that nearly 38 percent of all home care and home health care in 1992 was financed by Medicare, that 25 percent was financed by Medicaid, that nearly 6 percent was financed by private insurance and that 31 percent was financed directly out of pocket (Families USA Foundation 1993).

Home health care is covered by Medicaid in all states and 28 states also cover personal care services. In most states (48), home care and home health care is available as an alternative to nursing-home care. These programs are technically demonstration projects and therefore are often limited, both in geography and in who they serve. In Federal Fiscal Year 1990, 135,000 aged and disabled were assisted in these programs. Medicare will pay for home health care for beneficiaries confined to their home who need skilled nursing services on a less than full-time or intermittent basis or who need physical or speech therapy.

Home health care is the fastest growing line item in the national health-care expenditure accounts. While all personal health-care expenditures increased 38 percent, from 1988 to 1991 home health care increased nearly 123 percent. Expenditures on home health care from Medicare increased 144 percent. By comparison, Medicare's total expenditures increased only 34 percent. Medicare is now paying more for home health care than the entire nation purchased in 1988. Out-of-pocket payments for home health care increased 140 percent during this time. Expenditures for home health care from private insurance increased 133 percent, and expenditures from Medicaid increased 73 percent. By comparison, nursing-home care expenditures from 1988 to 1991 have been relatively stable. Overall, nursing-home expenditures increased 40 percent. But this was still nearly twice the rate of growth of all personal health-care expenditures. The rising cost of long-term care, generally, and home health care in particular is likely to be raised as a concern against expanding the financing.

What is Wrong with the Current Arrangements?

The current financing system is both symptomatic of and a perpetuator of the current delivery system. As indicated by the flow of dollars, the system is institutionally biased: financial assistance is more likely in a nursing home. Moreover, the financing is victim based, in that most of the cost, both direct and indirect, falls on the person who needs assistance and that person's family and friends. Medicaid requires that assets (other than the home) be liquidated and that income must be very low or in some states long-term care expenses must be relatively high before providing assistance.

The financing is not only biased, but it is fragmented across local programs making it difficult to put together a prudent and effective package of needed care. The lack of public funding for home- and community-based care has left such care to the private market and to voluntary philanthropic efforts. As a consequence, the availability of services varies tremendously by community. In part, the variation is dependent on the demand for care and the relative resources of that community.

To the extent there are home-and community-based services, the importance of Medicare in financing home health care has biased the structure of agencies towards the provision of relatively skilled care. As it becomes more difficult to provide care at home, it becomes easier to seek care in a nursing facility. Any prolonged nursing-home stay can be so costly, relative to family resources, that it can become financially difficult to leave the facility even if one is physically capable.

While public financing tends to encourage institutionalization, states have worked hard to limit the growth in nursing-home beds. Through certificate-of-need programs, changes in the tax treatment of the sale of nursing homes, and Medicaid nursing-home reimbursement policy, states have been very successful. Overall, the number of beds has not grown as fast as the growth in the elderly population. Perhaps, as a consequence, there is evidence that the average age of nursing-home residents has increased. Although Medicaid covers nursing-home care, not all nursing homes will accept Medicaid patients.

The complexity of Medicaid eligibility in conjunction with improved income and asset protection for spouses has encouraged legal specialization in this area. The increase in number of lawyers advertising this expertise has certainly made directors of state Medicaid programs very concerned. The evidence and the consequences of legal manipulation of asset ownership, however, have not been as thoroughly evaluated as other aspects of financing. Certainly the cost of securing one's rights by seeking legal advice is not usually considered a cost of long-term care, but perhaps it is. We do not know, however, how many people seek advice or establish the necessary trusts to transfer assets in such a manner as only to appear to have given up control for the purpose of being able to apply for state assistance from Medicaid.

Expanding the Public Financing of Long-Term Care

The public debate over long-term care has not only emerged on the national scene, it has also changed. A decade ago, the public policy discussions focused primarily on organizing and arranging services, access to care, and the quality of care. Before the 1992 Presidential election, the central part of the debate seems to have been over the degree to which the financing of long-term care should be privately or publicly financed. While this will ultimately be the center of the forthcoming congressional debate, the starting point has changed. Because of political promises and the desire to reform the entire health-care system, the question may have been changed to what is the minimal amount of public financing of long-term care necessary to obtain the support for health-care reform?

This bias is likely to lead toward a greater propensity to see the debate center on public financing of home- and community-based care and the public encouragement of private financing of nursing-home care. This bias is new. Most recently, the political debate had tended to be over the financing of nursing-home care. Home care was important because it was believed, or hoped, to be a cost-effective substitute for nursing-home care. What has changed is that home care has become a part of the debate as a needed service irrespective of its ability to save nursing-home expenses. People want to stay in their own homes.

As indicated previously, approximately 58 percent of long-term care is publicly financed; with the bulk of financing for nursing-home care financed through Medicaid. Most of the private financing is not insured. We really do not know how much is spent on long-term care. Part of our estimates of long-term care, especially those from Medicare and private insurance, might not really be for long-term care. Most are for post-acute or recuperative care. Moreover, there are expenditures that would have been for long-term care but were financed and therefore counted as acute care because a nursing-home bed was not available, or, because long-term care was not adequate to keep someone from requiring inpatient hospital care. Furthermore, missing entirely from these expenditures are the costs associated with caregiving.

Most long-term care is provided by family and friends. Neither the market value of these services, nor the indirect consequences of substituting caregiving for other forms of employment, are included. If a caregiver alters employment to provide care, there are likely to be changes in current income and retirement income, and consequently in tax revenues to the government. There is also a potential cost from lost productivity. Furthermore, if the economic security of that caregiver is sufficiently jeopardized by their caregiving decisions then, if they should become sick, their costs are more likely to be publicly financed than privately financed.

The distinction, then, between public and private expenditures gets somewhat confused. Because the private costs are only distributed among the victims and their family, there may be offsetting public costs. Furthermore, because current private and public funding does not provide adequate care for everyone, some of the long-term care costs get picked up as publicly financed acute care costs.

How long-term care is financed not only affects the distribution of public and private expenditures, but it can also affect the level of financing long-term care. There are three basic approaches: expand Medicaid; encourage private insurance; or establish a new program that is only based on long-term care needs. Building upon Medicaid to expand long-term care, for example, would increase the level of care, without changing the distribution of the costs. That is, need would be based on the need for care and a proof of insufficient resources to purchase that care. Options to increase private financing usually entail public efforts either by tax incentives (and therefore lower tax revenues), or by public expenditures for subsidies and the provision of information. The consequences of the third option depend on who is eligible for benefits and how much money is allocated to this care.

There are many ways to expand public coverage of long-term care and the variation in costs is infinite. In choosing the specific proposal, legislators are likely to try to maximize real benefits and political capital with a minimum increase in public expenditures. Finding the right combination of programs that will expand coverage and be politically acceptable requires an appreciation of alternative program costs, the distribution of benefits and a proper reading of the public opinion polls about long-term care.

Fairly comprehensive coverage of home- and community-based care and nursing-home care could easily start at $70 billion in new public expenditures, on top of the $60 to $70 billion currently spent. Comprehensive home and community care would easily cost over $30 billion. Comprehensive nursing-home coverage would exceed $44 billion.

Given that more than half of the new expenditures for a comprehensive program would be for nursing-home care, much of the public discussion over the past few years has been over the appropriate role for the government in paying for nursing-home care. To the extent there have been proposals to provide such coverage most has been for either "front-end" or "back-end" coverage. That is, non-means-tested public coverage for some initial front-end period (say the first three or six months) or after some extended back-end period (such as after two years).

A front-end approach reduces the public cost of nursing-home care by 70 percent since it covers a relatively small portion of the expected cost of a long nursing-home stay. Such an approach would completely cover about 55 percent of all elderly who enter a nursing home. It would also cover about 75 percent of the elderly who leave a nursing home alive. The Agency for Health Care Policy Research (AHCPR) estimates 8 percent of estimated lifetime costs would be covered by the front-end approach.

A back-end approach would cut the cost of comprehensive coverage nearly in half. As a consequence, the back-end approach would cover substantially more (59 percent) of the estimated lifetime cost (AHCPR 1993). Of course, only those with sufficient long-term care insurance or assets to sustain the first two years would be considered new costs. Proponents of "back-end" proposals recognize that by having the government take on the long-term risk, the price of private long-term care insurance is reduced and the need for private coverage for the first two years of nursing-home care not covered by the government is made more abundantly clear. Proponents of "front-end" approaches focus on the need to provide financial assistance for those most likely to physically be able to leave a nursing home to ensure their economic independence and feel that private insurance would be available for the risk of staying beyond the period covered by the public plan.

The Pepper Commission tried to bridge these two approaches by providing front-end protection (three months) without significant cost sharing and then substantial cost sharing after three months. The cost sharing was designed to provide full asset protection to most middle income persons, but to impose a substantial portion of the income towards the cost of care. Asset protection would parallel the spousal protection provided through the recent changes in Medicaid (through the Medicare Catastrophic Coverage Act of 1988) but would add similar protections to single individuals. Protecting non-housing assets up to $30,000 (in 1990) would have left 66 percent of the elderly free from the need of having to spend any of their assets for care. Greater proportions of income would be protected, to ensure that a spouse in the community would have income equal to twice the poverty threshold. Perhaps the most important component of the income protection was the housing allowance equal to 30 percent of income for one year for a single nursing home resident or for as long as there was a spouse remaining in the community. Income beyond these protections, less $100 a month for personal needs, would be applied toward the cost of the nursing-home care. Among those who stay in a nursing home beyond three months, the Pepper Commission estimated that 84 percent would have all of their assets protected, 18 percent would have all of their income protected, and 66 percent would have part of their income protected.

While proposals for long-term care differ on the role of government in covering nursing-home care, most of them would provide home- and community-based care, irrespective of the time in which nursing-home care was covered. Under the proposal by the Pepper Commission, program costs would be controlled by a uniform assessment of need and a coordinator of care who would have a budget. The overall agency budget would be based on level of dependency of each person under the care of that agency but the care coordinator would have the flexibility to purchase varying amounts of care based on need. That is, persons with five limitations in activities of daily living would bring the agency a greater budget, but there may be persons with three limitations who need more care purchased than some people with five limitations.

The approach taken by the Pepper Commission reflected an uneasiness many lawmakers have about the nature of the entitlement and consequently the ability to control costs. The recommendations were an attempt to make the entitlement an assessment and a care manager with a budget, rather than a list of benefits. Furthermore, the recommendations were intended to give care managers the greatest flexibility in formulating a care plan that made sense for each individual. At the time there were few models that would offer evidence that such an approach might work or that the extra cost of care management was necessary to maintain the budget. Perceptions about the ability to control costs are likely to dominate the structure of any serious proposal put before the Congress.

Opting to publicly encourage the purchase of private long-term care insurance includes clarifying the tax treatment of premiums and benefits at a minimum to providing tax credits and linking the purchase to offset eligibility for public assistance. The earnings on the long-term care insurance-policy reserves have already been clarified. Earnings on reserves are not subject to taxation by either the insurance company or the policy holders. Making the tax treatment of premiums and benefits similar to that of acute health-insurance benefits would enable individuals to purchase long-term care insurance with pre-taxed earnings and would ensure that all the benefits paid would be free from income taxes.

A more expensive step would be to provide tax credits to those who purchase insurance. The intent of such a subsidy would be to signal the importance of purchasing this insurance. Our experience with acute-care health-insurance subsidies, however, does not bode well for this as an effective policy tool. Relatively few people purchase health insurance if it is not provided by employers. Demonstration projects using subsidies or reduced health-care coverage by the Robert Wood Johnson Foundation and others have not yielded very many new purchasers of health insurance. The third approach, which has already begun in several states, is to link the purchase of long-term care insurance with special eligibility rules for public coverage. In the four states where this has begun, the link is to Medicaid, since this is the only public program in which states have any control.

The options to expand public coverage of home- and community-based care fall into three general approaches:

1 build upon Medicaid;
2 build upon Medicare; or
3 establish a completely new program.

Requiring Medicaid programs to provide personal-assistance programs without any other change would be a modest benefit expansion to those with few assets and very low incomes as long as they were categorically eligible (under age 6, over age 65, blind, disabled, receiving SSI or AFDC). Dropping the categorical eligibility requirement would add people who did not fit the disability definitions. Eliminating the categorical eligibility and the asset test would enable all low-income persons access, and raising the income thresholds would expand the definition of low income. All of these changes can be made by relatively small increments of new public spending. A much more significant increase in spending would be to mandate that Medicaid cover home- and community-based long-term care.

While these options could be exercised within Medicaid, they could also be exercised outside it. That is, if the intent of health-care reform is to absorb Medicaid under "mainstream" insurance coverage then all that may remain of Medicaid are benefits not included in the standard benefit package. This may call for the creation of a new means-tested long-term care program with Federal guidelines assuring eligibility standards that are the same nationally.

Medicare can also be expanded, but such changes would apply to all Medicare beneficiaries, irrespective of financial means. Among the more modest changes Medicare could undertake in its existing home health-care benefit are:

1 eliminate the intermittent requirement of home care,
2 increase the number of days home health care is covered, and
3 expand the list of services to included unskilled care.

The third approach would be to create a new program that is not means tested. Options that have been discussed include grants to states and the encouragement to apply for Medicaid waivers to expand home- and community-based programs. The grants would be available for direct care, to develop assessment and care-management centers, and to provide training for long-term care workers. The amount of the grants could, in effect, be arbitrarily determined by the amount Congress is willing to appropriate.

In 1993, President Clinton proposed somewhat of a compromise. States are encouraged, using a very high federal participation rate, to establish a home- and community-based program for persons of all ages who are severely functionally dependent on others. The entitlement is to an assessment and a care plan; the states are free to spend their money and the federal government matches this up to a capped amount to provide the care needed.

Reforming the Financing of Long-Term Care

When asked about their support for long-term care, most political leaders are in favor. Asking them to vote on legislation that would entitle all Americans to access to needed long-term care services, however, is another matter. The gap between rhetoric and action has been maintained because the cost of providing long-term care is so large. Comprehensive home and community care would easily cost over $30 billion in new public expenditures and comprehensive nursing-home coverage would exceed $44 billion. Obviously life could be improved for millions of people with less money. One does not need to finance it all, nor does one need to finance it all at once. But the issue of public cost is more than what it might cost today; there is concern that public programs that are not means tested will lead to cultural changes that encourage families to abandon their loved ones. That is, it is presumed that families provide so much care because they face the financial consequences of purchasing assistance directly. Such perceptions may be too difficult to counter on the merits of the argument, rather the proposal itself must contain assurances that costs are controlled.

Families and caregivers desperately work towards figuring out the "right thing to do." People struggle with formulating the right questions and then finding answers. Given the anxiety, guilt and denial associated with long-term care, it should not be surprising that people find this a difficult topic of conversation. However, as more people open up about their long-term care concerns, needs, and problems, more people will be aware of some of the problems inherent in the current financing system. Increasingly, many of those who are concerned about long-term care are in key management and decision-making positions; most are voters.

Public opinion surveys indicate that a sizable portion of voters are willing to pay additional taxes for expanded public coverage of long-term care. Not surprisingly, not everyone agrees. Furthermore, the dollar amounts people reveal they are willing to pay are not sufficient. When opinion polls inquire about specific taxes to finance long-term care, people tend to favor those taxes, such as "sin" taxes, that they are personally less likely to pay. Polling data on broader based taxes indicate that "earmarked" taxes are preferred. There is considerable information on the incidence of specific taxes and therefore we know the distributional consequences of a specific tax. It is fairly straightforward to evaluate the merits of particular taxes with how much is raised, who bears the burden of that tax, regardless of who writes the check for the tax, and how that tax is expected to grow with either the economy or the cost of long-term care over time. We also know about administrative costs.

Taxes tend to be evaluated in terms of how progressive or regressive they are; how fair or equitable the tax is on grounds other than progressivity; whether revenues from the tax will rise with the growth in expenditures; and the degree to which the tax relates to the benefits. There is no single tax that will be satisfactory on all accounts. Picking the "correct" combination of taxes to finance long-term care benefits requires finessing policy and politics.

No single tax is likely to be progressive, equitable, relate to the benefits, and grow with the benefit costs. Moreover, depending on the amount of new public dollars that need to be raised, it is not likely that one tax will be sufficient. The tax that is the most likely to come closest to these goals, the income tax, is the one that garners the least support. Public opinion consistently shows that people are willing to support taxes that "other people" pay.

In a recent Louis Harris & Associates survey for the Henry J. Kaiser Family Foundation, 76 percent of voters were willing to support taxes on liquor and cigarettes to finance health-care reform. More than half of the voters surveyed could support income taxes on those with incomes over $50,000; taxes on hospital charges, physician fees, and insurers; and taxes on the part of the employer's contribution to health insurance premiums. Less than half would support, in descending order of approval, a payroll tax on employers, a national sales tax, higher Medicare fees for upper income elderly, payroll taxes on employees, or income taxes for everyone above $25,000.

The tax that receives the least support is the one that does the best in terms of fairness, raising sufficient dollars, and growing with expenditures. Less than 29 percent said they would support higher income taxes on everyone. The tax that tends to receive the most public support, excise tax on cigarettes and alcohol, is regressive, of limited growth potential, and does not raise sufficient sums of money. The other "popular" taxes, with the exception of taxes on just the relatively wealthy, appear to be the only taxes that others would be willing to pay. Taxes on providers and employers are likely to fall back on employees, consumers, and insured persons in the form of higher health-care costs, higher insurance premiums, lower wage growth, and higher product prices. Some may fall on investors, with lower dividends, which not only includes the wealthy but all people of more modest means with retirement savings in equities and capital markets.

While 15 million or more people might be confronting long-term care issues at any one point in time; this is less than 10 percent of the voting public. Cumulatively, the constituency is bigger, but at any one point there will be more people who mistakenly presume that long-term care will not be an issue for their family; that it is covered, or that it is a manageable issue. There is, therefore, a constituency, but it needs to be brought forward. This will require political leadership and a public education. Opinion polls on willingness to pay more taxes for a specific public benefit will never be sufficient to bring about change of this magnitude. Leadership, emanating from the White House, within the Congress, and among key Governors is necessary to bring about new taxes. In the end, public support is necessary, but not sufficient to lead toward altering the financing of long-term care. Leadership from public officials is necessary and can be sufficient, for leaders can alter public opinion.

Notes

1 See for example, *A Message from the American Public: A Report of a National Survey on Health and Social Security*, A Report of the Advisory Council on Social Security, December 1991, Washington, D.C.
2 Data on long-term care is of very poor quality. Many aspects of care are simply not estimated because they are not captured in any of the data systems. In particular, care at home or in the community is very difficult to measure. The data systems are best for nursing-home care and have been evolving for home *health* care. Based on estimates from HCFA, private insurance financed 0.98 percent of nursing-home care in 1980 and 1.0 percent in 1991. Private insurance financed 7.69 percent of home health care in 1980 and 7.14 percent in 1991.
3 This is actually the number of policies sold, not the number of people with policies.
4 The Gallup poll indicated that among those who said they would buy long-term care insurance, the median response was $500 a year. Among those who said they would be willing to pay more in income taxes for a government program, the median was $200 a year.
5 This is based on a policy that is not indexed for inflation or includes any vaue if premiums are stopped. Nonforfeiture and inflation protection raise the premiums considerably. The benefit is capped at $100 a day if in a nursing home and $50 a day for care at home and the premiums vary with the initial age of purchase, ranging from a low of $254 per year for those who purchased at age 45 to a high of $1,680 if initially purchased at age 70. The cost if initially purchased at age 60 is $787 per year.

References

Agency for Health Care Policy and Research (AHCPR). 1993. *Intramural Research Highlights, Long-Term Care Studies Program*, No. 23. US Department of Health and Human Services, Washington, D.C.

Families USA Foundation. 1993. *The Heavy Burden of Home Care.* Washington, D.C.

Feder, J., M. Moon, and W. Scanlon. 1987. Medicare Reform: Nibbling at Catastrophic Costs. *Health Affairs* 6: 6–19.

Health Insurance Association of America (HIAA). 1993. *Long-Term Care Insurance in 1991, Policy and Research Findings.* Washington, D.C.

Liu, K., M. Perozek, and K. Manton. 1993. Catastrophic Acute and Long-Term Care Costs: Risks Faced by Disabled Persons, *The Gerontologist* 33(3): 299–307.

The Pepper Commission. 1990. *A Call For Action: Final Report.* Washington, D.C.: Government Printing Office.

Rice, T. and J. Gabel. 1986. Protecting the Elderly Against High Health Care Costs. *Health Affairs* 5: 5–21.

Somers, A.R. 1993. Lifecare: A Viable Option for Long-Term Care for the Elderly. *Journal of the American Geriatrics Society* 41(2): 188–91.

Stone, R. and P. Kemper. 1989. Spouses and Children of Disabled Elders: How Large a Constituency for Long-Term Care Reform. *Milbank Quarterly* 67(3–4): 485–506.

Zedlewski, S.R., and T.D. McBride. 1992. The Changing Profile of the Elderly: Effects on Future Long-Term Care Needs and Financing. *Milbank Quarterly* 70(2): 247–75.

8

Labor Market Issues in Home Care
Penny Hollander Feldman

Although home care represents a tiny fraction of the $900 billion US health-care industry, it is the fastest growing segment. Annual home health expenditures rose from $1 billion in 1980 to $7 billion in 1990, and are expected to exceed $30 billion in 2000 – an average annual growth rate of over 15 percent (Burner, Waldo, and McKusick 1992). Supporting this growth, "home health aide" – the largest occupational category in the home-care workforce – is projected to be the fastest growing occupation in the US between 1992 and 2005 (Silvestri 1993). Registered nurses (RNs), licensed practical nurses (LPNs), physical therapists (PTs), and occupational therapists – all employed in significant numbers by home health agencies – are also among the occupations with the largest numerical and/or fastest projected rates of job growth over the next decade (Silvestri 1993).[1]

Because the home-care industry is rapidly growing, highly labor intensive and heavily reliant on relatively low-skilled paraprofessional workers to provide care to especially vulnerable populations, workforce issues have been of considerable interest. During the late 1980s, labor shortages became a focus of public concern as service demand increased dramatically and many home-care agencies reported difficulties in recruiting and/or retaining nurses, therapists and aides in a tight labor market (Jones 1988;

MacAdam 1993). During the same period, reported incidents of poor quality care, attributed to the high concentration of part-time "contract" and paraprofessional workers, became more numerous (Eustis, Kane, and Fischer 1993). Concerns about the availability of an effective and caring workforce (Bayer, Stone, and Friedland 1993) created pressures to improve wages and working conditions (Barnow et al. 1988; Feldman, Sapienza, and Kane 1990; Feldman 1993). At the same time, however, pressures for cost containment appeared to constrain industry attempts to fund work-life improvements (Szasz 1990; Feldman 1993).

As the industry's diverse constituencies attempt to sort out the implications of these two apparently contradictory sets of pressures and to develop workforce policies for the coming decade, they have been preoccupied with two main questions: (1) will the home-care industry be able to attract sufficient labor to meet the projected demand for service, and (2) will the workforce employed by the industry have the capacity to deliver high-quality services? This chapter addresses these questions by describing the home-care labor market and reviewing what is known about the linkages between quality of work life, labor supply, and quality of care. In addition, it examines evidence on two important contextual questions: (1) how have efforts to improve quality of work life affected the affordability of care, and (2) how have efforts to constrain costs affected quality of work life and quality of care.

The chapter draws three conclusions. First, although the home-care industry – particularly the sector delivering skilled nursing services – is heavily reliant on government funds, and its freedom to control wages and working conditions is therefore constrained by government policies as well as market forces, it has shown some capacity over the last few years to respond effectively to labor shortages. Second, precisely because the industry is so heavily reliant on government dollars, its future adaptability will be heavily dependent on the relative generosity of government benefit and payment policies and on the incentives embodied in them. Third, to avert recurrent or persistent labor shortages, those policies should allow employers significant flexibility to determine the compensation package, the skill mix and the deployment of their workforce within the constraints of public accountability and affordability.

The Home-Care Labor Market

Any attempt to meaningfully describe the home-care labor market faces two impediments. First, the home-care industry consists of several distinct but overlapping segments: (1) a home *health* segment that emphasizes short-term, post-acute "rehabilitative" and "skilled" services; (2) a chronic-care segment that emphasizes long-term, social-supportive, "custodial" or "unskilled" services; and (3) a newer, "high-tech" segment that specializes in home infusion therapy, home renal dialysis, and respiratory and life support services (Kane 1989).[2] While all three segments employ nurses, aides and other paraprofessionals, their labor needs, reimbursement and regulatory constraints, and market conditions differ in some respects. Yet available data do not facilitate cross-segment comparisons. Second, information on Medicare/Medicaid-certified agencies that provide short-term post-acute skilled care is more plentiful and more reliable than information on agencies in the chronic or high-tech markets. Yet anecdotal evidence suggests that employment conditions in the skilled market may be better than in the unskilled market (National Aging Human Resource Institute 1994). Thus analyses based on data from certified agencies may yield more favorable conclusions than analyses based on a broader set of data, were it readily available.

Whenever possible, this chapter draws on broader data sources encompassing both certified and uncertified, skilled and unskilled market segments. Nevertheless, certain vital pieces of information, especially Bureau of Labor Statistics data on worker hours and earnings, are available only for agencies providing skilled services. The generalizations made in the chapter should be judged accordingly. Furthermore, in the discussion that follows, the reader should be sensitive to the distinction made between the terms "home-care industry," "home-care services," and "home-care agency," which encompass all market segments and provider types, and the terms "home *health* services" and "home *health* agency," which refer primarily to the certified and skilled segment of the industry.

Employers

Home-based services are provided by visiting nurse associations (VNAs) and other private nonprofit agencies; by for-profit agencies, many of them affiliated with large national chains; by hospital- and nursing-home-affiliated agencies; by local government-sponsored agencies; and by independent workers employed directly by elderly or disabled clients. Estimates of the number and types of agencies are imprecise. According to the National Home and Hospice Care Survey (NHHCS), there were approximately 7,000 home health agencies (HHAs) in the US in 1992, about 85 percent of them Medicare and/or Medicaid-certified (Strahan 1993). However, some experts believe that the NHHCS missed a substantial number of both "high-tech" and "low-tech" home-care providers that did not require Medicare certification for reimbursement (Estes and Binney 1993). Using a broader definition including private duty nursing agencies, firms providing homemakers and aides, and home infusion therapy providers, Marion Merrell Dow (1993) estimated that there were 9,982 home-care agencies in 1992, up from 5,283 in 1986.

Once a negligible part of the home-care industry, for-profit agencies are now a significant presence. They constituted about 38 percent of home health agencies included in the NHHCS (Strahan, 1993) and 49 percent of agencies in the 1992 Marion Merrell Dow survey (Marion Merrell Dow 1993). Most for-profit agencies are part of large national or regional chains, and ten of these chains employed approximately a fifth of the entire home-care workforce in 1992 (Marion Merrell Dow 1993).

Overall, the industry – particularly the certified sector providing skilled nursing services – is heavily reliant on government funding. According to national health accounts, almost 75 percent of US home health expenditures came from public coffers in 1992; the comparable figure for nursing-home expenditures was only 57 percent (Burner, Waldo, and McKusick 1992). VNAs and hospital-based home health agencies were most dependent on government funds: approximately 80 percent of their revenues came from Medicare, Medicaid and state or local governments. In contrast, only about 55 percent of for-profits' revenues came from government sources (Marion Merrell Dow 1993).

Home care is a highly labor-intensive industry that makes extensive use of paraprofessional and part-time or "contract" workers. Wages and fringe benefits are estimated to account for 70 to 90 percent of an agency's budget, compared to approximately 60 percent for hospitals (Szasz 1990; Donham, Maple, and Cowan 1992). Low-skilled homemakers and home health aides are the largest contingent of the home-care workforce (42 percent in 1992), and most of them work part-time (70 percent in 1992) (Marion Merrell Dow 1993). Overall, almost 60 percent of the home-care workforce was part-time in 1992 (Marion Merrell Dow 1993), and, according to BLS establishment data, nonsupervisory home health services employees worked on average only 27.4 hours per week (US Bureau of Labor Statistics 1993a). This workweek was significantly shorter than the 32.2 hours reported for nursing-home workers, 34.4 hours reported for hospital workers, and 31.4 reported for social-service workers (US Bureau of Labor Statistics 1993a).[3]

Employment practices vary by agency type. For-profit agencies make greatest use of part-time employees, who comprise on average two-thirds of their workforce (Marion Merrell Dow 1993). Among the major provider types, they are most reliant on less skilled LPNs and homemaker/home health aides. In contrast, hospital-based agencies are least reliant on part-time employees, who comprise little more than a third of their workforce, and most reliant on skilled labor (nurses and PTs) (Marion Merrell Dow 1993). Hospital wage ranges in 1992 were somewhat lower on average than those of for-profits and VNAs; however, benefits were probably better, inasmuch as proportionately fewer workers were employed on a part-time, temporary basis. VNAs and other nonprofit agencies generally fall between for-profit and hospital-based agencies in their reliance on part-time workers and skilled labor.

Employees

Just as employer estimates are imprecise, so are estimates of the home-care workforce. Bureau of Labor Statistics (BLS) 1992 payroll data indicated an average of 386,000 employees working in "establishments primarily engaged in providing skilled nursing or medical care in the home, under supervision of a physician (SIC code 8082, US Bureau of Labor Statistics 1993b). Based on its broader definition of home-care agency, Marion Merrell Dow (1993) estimated that the industry employed approximately 650,000 people in 1992, up 10 percent from the previous year. Estimates of the home aide portion of the workforce range from a low of 146,000 (13 percent of all nursing aides, orderlies and attendants identified by the 1992 Current Population Survey) to a high of 408,000 (based on a 1988 BLS estimate of 327,000 aides, trended forward at a compound annual growth rate of 5.68 percent [Outlook 2000 1990]). The latter estimate includes some number of self-employed or independent providers (IPs), who are hired directly by consumers, although they may be funded by state or local governments (MacAdam 1993). Thirty-one states funded IPs in the late 1980s (Litvak et al. 1987; Riley 1989), and a telephone survey of state programs indicated that approximately 145,000 workers served as IPs in 1986 (Feldman, Sapienza, and Kane 1990).

Although there has been no national survey of the home-care workforce, several area studies, as well as an analysis of the Current Population Survey (CPS), have produced descriptive data on individuals working as aides (Donovan 1989; Cantor and Chichin 1990; Feldman, Sapienza, and Kane 1990; Crown et al. 1992a and b). With the exception of race and ethnicity, which vary by local market area, and family income, which varies with race and ethnicity, the findings are remarkably consistent. They describe a middle-aged, predominantly female, disproportionately minority workforce with low education, low pay, and a high degree of part-time employment. Few aides have health insurance through their employer or union, and a large proportion have low personal and family income (Feldman, Sapienza, and Kane 1990; Crown et al. 1992a, b).

Unions
Scattered across multiple work sites, home-care workers are far more difficult to unionize than health-care workers in institutional settings. The vast majority of professional and paraprofessional employees do not belong to unions. Nevertheless, in some large cities, unions have successfully organized the aide workforce, principally in agencies that contract with state and local governments to provide publicly financed services. Independent providers working in state and county home-care programs have also been a target of union organizing. Because IPs cannot be reached through their immediate employer (the client), and the government agencies that issue their paychecks will not release their names, IPs must be identified and recruited through grass-roots contacts.

The major unions in the home-care market are the Service Employees' International Union (SEIU); the American Federation of State, County and Municipal Employees (AFSCME); Local 1199 of the Retail, Wholesale Department Store Union, based exclusively in New York City; and the United Domestic Workers' Union, based exclusively in California. Altogether, these unions probably have a home aide membership of about 60,000 to 75,000 dues-paying members.[4]

Factors affecting labor demand and supply
Traditional economics views labor-market outcomes as the result of demand and supply, mediated by wages (Burbridge 1993). In the home-care labor market, factors affecting the demand for service and therefore the demand for paid labor include the number of consumers, their health and functional status, the intensity of use, the availability of informal caregivers (family and friends), and the

cost of services (Burbridge 1993). Major trends that have fueled demand are growth in the numbers of elderly requiring both post-acute and chronic care; growing limitations on families' ability to provide informal care to family members; expanding Medicare and Medicaid benefits; constraints on hospital inpatient payments and lengths of stay, leading to increased use of post-acute, skilled home care (US General Accounting Office 1986; Silverman 1990); and technological developments allowing more sophisticated treatment at home. These trends are reflected in Medicare statistics for the period 1987–92, showing a 9.9 percent average annual increase in the number of home health users and an 18.2 percent average annual increase in the number of visits per person served (Health Care Financing Administration, Bureau of Data Management and Strategy 1993b).

While most experts expect that the demand for home-care services will continue to rise over the coming decades, several factors could moderate the rate of growth. Effective health promotion and disease-prevention programs (e.g., the development of new pharmaceutical agents for the prevention and management of Alzheimer's disease) could have a fundamental effect on the level and type of chronic services consumed by the elderly (Manton and Suzman 1992). Continued growth of cost-conscious managed-care systems could lead to reductions in the number of visits per person served. And continued federal and state budget pressures could lead to the growth of alternative programs such as elder foster-care or adult day-care centers.

Factors affecting the supply of labor include the size and composition of the personnel pools from which workers are drawn; wages, benefits, and working conditions in the home-care industry; and alternative sources of employment and income (Burbridge 1993). The relevant labor pools for home care – RNs, LPNs, therapists, and low-skilled service workers – all grew faster than the US population in the 1980s, albeit somewhat unevenly (Clare et al. 1987; Pope and Menke 1990. The pool of middle-aged and minority women who supply the aide workforce also grew rapidly during the 1980s, as the baby boom generation entered middle age (Fullerton 1990). By 2010, as baby boomers reach old age and begin to require assistance themselves, the pool of middle-aged women available to provide low-skilled basic services will be substantially smaller (Committee on Ways and Means 1992). However, increasing cost-containment pressures may force hospitals to reduce their workforce and change their occupational mix, thereby "freeing up" a pool of nurses, aides, and perhaps therapists to work in the home-care industry.

Even as labor pools grew over the last decade, home-care agencies perceived themselves at a disadvantage in offering wages, benefits, and working conditions competitive with other health-care and service employers. In particular, quality of work life for aides was identified as the least tractable problem. During the period 1985 through 1990, home aide wages were 30 to 60 percent lower than those of aides employed by hospitals (Feldman, Sapienza, and Kane 1990; Crown et al. 1992b). They also lagged behind the wages of nursing-home aides and of unskilled, non-supervisory workers in restaurants, hotels, laundries, etc. (Kane 1989). In addition to inferior pay rates, agencies offered aides minimal benefits, irregular hours of work, and limited opportunities for advancement (Massachusetts Rate Setting Commission 1987; Long Term Care Policy Coordinating Council (LTCPCC) 1990; Donovan 1989; Barnow et al. 1988; Feldman, Sapienza, and Kane 1990). Although attitude surveys found high worker satisfaction with the intrinsic characteristics of the job, such as helping, doing "worthwhile work," learning new things, and doing work "suited to their abilities," they found high dissatisfaction with objective employment conditions. Higher rates of dissatisfaction with pay and benefits were, in turn, linked with stronger intent to leave the job and with higher turnover (Cantor and Chichin 1990; Feldman, Sapienza, and Kane 1990; LTPCC 1990; Gilbert 1991).

The situation was less bleak for nurses and physical therapists. In 1989, average hourly earnings for RNs employed in home care were $12.90 (Marion Merrell Dow 1989), almost 15 percent lower than the $14.83 hourly pay of general-duty RNs in hospitals (Pope and Menke 1990). Nevertheless, anecdotal accounts suggested general nurse satisfaction with other aspects of home-care employment, especially the opportunity to work part-time and the high degree of professional autonomy (Maraldo 1988). Available data for physical therapists suggest that home-care agencies offered higher hourly wages than hospitals (Marion Merrell Dow 1989; Pope and Menke 1990) and that during the earlier part of the decade PTs gravitated toward home care. Between 1979 and 1983, the percentage of all PTs working in home care increased from 5.8 to 8.3 percent (Laxton 1988).[5]

Applicability of Classical Labor Market Theory to Home Care

According to traditional economic theory, labor shortages in competitive markets should not exist in the long run. Employers who experience difficulty in hiring workers to meet increasing demand for their products or services will increase wages, alter the skill mix of their workforce, and/or substitute non-labor inputs. Increased wages will attract additional workers to the market. At the same time, wage increases will induce suppliers to substitute other factors of productivity and will also raise the price of service to consumers, who will then demand fewer services. The combination of increased worker supply and decreased employer and consumer demand will restore equilibrium to the labor market (Barnow et al. 1988).

Labor shortages may persist, however, where market "imperfections" impede competitive behavior. For example, government licensing regulations might impose specialized training requirements that prevent workers from rapidly entering a field or employers from substituting one type of worker for another. Government price controls or payment regulations might depress wage rates below the market-clearing level. Conversely, government entitlement policies insulating consumers from the cost of service might sustain high and increasing demand in the face of rising prices that would otherwise dampen use.

A number of providers, policymakers, and home-care experts have argued that the home-care labor market deviates significantly from the prototypical competitive labor market and that all of the imperfections cited above apply to the field. Federal and state statutes and regulations governing professional and paraprofessional practice and training constrain employers' ability to adjust their occupational mix to meet changing volume and quality demands. State practice acts, for example, prevent agencies from training and deploying aides to administer medication or provide simple elements of physical therapy unless they become fully licensed nurses or therapists. Programmatic differences in job titles and training requirements (e.g., for Medicare "home health aides," Medicaid "personal care attendants," and county "homemaker/chore workers" – all of whom carry out similar tasks) further impede flexibility in worker employment and assignment (Lombardi 1988).

Far more expansive than its licensing role is the government's role as the major purchaser of home-care services. Because government entities account for the bulk of industry revenues, their benefit and payment policies exert considerable influence on both the demand for services and the industry's capacity to deliver them. Decisions to liberalize benefits – for example, by eliminating the 20 percent co-insurance rate, the 100-visit per year limit and the three-day prior hospitalization requirement for Medicare home health visits – can rapidly increase consumer demand (Silverman 1990) and create upward pressure on employee compensation, which may or may not be reflected in reimbursement policies. Conversely, decisions to limit utilization – for example, by increasing claims denials, as Medicare intermediaries did in 1986 and 1987, or by cutting service hours, as many states and counties have done to reduce budget deficits (MacAdam 1993) – constrict both the demand for workers and the revenues to sustain competitive wages, benefits and working conditions.

Moreover, because labor is the largest component of home-care costs, regulating reimbursement rates is virtually tantamount to regulating wages directly (Barnow et al. 1988). Medicare, Medicaid, and other state or local home-care programs use widely disparate reimbursement methods and often provide widely disparate levels of payment for essentially the same services (MacAdam 1993). Strict price regulation and low levels of payment typical of many state and county programs leave employers little if any flexibility to increase wages in the face of labor shortages. In fact, a number of states and counties with tight reimbursement policies (e.g., low, flat rates or competitive bidding) have found it difficult to attract provider agencies to offer services in high-cost areas, and a few have had to institute emergency rates or exceptions to ensure provider availability (MacAdam 1993). In theory, Medicare's retrospective cost-based, per visit reimbursement rates should allow employers relative flexibility to increase wages when necessary to meet service demands. However, Medicare has not been immune from periodic efforts to tighten reimbursement caps and restrict providers' freedom to shift costs among various labor categories (Szasz 1990; Benjamin 1993).

The 1980s Home-Care Labor Shortage

During the period 1985 through 1990, many home-care employers, policymakers, and outside experts observed the signs of home-care labor shortages and raised alarms about the industry's ability to respond competitively to meet accelerating demand. A 1988 survey of the National Association for Home Care reported that half or more of responding agencies were having difficulty recruiting and keeping nurses and aides; many respondents said they would like to employ LPNs to address service gaps, but could not do so because Medicare would not pay for skilled care provided by an LPN (Jones 1988). Indicators of shortage included high and increasing turnover, increased vacancy rates for job openings, increased time required to fill vacancies, reduced quality of applicants for jobs, and increasing gaps between authorized and delivered service hours in publicly funded home-care programs (Barnow et al. 1988; Lombardi 1988; Crown et al. 1992b; Feldman 1993). Reported shortages were most acute in East and West Coast states and in large metropolitan areas (Jones 1988). Surveys indicated that agencies were relying more heavily on part-time, temporary workers and extracting a higher volume of care from all employees (Szasz 1990). Resulting alienation was identified as a problem among both professional and paraprofessional employees (Szasz 1990). However, attention focused most sharply on the aide workforce and its pivotal role in providing basic services to both post-acute and chronic patients. High turnover among home aides, attributed to inferior working conditions and associated worker dissatisfaction, was judged a major barrier to reliability and consistency of service (Surpin 1988). Poor quality of work life was blamed for a variety of additional quality-of-care problems, including deficiencies in basic knowledge and skills, failure to perform or complete tasks, failure to conform to physicians' orders, unintentional or intentional client injury or abuse, theft and financial exploitation, tardiness, and absenteeism (Eustis, Kane, and Fischer 1993).

Interventions Designed to Improve Recruitment, Retention, and Quality of Care

Although there was little "hard" evidence linking job improvements to improvements in employee recruitment, retention, or quality of care, most employers and many policymakers believed that upgrading the job – particularly the job of the home aide – would ameliorate both the labor shortages and the quality problems that seemed to be on the upswing in the late 1980s. They recommended a variety of work-life improvements, including higher wages, more comprehensive benefits, more specialized training, increased supervisory and peer support, guaranteed hours, enhanced status, and greater opportunity for advancement along a career ladder (Lombardi 1988; Surpin 1988; Feldman 1993). To support such improvements, they also recommended changes in state and county reimbursement policies, including specification of minimum wage and benefit floors, modification of competitive bidding practices, and incentives for employers to institute optional work-life improvements (MacAdam 1993).

Building on expert consensus that effective action could and should be taken, the Ford Foundation and the City of New York launched several demonstration projects to test the feasibility and impact of work-life improvements designed to reduce turnover in the home aide workforce. Research on these demonstrations provided support for the proposition that upgrading wages, benefits, training, and support could increase job satisfaction and significantly reduce worker turnover. It also suggested that improved worker retention would increase continuity of care, a key dimension of quality (Feldman 1993). At the same time, the research documented substantial financial and political barriers impeding the adoption of work-life improvements (Feldman, Sapienza, and Kane 1990; Feldman 1993).

Efforts to modify state and local reimbursement policies in support of work-life improvements were also limited. A few states enacted wage pass-through legislation in the 1980s, requiring that rate increases be passed along to workers. A few others either required that a specified percentage of the total rate be allocated to the wages and benefits of direct care workers or specified a minimum average compensation package (MacAdam 1993). In addition, at least one state (Massachusetts) established an optional incentives program allowing employers to add as much as $0.93 per hour to the payment rate to cover the costs of special initiatives such as paid vacation and sick leave, travel reimbursement, specialized training programs, and health insurance bonuses (MacAdam 1993). However, wage pass-through provisions were established less frequently for home-care workers than for nursing-home staff, perhaps because of the lower level of unionization in the home-care industry (Bayer, Stone, and Friedland 1993). Moreover, as state budget deficits rose in the late 1980s, home-care authorizations were cut in many areas, and funding for special work-life improvement programs dwindled (Bayer, Stone, and Friedland 1993).

Congress addressed worker-training issues in the Omnibus

Reconciliation Act of 1987. Starting January 1990, Medicare-certified home health agencies were prohibited from hiring aides on a full-time, part-time or per diem basis unless they had completed a 75-hour training program or passed a competency evaluation requiring proficiency in all tasks to be performed on the job, including taking a patient's temperature, providing grooming and hygiene assistance and moving a patient safely from one setting to another. The extent to which these requirements resulted in increased training is unknown but probably limited (Bayer, Stone and Friedland 1993). They applied only to certified agencies providing Medicare or Medicaid-reimbursable services, and many such agencies had paraprofessional training programs prior to passage of the amendments. Nor is there readily available evidence on cost increases or quality improvements associated with increased regulation.

New Evidence on the Responsiveness of the Home-Care Labor Market

The experience of the late 1980s led many experts to conclude that structural features of the home-care industry would produce labor-supply and labor-quality problems over the long term, regardless of short-term fluctuations in the business cycle (MacAdam 1993; Bayer, Stone, and Friedland 1993). Yet current data on home-care workers' employment and earnings suggest that, despite a time lag between market changes and industry response, agencies' capacity to respond to an increased demand for labor may have been greater than anticipated. Because the available data are drawn principally from the home health segment of the industry, cover a short period of time, and are aggregated in such a way that it is difficult to disentangle increases in wages from increases in the skill mix of employees, they must be considered as suggestive rather than conclusive. Nevertheless, figures from two separate sources suggest that starting in 1988, home-care agencies were able to increase wages and/or adjust their skill mix more rapidly than nursing homes or hospitals to respond to the apparent imbalance between labor demand and supply in the industry.[7]

Table 8.1 presents BLS data on average hourly and weekly earnings of non-supervisory employees in home health agencies (HHAs), nursing homes, and hospitals for the years 1988–92. (Data for HHAs were not collected prior to 1988.) These data indicate that average

Table 8.1 Average hourly and weekly earnings of non-supervisory employees in home health agencies, nursing homes, and hospitals: 1988–1992

Average Hourly Earnings	1988	1989	1990	1991	1992	Avg. Annual % Growth
HHAs[1]	$7.31	$7.88	$8.77	$9.40	$10.01	+8.2
% annual change[3]		7.8	11.3	7.2	6.5	
NHs[2]	6.33	6.79	7.24	7.56	7.66	+4.9
% annual change[3]		7.3	6.6	4.4	1.3	
Hospitals	10.51	11.21	11.79	12.51	13.03	+5.6
% annual change[3]		6.7	5.2	6.1	4.2	

Average Weekly Earnings	1988	1989	1990	1991	1992	Avg. Annual % Growth
HHAs[1]	$193.72	$200.15	$222.76	$245.34	$274.27	+9.1
% annual change[3]		3.3	11.3	10.1	11.8	
NHs[2]	200.03	215.92	232.08	242.68	253.85	+6.1
% annual change[3]		7.9	7.5	4.6	4.6	
Hospitals	357.34	381.14	403.22	427.84	448.23	+5.8
% annual change[3]		6.7	5.8	6.1	4.8	

[1] HHA: Home health-care services establishment.
[2] NH: nursing and personal care facility.
[3] Percentage change from previous year.
Sources: U.S. Bureau of Labor Statistics, *Employment, Hours, and Earnings, U.S., 1909–1990*, Vol. 2, March 1991, Bulletin 2370; U.S. Bureau of Labor Statistics, *Employment and Earnings*, June 1992, June 1993, Table C-2.

hourly earnings in HHAs increased 8.2 percent per year between 1988 and 1992, compared with only 4.9 percent in nursing homes and 5.6 percent in hospitals. Average weekly earnings in HHAs also rose more rapidly (9.1 percent per year for HHAs, compared with 6.1 percent for nursing homes and 5.8 percent for hospitals), indicating that increased hourly earnings were not undercut by reductions in hours worked. Because average earnings will rise if organizations upgrade the skill mix of their employees as well as if they increase compensation for workers at a given skill level, it is impossible to tell from the BLS data what proportion of the respective increases is attributable to which factor. The figures for HHAs, however, do suggest a more dynamic situation in the skilled segment of the home-care industry than in hospitals or nursing homes.

Available occupation-specific data collected for Marion Merrell Dow's broader sample of home-care agencies suggest that increases in average hourly earnings were not limited to the home health segment of the market and were not simply the product of a rising skill mix but also of improvements in home-care compensation (table 8.2). Thus the rate of increase in both RN and aide hourly wages was more than twice as fast in the home-care industry as in the nursing-home industry between 1990 and 1992. LPN wages also grew more rapidly in home care than in nursing homes during this period, though the disparity was not as great as for RNs and aides. (Comparable data for PTs and for hospitals were not available.)

Impact of Employment Practices on Home-Care Costs and Quality

How did employers' response to perceived labor shortages affect the affordability and quality of care? As discussed above, in purely competitive markets, wage increases should be passed on to consumers through higher prices, leading to reduced demand. However, in regulated and subsidized markets such as home care, prices may be limited, while volume may be relatively unconstrained. Facing price constraints, employers could have offset the cost of higher wages by shifting costs to unregulated services, reducing non-labor costs, imposing heavier workloads on employees, delivering a higher volume of care, and/or reducing service quality. Alternatively, they could have internalized rising labor costs by reducing margins. How then did they respond? Available Medicare data confirm that home health wage increases

Table 8.2 Average hourly wages for home-care agencies and nursing homes: 1990–1992

	1990	1991	1992	Avg. Annual % Growth
RNs				
HCAs[2]	$14.62	$15.33	$16.39	+5.9
% annual change[1]		4.9	6.9	
NHs[3]	13.15	13.52	13.77	+2.3
% annual change[1]		2.8	1.8	
LPNs				
HCAs	10.51	10.95	11.57	+4.9
% annual change[1]		4.2	5.7	
NHs	9.63	9.97	10.21	+3.0
% annual change[1]		3.5	2.4	
AIDES				
HCAs	5.65	5.91	6.06	+3.6
% annual change[1]		4.6	2.5	
NHs	5.71	5.77	5.87	+1.4
% annual change[1]		1.1	1.7	

[1] HCA: Home-care agency.
[2] Percent change from previous year.
[3] NH: nursing and personal care facility.

Source: Marion Merrell Dow, *Managed Care Digest: Long Term Care Edition*, 1991, 1992, 1993.

granted between 1989 and 1992 were not fully reflected in increased Medicare charges and that per visit price increases were not a primary cause of Medicare home health expenditure growth (Bishop and Skwara 1993). Medicare charges per visit increased only 5 percent per year between 1989 and 1992 (Health Care Financing Administration 1993b), less than the 6.2 percent average annual increase in the HCFA price index of home health wages and salaries and considerably less than the 8.2 percent per year annual increase in average hourly earnings reported by BLS (see table 8.1).

It is possible that home health agencies shifted some of their rising wage costs to non-Medicare payers. However, data to compare Medicare visit charges with non-Medicare visit charges are not available. In any case, opportunities for cost-shifting and cross-subsidization were limited to some extent by Medicare rules requiring the segregation of certified and non-certified operations.

Evidence on the pursuit of non-labor savings by employers suggests that they did try to reap some economies of scale in the areas of administration, purchasing, and the like. For example, one survey of 166 home health agencies in nine SMSAs found that the overwhelming majority of changes in organizational structure over a fifteen-month study period were toward greater affiliation with chains or multifacility systems (Estes et al. 1992). However, HCFA price index data show that cost increases for categories other than wages and salaries were about the same for home health agencies as for skilled nursing facilities between 1989 and 1992, and lower for hospitals (table 8.3). Furthermore, given the labor-intensive nature of home care, it would be difficult for savings in this area to completely offset wage and salary price increases.

Given a history of weak management, employers could have expected significant gains from tightening labor processes to increase workers' productivity (Szasz 1990). Data on management practices in the industry are sparse but do suggest that the cost of wage increases was offset to some extent by imposing heavier workloads and increasing volume. The same survey of agencies in nine SMSAs cited above documented widespread efforts to increase labor output through imposition of explicit standards for visit numbers and time per visit, reductions in allowable travel time, and increased monitoring of the amount, pace, and rhythm of work (Szasz 1990). In addition, HCFA data indicate that the volume of reimbursable care increased dramatically between 1988 and 1992, as home health agencies increased their penetration of the Medicare market and greatly increased the number of visits per person served (Bishop and Skwara 1993). This growth in volume was accomplished principally through growth in the numbers of visits per agency, which increased about 17 percent per year between 1986 and 1990 (Bishop and Skwara 1993).[8,9]

Whatever combination of strategies employers may have used to offset rising wages, there is no evidence to suggest that they absorbed increased labor costs by reducing their margins.[10] Home-

Table 8.3 Percentage change in four-quarter running averages: total expenses excluding wages and salaries

	1989 Qtr. I	1990 Qtr. I	1991 Qtr. I	1992 Qtr. I	Avg. annual change 1989–1992
HHAs[1]	5.1	5.2	5.3	4.3	5.0
SNfs[2]	4.9	5.5	5.7	3.6	4.9
Hospitals	6.0	5.2	4.6	2.5	4.6

[1] HHAs: Home Health Agencies.
[2] SNfs: Skilled Nursing facilities

Source: Figures calculated from *Health Care Financing Review*, Fall 1992, "Health Care Indicators", Tables 8, 10, 12.

care agency margins rose from an average 6.3 percent loss in 1989 to an average 7.2 percent profit in 1992 (Marion Merrell Dow 1989–93). Concomitantly, Medicare home health payments tripled, even though per visit charges increased only 5 percent per year.

How job satisfaction, turnover, and quality of care were affected by changes in wages, skill mix, workload, and volume is not known. Valid, reliable, industry-wide data on worker attitudes, turnover, and performance do not exist, and measurement of home-care quality, including clinical outcomes and client satisfaction, is at an early stage (Eustis, Kane, and Fischer 1993; Weissert 1991; Kramer et al. 1990). On the whole, studies linking quality of work life to worker performance and efficacy of long-term care have been characterized as "chronicles from the frontier of analysis" (Brannon 1992). Given the state of the art, it is not surprising that the link between quality of work life and quality of care is "still an undertested, though reasonable, assumption" (Eustis, Kane, and Fischer 1993: 67).

Current Policy Proposals and their Implications for the Home-Care Labor Market

The rapid rise in home health expenditures, the recent debate over benefits to be included in national health reform, and the current move to cut Medicare and Medicaid costs have all intensified concerns over home-care cost and quality. Although rising labor costs and increases in visit charges are not primarily responsible for the dramatic growth in home health expenditures (Bishop and Skwara 1993), high on the policy agenda are proposals to move from retrospective to prospective Medicare payment, on a per visit, per episode or per capita basis. Greater integration of acute and chronic care and greater reliance on case-management systems are also being considered as ways to control service use and costs. Although most policymakers, concerned about accountability and quality of care, continue to support the provision of home-care benefits through licensed or certified agencies, some states are making extensive use of independent provider programs to save program dollars (Commonwealth Fund 1993). In addition, the disability community and elder advocacy groups, concerned with consumer choice and autonomy, are actively promoting "consumer-driven" service models that would reduce the role of home-care agencies as employers. What do these varied proposals portend for future labor supply and service quality?

Prospective payment and capitation

Analysis of the financial incentives created by various payment methods suggests that the retrospective cost-based reimbursement approach currently employed by Medicare is more conducive to maintaining quality of work life and quality of care than most other methods being considered, including prospective per visit or per episode payment, "bundling," and capitation (Schlenker and Shaughnessy 1992). Under current Medicare rules, home health agencies can be fully reimbursed for the costs of wage increases and service quality improvements, so long as their overall visit costs remain below the aggregate cost limit. In past years, only a modest proportion of certified agencies (approximately 25 percent in 1992) presented visit charges that exceeded the Medicare cost ceiling (Bishop and Skwara 1993). However, the proportion has been rising, and further ratcheting down of the limit would reduce the opportunity to pass through the costs of wage or quality improvements and cause the retrospective-payment approach to resemble more closely a prospective system.

Current Medicare payment policy also provides positive access and quality incentives by allowing agencies relative flexibility to determine a service "package" for a given client and deploy a mix of personnel appropriate to deliver that package. If one patient, for example, requires more PT visits than another, the agency can provide them and be reimbursed by Medicare, so long as the care is provided by a licensed PT. A major advantage of this method is that, providing there is an adequate supply, higher skilled (and thus more costly) personnel can be used, presumably with positive quality effects (Schlenker and Shaughnessy 1992). (Should higher-skilled personnel be in short supply, however, neither Medicare nor most state licensing agencies will permit the substitution of non-licensed for licensed personnel, even if non-licensed staff have been trained to perform equivalent tasks.)

The major disadvantage of retrospective payment is, of course, the lack of cost-containment incentives. In the absence of a tight cost limit or supplementary policies limiting the number of visits (e.g., by narrowly proscribing eligibility requirements or range of covered services), retrospective cost-based per visit payment constrains neither unit price nor service volume. Hence the current interest in various forms of prospective payment.

Because number of visits – not cost per visit – is principally responsible for the dramatic growth of national home-care expenditures, any new payment system that seriously hopes to control rising expenditures will have to provide incentives for agencies to constrain service volume. Prospective per visit payment would encourage agencies to minimize cost per visit, but it would not address the volume problem. Moreover, it could exacerbate labor supply, service quality, and cost problems by putting downward pressure on wages while encouraging employers to further increase workloads, cut visit time, and maximize the number of visits.

Other forms of risk-based payment might or might not be preferable. Compared to per visit payment, "bundling" (e.g., including home health as an add-on to hospital DRGs), per episode, and per capita payment embody stronger incentives for constraining volume (although agencies paid per episode rather than per visit might simply seek to maximize the number of episodes). Adjusted for patient case mix and combined with quality monitoring, these payment methods might give agencies the incentive to integrate and allocate skilled and unskilled labor more efficiently and effectively (Bishop and Skwara 1993). Pending modifications in federal Medicare and state practice regulations, one result might be increased reliance on lower-cost paraprofessional workers to assume case-management or patient-care responsibilities currently restricted to RNs. Assuming that these paraprofessionals received appropriate training, supervision and compensation, this substitution of unskilled for skilled labor would be likely to benefit the paraprofessional workforce without jeopardizing quality of care. This is clearly one of the expectations motivating experimentation with risk-based integrated-care models such as social HMOs and the new PACE demonstrations (Vladeck, Miller, and Clauser 1993). Underfunded or poorly monitored, however, risk-based payment might simply encourage providers at financial risk to minimize costs by lowering their skill mix, skimping on training and supervision, or eliminating possibly beneficial visits.

Ideally, policymakers and third-party payers could specify desired client outcomes, provide reimbursement adequate to produce those outcomes in an efficient manner, hold home-care providers accountable for the outcomes, and leave the details of service delivery to the industry. However, until valid and reliable patient classification systems are fully developed and outcome studies yield their results, some specification of labor inputs and processes is probably necessary to deter agencies from reducing the quality of personnel or the quality of care in response to cost-containment incentives embodied in various forms of risk-based reimbursement (MacAdam 1993). The problem is that the input regulations currently imposed by Medicare and other public programs sometimes prevent employers from making appropriate labor substitutions and/or providing stable employment for workers whose job descriptions vary across categorical programs. One challenge for rational policy, then, is to modify rigid professional practice acts and categorical program restrictions in ways that preserve public accountability while allowing HHAs greater freedom to respond to changes in labor-market conditions.

Case management

A second challenge for rational policy is to develop home-care eligibility criteria, reinforced by case-management and claims review mechanisms, that promote appropriate access while deterring unnecessary utilization (and thus unnecessary costs). This will be difficult under any circumstances but virtually impossible at the macro or national level until a workable consensus emerges on government's responsibility in balancing its citizens' short-term, post-acute home-care needs with their chronic needs for less skilled, supportive services (Benjamin 1993; Bishop and Skwara 1993). In the meantime, there is active debate about the propriety and efficacy of allowing home-care agencies to exercise case-management functions within various categorical programs. If case management is confined to certification of clients for home-care eligibility, lodging such functions outside the service-delivery agency would seem to promote public accountability with little adverse impact on employment practices or quality of care. However, if case management is defined to include micro-management of the content of client-care plans, lodging control in bodies with less intimate knowledge of clients and no responsibility for service delivery could both compromise quality and significantly constrain the rational allocation of human resources.

Independent provider programs and consumer-driven service models

IP programs and other forms of consumer-directed care would reduce or eliminate altogether the role of home-care agencies as employers and service providers for "self-directing" clients. Advocates of consumer-directed models have rarely addressed worker interests or quality of work life as goals in themselves or even as a means to achieve quality care. Perhaps because they are concerned primarily with the delivery of chronic supportive services, choice advocates emphasize consumer satisfaction as the key dimension of service quality and pay relatively little attention to the technical aspects of care. Their literature focuses on the importance of giving clients control over the hiring and firing, scheduling, supervision, and payment of direct-care workers (Alliance for Aging Research 1993). And recent survey data show a strong relationship between degree of control over these aspects of care and consumer satisfaction (Commonwealth Fund 1993). Because IP programs often allow service recipients to hire relatives, friends and neighbors (for example, two-thirds of providers in Michigan's IP program fall in one of those categories [Commonwealth Fund 1993]), this finding is not surprising.

While IP programs were quite common in the late 1970s, during the next decade many states, seeking to reduce fraud, avoid liability, and improve administrative and substantive oversight of services, phased them out and began to channel funds through contract or vendor agencies. To date, those states that have maintained large IP programs have done so more out of a desire to minimize unit costs per hour of service than respond to consumer demands for choice or control. The California In-home Supportive Services program (IHHS) is the most prominent example. A comparison of alternative service modes conducted in the early 1980s found that hourly service costs for independent providers (IPs) in that program (including both labor and administrative costs) were approximately 55 percent lower than the hourly costs of vendor agencies in counties that used both IPs and contract agencies (Program Review Bureau 1983). Much of the difference was accounted for by IP wages and benefits, which were 45 percent lower than wages and benefits in the contract sector. In addition, IP programs avoided the overhead costs associated with worker recruitment, training and supervision, and with contract monitoring. California counties that use both IPs and contract agencies generally channel their sicker and more disabled clients, requiring larger amounts of service, to the cheaper IP sector to keep down program costs. Thus clients requiring more intensive care may be served by untrained and unsupervised workers (Feldman, Sapienza, and Kane 1990).

Depending on the perspective from which they are viewed, IP programs can be seen as either a relatively safe and inexpensive way to satisfy consumer needs and allow payment of relatives and friends for useful services or a vehicle for depressing wages, exploiting workers, and possibly harming vulnerable consumers who may be unable to exercise adequate supervision of their care.[11] Given the paucity of research to support either perspective, development of consumer-choice models should be accompanied with careful monitoring and evaluation to identify the appropriate candidates for consumer control, and to assess the impact of particular models on quality of work life and quality of care. To better serve both consumer and worker interests, existing IP programs should be monitored as carefully as contract or "vendor" programs. Finally, to allay the concerns of worker advocates and responsible employers, policymakers should promote wages, benefits, and standards of care commensurate with the organized sector of the industry.

Conclusions

Despite concerns that government regulation would preclude employers from responding effectively to changing market conditions, the evidence presented in this chapter suggests that the home-care industry – in particular, the home health segment most heavily nourished by Medicare and Medicaid payments – was able to bid up wages to attract workers in a period of increasing demand. Some portion of increased labor costs was probably offset by reducing non-labor costs and increasing employee workloads – with unknown effects on job satisfaction or quality of care. In addition, some portion was passed on to Medicare and other payers through rising prices and much more rapidly rising volume. Indeed, during the period under consideration, expanding Medicare benefits and retrospective cost-based Medicare reimbursement created both increased demand for labor and the conditions to pay for it.

Precisely because the industry is so heavily reliant on government dollars, its future adaptability will be heavily dependent on the relative generosity of government eligibility and payment policies and on the incentives embodied in them. In light of the "Contract with America" and the prospect of shrinking public coffers, it is probably safe to assume that the future will bring increased pressure to improve the efficiency and affordability of home-based services (Weissert 1991). Experimentation with prospective risk-based methods of payment is likely to accelerate in both the post-acute and chronic-care segments, providing incentives to cut both unit costs and service volume. Cost-containment pressures, in turn, may exacerbate quality-of-work-life and quality-of-care problems.

Yet cost-containment pressures, which certainly will not be confined to the home-care industry, may be two edged. First, projected cuts in the acute-care sector may lead to sharply reduced demand for hospital labor and to further abatement of hospital wage increases. Should wage increases continue to moderate in the rest of the health-care system, wage disparities are likely to be less of a problem for home-care employers in the future than they have been in the past. (Had national health reform resulted in universal insurance coverage, benefits disparities would also have diminished in importance.) Second, as argued above, cost-containment incentives embodied in certain forms of risk-based payment could conceivably improve rather then detract from quality of work life (and quality of care) to the extent that less skilled, paraprofessional workers are better integrated into the service system, vested with greater responsibilities, and provided with training, compensation, and support commensurate with those responsibilities.

Given the variability in estimates of service needs, the rapid evolution of service-delivery and payment systems, and the uncertain future of health-care reform, home-care labor force requirements may change dramatically over the coming decades. Given the dynamics of labor supply and demand and the length of time involved in the policymaking process, direct government intervention in the home-care labor market (e.g., in the form of a national training program or an across-the-board wage increase) might well promote rather than prevent a market imbalance. Thus the most effective government policy may be one that conceives of worker shortages (or surpluses) as a function of delayed market response and that aims not to bypass the market but to facilitate its movement toward equilibrium (Newschaffer and Schoenman 1990). To avert recurrent or persistent labor shortages on the one hand, or a glut of workers on the other, employers must be allowed, even encouraged, to alter employment practices to respond to fluctuations in market conditions. It follows that policies designed to promote efficient and affordable home care should avoid rigid constraints on worker classification, compensation, or deployment and offer rewards for employer initiatives designed to upgrade worker skills, enhance productivity, and improve performance on the job.

Notes

1. RNs and LPNs are listed among the 20 occupations with the largest projected growth in absolute numbers of jobs between 1992 and 2005. PTs and OTs are listed among the 20 occupations with the highest growth rates (Silvestri 1993).
2. For the purposes of this chapter, I exclude a fourth segment – companies (including a growing number of home health agencies) that distribute durable medical equipment such as beds and wheelchairs, as well as medical supplies such as ostomy, incontinence, and pressure sore products.
3. Although home health establishments reported a workweek of only 27.4 hours per non-supervisory worker, data from the Current Population Survey indicate that individual home-care aides worked on average 35.18 hours per week, not significantly different from hospital aides (35.66 hours) or nursing-home aides (35.91) (Crown 1992a). Two factors may account for the seeming disparity in findings: (1) the BLS data are for all non-supervisory employees, not just aides; and (2) the BLS data are "per establishment," while the CPS data reflect hours at more than one establishment.
4. Personal communication from David Snapp, SEIU, 8/13/93.
5. Although current quantitative data are not available, anecdotal accounts suggest that HHAs are currently experiencing a significant shortage of PTs.
6. Medicare pays HHAs the lower of reasonable costs or charges per visit. Costs are paid up to a ceiling, which was originally 120 percent and is now 112 percent of the wage-adjusted mean for all free-standing agencies in a prior year, trended ahead to the current year using an inflation factor. Hospital-based agencies are allowed an add-on reflecting their higher administrative and general costs. (This add-on was eliminated by the recent Clinton budget agreement.) Except for a short period in the mid-1980s, ceilings have been applied in the aggregate, rather than by type of visit (Bishop and Skwara 1993).
7. The fact that home-care wages continued to increase more rapidly even in 1991 and 1992, despite the fact that the country was by then in a recession and the labor market was slackening, provides further evidence of a time lag between market signals and industry response.
8. Industry-wide data including both Medicare and non-Medicare visits indicate a similar but somewhat smaller average annual increase (13.5 percent) in visits per agency over the period 1988–92 (Marion Merrell Dow 1993).

9 In the absence of reliable data on trends in full-time equivalent workers over time, it is not possible to assess changes in workload as a function of increased agency volume.
10 Margins here are calculated as net income (or loss) from services divided by total patient revenues.
11 Critics of IP arrangements also express concern about moral hazard involved in allowing relatives to be paid as independent providers. Their concern is that government will end up paying for services which were previously provided at no charge to the public sector.

References

Alliance for Aging Research. 1993. Providing Choice in Home Care Services: The Michigan Approach to Personal Care Services. Washington, D.C.

Barnow, B., J. Constantine, et al. 1988. The Home Care Labor Market in New York State: An Analysis of the Issues and Projections through 2000. Washington, D.C.: Lewin/ICF.

Bayer, E., R. Stone, and R. Friedland. 1993. *Developing an Effective and Caring Long-Term Care Workforce*, Washington, D.C.: Project Hope.

Benjamin, A. 1993. An Historical Perspective on Home Care Policy. *Milbank Quarterly* 71(1): 129–66.

Bishop, C., and K. Skwara. 1993. Recent Growth of Medicare Home Health: Sources and Implications. *Health Affairs* 12(3): 95–110.

Brannon, D. 1992. Toward Second-Generation Nursing Home Research. *The Gerontologist* 32(3): 293–4.

Burbridge, L. 1993. The Labor Market for Home Care Workers: Demand, Supply and Institutional Barriers. *The Gerontologist* 33(1): 41–6.

Burner, S.T., D.R. Waldo, and D.R. McKusick. 1992. National Health Expenditures Projections Through 2030. *Health Care Financing Review* 14(1): 1–29.

Cantor, M., and E. Chichin. 1990. Stress and Strain among Homecare Workers of the Frail Elderly. New York: Fordham University, Brookdale Research Institute on Aging, Third Age Center.

Clare, F.L., E. Spratley, P. Schwab, and J. Iglehart. 1987. DataWatch: Trends in Health Personnel. *Health Affairs* 6(4): 90–103.

Committee on Ways and Means. 1992. *Green Book*. Washington, D.C.: US House of Representatives, 102nd Congress, 2nd Session.

Commonwealth Fund, Commission on Elderly People Living Alone. 1993. The Importance of Choice in Home Care Programs: Maryland, Michigan, and Texas. New York: Commonwealth Fund, June 9, 1993.

Crown, W., et al. 1992a. Home Care Workers: A National Profile. *Caring* April: 34–8.

Crown, W., et al. 1992b. *Health Aides: Characteristics and Working Conditions of Aides Employed in Hospitals, Nursing Homes, and Home Care*. Report to the Health Care Financing Administration, Contract Number HCFA 500-89-0056. Waltham, MA: Brandeis University, Institute for Health Policy.

Donham, C., B. Maple, and C. Cowan. 1992. Health Care Indicators. *Health Care Financing Review* 14(2): 177–98.

Donovan, R. 1989. Work Stress and Job Satisfaction: A Study of Home Care Workers in New York City. *Home Health Services Quarterly* 10(1/2): 97–114.

Estes, C., and L. Binney. 1993. The Restructuring of Home Care. San Francisco, CA: Institute for Health and Aging. Unpublished paper.

Estes, C., J. Swan, L. Bergthold, and P. Spohn. 1992. Running as Fast as They Can: Organizational Changes in Home Health Care. *Home Health Care Services Quarterly* 13(1/2): 35–69.

Eustis, N., and L.R. Fischer. 1991. Relationships Between Home Care Clients and Their Workers: Implications for Quality of Care. *The Gerontologist* 31: 447–56.

Eustis, N., R. Kane, and L. Fischer. 1993. Home Care Quality and the Home Care Worker: Beyond Quality Assurance as Usual. *The Gerontologist* 33(1): 64–73.

Feldman, P. 1993. Work Life Improvements for Home Care Workers: Impact and Feasibility. *The Gerontologist* 33(1): 47–54.

Feldman, P., A. Sapienza, and N. Kane. 1990. *Who Cares for Them: Workers in the Home Care Industry*. New York: Greenwood Press.

Freeland, M., G. Chulis et al. 1991. Measuring Hospital Input Price Increases: The Rebased Hospital Market Basket. *Health Care Financing Review* 12(3): 1–14.

Fullerton, H. 1990. New labor force projections, spanning 1988 to 2000. In *Outlook 2000*. Washington, D.C.: US Department of Labor, Bureau of Labor Statistics. Bulletin 2352, April.

Gilbert, N. 1991. Home Care Worker Resignations: A Study of the Major Contributing Factors. *Home Health Services Quarterly* 12(1): 69–83.

Health Care Financing Administration, Bureau of Data Management and Strategy. 1993a. Number of Providers, Persons Served, Visits, and Program Payments, for Medicare Home Health Agency Vendors, by Type of Agency: Calendar Year 1990. Unpublished data, Baltimore, MD.

Health Care Financing Administration, Bureau of Data Management and Strategy. 1993b. Trends in Persons Served, Visits, Total Charges, Visit Charges, and Program Payments, for Medicare Home Health Agency Services, by Year of Service: Selected Calendar Years 1974–1992. Unpublished data.

Jones, P. 1988. Nursing Shortage: A Caring Shortage. *Caring* 7(5): 15–18.

Kane, N. 1989. The Home Care Crisis of the Nineties. *The Gerontologist* 29(1): 24–31.

Kramer, A., Shaughnessy, P., et al. 1990. Assessing and Assuring the Quality of Home Health Care: A Conceptual Framework. *Milbank Quarterly* 68(3): 413–44.

Laxton, C. 1988. The Home Care Personnel Shortage: Its Effect on the Supply of Physical Therapists. *Caring* 7(5): 32–5.

Litvak, et al. 1987. *Attending to America: Personal Assistance for Independent*

Living: A Survey of Attendant Service Programs in the US for People of All Ages with Disabilities. Berkeley, CA: World Institute on Disability.

Lombardi, T. 1988. Recruitment, Training, and Retention of Home Care Paraprofessionals. *Caring* 7(5): 24–5, 54–8.

Long-Term Care Policy Coordinating Council (LTCPCC). January 1990. Strengthening the Home Care Work Force in New York State: A Study of Worker Characteristics, Recruitment and Retention. Albany, New York: New York State Department of Social Services, Office of Program Planning Analysis and Development and the Division of Medical Assistance.

MacAdam, M. 1993. Home Care Reimbursement and Effects on Personnel. *The Gerontologist* 33(1): 55–63.

Manton, K., and R. Suzman. 1992. Forecasting Health and Functioning in Aging Societies: Implications for Health Care and Staffing Needs. In *Aging, Health, and Behavior,* ed. M. Ory, R. Abeles, and P. Lipman. Newbury Park, CA: Sage.

Maraldo, P. 1988. Nursing Supply Crisis: How Does Home Care Compare to Other Sectors? *Caring* 8(5): 10–14.

Marion Merrell Dow. 1989. *Long Term Care Digest, Home Health Care Edition.* Kansas City, Missouri.

Marion Merrell Dow. 1991. *Managed Care Digest, Long-Term Care Edition.* Kansas City, Missouri.

Marion Merrell Dow. 1992. *Managed Care Digest, Long-Term Care Edition.* Kansas City, Missouri.

Marion Merrell Dow. 1993. *Managed Care Digest, Long-Term Care Edition.* Kansas City, Missouri.

Massachusetts Rate Setting Commission. 1987. *The Homebound Elderly: Who Cares.* Boston.

National Aging Human Resource Institute. 1994. The Home Care Labor Market: Policy Issues for the Aging Network. New York: Brookdale Center on Aging. Unpublished paper.

Newschaffer, C., and J. Schoenman. 1990. Registered Nurse Shortages: Appropriate Public Policy. *Health Affairs* 9(1): 98–106.

Pope, G., and T. Menke. 1990. DataWatch: Hospital Labor Markets in the 1980s. *Health Affairs* 9(4): 127–37.

Program Review Bureau. 1983. Evaluation of In-Home Supportive Services Program. CA: Department of Social Services, Adult Services Branch. Unpublished paper, Sacramento.

Riley, T. 1989. Quality Assurance in Home Care. Washington, D.C.: AARP Public Policy Institute.

Schlenker, R., and P. Shaughnessy. 1992. Medicare Home Health Reimbursement Alternatives: Access, Quality and Cost Incentives. *Home Health Services Quarterly* 13(1/2): 91–115.

Silverman, H. 1990. Use of Medicare-Covered Home Health Agency Services. *Health Care Financing Review* 12(2): 113–26.

Silvestri, G. 1993. Occupational Employment: Wide Variations in Growth.

Monthly Labor Review, November, 58–86.
Strahan, G. 1993. *Overview of Home Health and Hospice Care Patients: Preliminary Data from the 1992 National Home and Hospice Care Survey.* Advance Data, DHHS Publication No. (PHS) 93–1250. Washington, D.C.: National Center for Health Statistics.
Surpin, R. 1988. Improved Working Conditions Lead to Improved Quality. *Caring* 7(5): 26–31.
Szasz, A. 1990. The Labor Impacts of Policy Change in Health Care: How Federal Policy Transformed Home Health Organizations and Their Labor Practices. *Journal of Health Politics, Policy and Law* 15(1): 191–210.
US Bureau of Labor Statistics. 1993a. Establishment Data: Hours and Earnings. In *Employment and Earnings*, June, Table C-2. Washington D.C.
US Bureau of Labor Statistics. 1993b. Establishment Data: Employment Not Seasonally Adjusted. In *Employment and Earnings*, March, Table B-2. Washington, D.C.
US Bureau of Labor Statistics. 1993c. Household Data. In *Employment and Earnings*, January, Table 56. Washginton, D.C.
US Department of Labor, Bureau of Labor Statistics. *Outlook 2000.* Bulletin 2352, April. Washington, D.C.
US General Accounting Office. 1986. Medicare: Need to strengthen home health care payment controls and address unmet needs. Report to the chairman, special committee on aging, United States Senate. Washington, D.C. GAO/HRD-87-9. December.
Vladeck, B., N. Miller, and S. Clauser. 1993. The Changing Face of Long-Term Care. *Health Care Financing Review* 14(4): 5–24.
Weissert, W. 1991. A New Policy Agenda for Home Care. *Health Affairs* 10(2): 67–77.

9

Housing Policy and Home-Based Care
Sandra J. Newman

Several prominent social and demographic trends – women's increased attachment to the labor force, changes in the nature of the family, and the growth of the elderly population – have stimulated new interest in home- and community-based services. Despite the continued responsiveness and durability of family support systems, interest in formal services has been particularly strong for at least two reasons: the often substantial social costs of family care, and the service gaps experienced by those with no viable family caregiving systems.

Partly in response to these concerns, researchers have attempted to gain a better understanding of the need and demand for formal services in the home. Studies have addressed such questions as who uses in-home services, what conditions precipitate their use, and what effects they have on users (e.g., Noelker and Bass 1989; Mathematica Policy Research, Inc. 1987; Berkeley Planning Associates 1985; Tennstedt and McKinlay 1987; Wan 1987; Mindel et al. 1986). But little attention has been paid to the question of *how* the formal service system functions or, more particularly, what factors *enable* this system to function successfully. Public policy can do little to alter family demographics or the amount of affection and caring within families. But exogenous factors that either facilitate or impede home- and community-based care access and quality are appropriate targets for policy consideration. One such enabling factor may be the housing environment in which the individual in need of care lives. Because, by definition, the individual's home is the setting in which home-based long-term care services are delivered, it is plausible to expect that characteristics of that setting may affect how, or what, care is provided, or even whether it is feasible to provide it at all. For example, features of the housing environment, such as the size and configuration of the dwelling and the characteristics of its neighborhood, may either facilitate or prevent linkages to needed home-based services. Even more fundamentally, housing can have a dramatic effect on the ability of a chronically ill or disabled person to continue to live independently in the community (Thomas 1983). In some cases, the ability to make physical modifications to the dwelling or property may determine whether a person with severe mobility problems can remain at home (Struyk and Katsura 1988; Pynoos et al. 1987). Thus, housing arrangements can be an important element in designing cost-effective policies to help sustain the chronically ill or disabled in the community.

The premise that housing can affect functioning and continued community living has already had a substantial impact on decisions in the public and private housing sectors, such as the development of housing design standards for the disabled and a range of special design features both in the federally subsidized Section 202 Housing Program for the Elderly and Handicapped and in private-sector life-care and assisted-living community developments. Even more broadly defined, the nation's housing policies – and particularly those designed to meet the needs of low-income or otherwise vulnerable households – are relevant to home-based long-term care policy. Because housing policy often has a direct impact on the structural and neighborhood characteristics of the housing stock, it is important to consider the role such policy may play in the delivery of home-based care to those in need.

This chapter presents a critical review of housing policies that are relevant to home-based care – the range of health and social services delivered to disabled persons in their homes or communities. The next two sections establish the context for this review, the first by highlighting research findings on the linkage between housing and home-based care, and the second by providing a brief legislative history of how housing policy has viewed health issues over time. The subsequent three sections examine three primary ways in which housing policy affects home-based care: financing mechanisms, regulations and statutes, and coordination. The final section offers some broad targets for policy that might foster greater coherence between housing and home-based care policies with the ultimate goal of increasing home-based care access, quality and options.

Housing and Home-Based Care: A Review of the Research Evidence

Knowledgeable observers make a strong case for the effects of housing on home-based care. For example, Eustis et al. (1993) offer the hypothesis that "structural features of the job" may affect the quality of care provided by home-care workers; one plausible structural feature is the housing setting. Using their experience with the Chelsea Village Home Care Program in New York City, Scharer et al. (1990) support this hypothesis: "Providers are increasingly concerned about their ability to deliver good quality care in unsafe neighborhoods and deteriorating home environments" (p. 518). Unfortunately, very little research has been done to systematically examine whether particular housing attributes affect either the probability of arranging for home-based care services or the effectiveness of these services. The scant research that has been done focuses on two population groups: the elderly, and persons with severe mental illness.

Sussman (1979) and Noelker (1982) provide empirical evidence on the effects of housing on family caregiving to the elderly. Sussman (1979) found that situational variables, including a small number of housing characteristics, appeared to facilitate a family's willingness to care for an elderly relative (also see Sangl 1983). Noelker (1982) also highlighted the potential modifier effects of housing primarily by emphasizing features that may impede family care, such as lack of privacy or insufficient space.

Newman's (1985) study of the suitability of dwellings and neighborhoods for the delivery of in-home care extended this hypothesis to the purchase of formal services, such as home-based care. She found that roughly 17 percent of the elderly population who might be able to remain in the community and receive in-home and community-based services are living in housing units and neighborhoods that either impede the efficient delivery of these services or preclude their delivery altogether. These impediments include physical features of the dwelling, such as lack of space or special modifications, that would make it difficult, if not impossible, to accommodate long-term care service delivery in the home; and features of the building (number of units in structure) or neighborhood (low density of dwellings) that are likely to increase the cost of service delivery because of the absence of economies of scale.

This finding was tested more rigorously in later research (Newman et al. 1990). Two key hypotheses tested were whether housing and neighborhood attributes have a *direct* effect on the chances that a frail older person will enter a nursing home, or an *indirect* effect, by influencing the ability to provide informal or formal care to the older person in the community. The researchers found that some informal caregivers – spouses, for example – appear to be aided in their caregiving by the presence of special dwelling modifications in the home. These modifications include such features as grab bars, ramps or specially equipped bathrooms. In addition, a small number of environmental features played a significant role in the efficacy of formal, paid home-based care. Adequate space in the dwelling, for example, appeared to be an enabling factor that strengthened the deterrent effects of formal care on the impaired person's institutional risk. Thus, while environmental features did not directly affect institutionalization, a subset of such features did have indirect effects.

Recent research on another population group – persons with severe mental illness – suggests a relationship between utilization of home- and community-based care services, residence in affordable and physically sound housing, and beneficial outcomes (Newman et al. 1994). Using data from a longitudinal survey of severely mentally ill persons who were using Section 8 rental housing certificates, the researchers found that the combination of affordable, decent housing and the availability of support services increased residential stability, and decreased the average number of hospital days per year and service needs.

Taken together, this body of work, albeit limited, suggests that the effects of informal or formal care – including home-based care – on a host of outcomes such as institutionalization, hospital length-of-stay, and residential stability, may depend in part on the presence or absence of an accommodating environment. For the frail elderly, for example, a spacious, flexible, or convenient setting may simply make it easier to deliver long-term care services, or may increase their quality and effectiveness. For persons with severe mental illness, access to a decent, safe and sanitary dwelling was found to be significantly associated with a decline in gaps in needed home- and community-based services, and both decent housing and supportive services were associated with beneficial outcomes.

By providing some empirical basis for the relationship between housing and neighborhood characteristics and home-based care, this research literature also provides some justification for examining how housing policies may encourage, or discourage, home-based care. But further research on such issues as whether housing or other contextual characteristics play a role in the decision to utilize home-based care services, the quality of those services, and their cost could strengthen this justification substantially. The practical importance of learning more about housing and home-based care is that if particular housing attributes are found to contribute to continued residence in community settings in part because of their effects on home-based care feasibility, quality, or costs, then it may be possible to reproduce these features for other members of the "at risk" population (Struyk and Zais 1982; Newman 1985).

Before turning to specific housing policies that are most relevant to home-based care, it is useful to first provide a broader context for this review. Therefore, the next section describes one facet of the evolution of housing policy, namely, how it has historically viewed concerns about the health of occupants.

Housing and Health: A Historical Perspective

The relationship between housing policy and health policy in the US has had a checkered history. Perhaps the strongest linkage existed in the earliest years of housing policy development in the 1920s and 1930s when the deleterious effects of substandard housing were used as a primary rationale for developing a national housing policy. Such specific programs as slum clearance, the production of public housing, and the introduction of standard building codes can all be traced to the underlying notion that housing affects health. Frequent references to "healthful living conditions," particularly for families with small children, can be found in early iterations of the National Housing Act and associated regulations. There is also some evidence of collaborative efforts in these early years between health professionals (e.g., the American Public Health Association) and housing professionals (e.g., the National Association of Housing and Redevelopment Officials). For example, at the national level, health and housing groups worked together to develop broad policy goals regarding healthful housing, while in some states and localities, inter-agency groups created mechanisms to implement these goals.

Until very recently, it would have been fair to say that this shared vision of the early years has been on the decline ever since. As in many areas of social welfare policy, after World War II housing policy entered a period of specialization, regulatory complexity and bureaucratic expansion. Undoubtedly, the most significant benefit associated with this evolution was the steady improvement in physical housing conditions over time to the point where only a nominal fraction of the housing stock is generally considered inadequate (Weicher 1980). But one clear cost was the disincentive for coordination with other agencies or policies including those pertaining to health.

There have been a few intermittent exceptions to this pattern. Perhaps the most prominent example is the investigation of the deleterious effects of lead-based paint on children's health, which led to legislation governing the use of lead-based paint in residential settings. Another example is the development of dwelling modification standards for the physically handicapped (Steinfeld 1975).

Recent shifts in the tenor of the housing policy debate, and in some features of recent housing legislation, suggest that we may now be on the threshold of a third phase of housing policy. There are two key aspects to this rethinking. The first is the need to return to "first principles" regarding the justification for government involvement in housing assistance for the poor. The focus seems to have been lost or diluted over time as emphasis on causes was replaced by emphasis on symptoms. In addition, there is increasing recognition that housing policy alone, as it has been narrowly defined in the last 40 years solely in terms of "bricks and mortar," is simply inadequate to meet the fundamental goals of most social welfare policy, namely, assisting the nation's citizens to reach their maximum potential. For various population groups – the elderly, the handicapped, and vulnerable families with children – housing policy is increasingly emphasizing the goal of independence. Few would argue that this goal can only be achieved if it is explicitly shared by the housing, health, and related sectors, and if policies in these different arenas are consistent. Both of these new directions will also require closer coordination between housing interests and other spheres including, prominently, the health sector.

Housing Policies and Home-Based Care

Housing policy can influence home-based care in at least three ways: (a) through the design of *financing mechanisms* for housing subsidy programs that discourage, tolerate or support the provision of home-based assistance; (b) through *regulations* and *statutes* that either encourage or discourage home-based care; and (c) through statutory and regulatory provisions, as well as informal mores, that facilitate or obstruct the *coordination* of housing policy and programs with those in the health-care arena.

Financing

Housing subsidy programs are directed mainly at rental housing. There are more than four million rental housing units in the nation that are part of the federally assisted or subsidized housing inventory. Assistance takes one of two forms: supply-side (or "project-based") subsidies, which underwrite housing development, and in some cases operating, costs; and demand-side (or "tenant-based") subsidies, which provide assistance to the tenant recipient in the form of a rent write-down. Each of these two generic types of assistance has taken numerous forms over the roughly 60-year history of assisted-housing policy. All of these designs focused solely on financing physical structures or rental payments; supporting home-based care was never a consideration. Throughout all of these variations, however, there is little to suggest that the inherent design of any of these housing subsidy financing schemes has either encouraged or discouraged home-based care. Their effects appear to be neutral.

One general feature of current domestic policy fragmentation has proved to be problematic to housing providers attempting to serve tenants with needs for both housing and supportive services, however. Essentially all housing subsidy programs – be they for supply or demand – represent multiyear commitments of federal revenues. Development subsidies typically commit a stream of funding over 20, 30 or even 40 years, while tenant subsidies have generally been for 15 years, recently reduced to five years but with the possibility of renewal. But in almost all cases, home- and community-based services are funded annually, introducing the element of risk of losing funding – a risk that does not exist with federally guaranteed, multiyear housing subsidies. This inconsistency in funding terms has discouraged developers with an interest in providing housing for individuals needing supportive services from acting on that interest.

Perhaps surprisingly for some, there are a number of ways in which the financing of assisted housing actually encourages home- and community-based care. As noted earlier, federal housing policy has begun to recognize the legitimacy of broadening its scope beyond traditional housing boundaries. Although the Department of Housing and Urban Development (HUD) is a housing, not a service agency, a growing body of convincing evidence indicates that the ability of some individuals to maintain – and retain – housing is closely connected to, and in some cases determined by, availability of appropriate services. This has led to the somewhat ironic conclusion that a key *housing* policy issue is ensuring that the service needs of residents are being met (Newman 1992). This evolution in the definition and boundaries of housing policy is reflected in various features of a number of housing programs, including their financial structure, a topic that is reviewed in the next section. Because the connection between housing policy and home-based care is embodied in programs designed for two population groups – the frail elderly, and disabled persons, some proportion of whom are homeless – this review treats separately the programs that address each of these groups. Key features of each program are summarized in Appendix Table A.

1. The Frail Elderly

Supply-side programs. Four supply programs that serve the frail elderly have funding mechanisms designed in part to facilitate service access and utilization. Section 202 subsidized developments are required to be designed to enable the provision of services. To meet this requirement, properties must be barrier free and developers are able to use a portion of their subsidy to provide common rooms, such as dining areas for congregate meals, recreation rooms, and offices. Under recent legislation, a predetermined proportion of the subsidies received from HUD can now also be used to cover the cost of a service coordinator whose primary role is to link the frail elderly tenant to needed supportive services that are available in the community. A similar service-coordinator funding provision has also been extended to other housing programs, including public housing and other supply-side programs that have served the frail elderly. The fourth program represents the most significant acknowledgment of the frail elderly's need for supportive housing, though this acknowledgment is stronger in concept than in numbers of persons assisted. Prior to 1990 legislation, the only housing program for the elderly that allowed – and in fact required – the provision of supportive services was the federal Congregate Housing Services Program (CHSP) administered by HUD in urban areas, and the Farmers Home Administration (FmHA) in rural areas. The distinguishing feature of CHSP is that funding for *both* housing and support services comes from HUD or FmHA. However, CHSP is a very small program that has operated in only about 60 public housing and Section 202 projects, with about 1800 persons receiving housing and support services annually. HUD and FmHA recently announced awards to 45 new sites – the first new awards in over a decade.

The nature of HUD financing under the Section 8 New Construction (NC) and Substantial Rehabilitation (SR) programs suggests that many developments are likely to have sufficient excess income to afford some level of expenditure on services above and beyond any increased funding they may receive from HUD or other sources. This excess income is a direct result of the way in which the subsidy they received from HUD was structured. As a result of the application of an annual adjustment factor (AAF) designed to account for inflation in costs over time, surplus cash accumulates in the project over time.

A major reason for the growth in surplus cash is that the AAF is applied to both the variable costs of operating expenses (utilities, insurance, and the like) and the stable costs of debt service. This issue is one, among many, now being examined by HUD and Congressional committees. Obviously, if the AAF is redesigned so that it can only be applied to variable operating expenses, the pool of surplus cash will not grow at nearly the same rate as it has historically. Nonetheless, all developments currently in operation were developed and have functioned under the original system so that many have generated at least some level of surplus cash. Thus, if services were recognized by HUD as a legitimate operating expense, it is likely that a significant number of developments could leverage at least some of their surplus cash to cover the cost. Because the relevant regulation currently states that HUD must approve the uses of surplus cash, this recognition would not require a change in HUD regulations, but would require that HUD approve supportive services as an operating cost. (One component of the Robert Wood Johnson Foundation's Support Services in Senior Housing demonstration program has been testing the use of surplus cash to cover service costs, as described later.)

In the event that surplus cash is not available, an alternative method that could be pursued to fund supportive services is a liberalization of the "special rent adjustment" (SRA) provision in the Section 8 law. Currently, SRAs are limited to increased costs for security, insurance, real estate taxes, and utilities that exceed the growth accounted for by the AAF. Congress could expand these categories to include supportive services. It is important to emphasize that the SRA does *not* affect the amount of rent paid by the elderly tenant. This remains at 30 percent of the household's adjusted income.

If HUD gave approval to all private developments such as Section 8 NC and SR to use operating reserves for supportive services, a rough estimate of the number of elderly households who would be affected is more than 600,000 (based on US Department of Housing and Urban Development 1993, and Casey 1992).

Demand-side programs. In contrast to the long history of, and high participation rates in, supply-side supportive housing sponsored by HUD, accommodating the frail elderly in demand-side programs (Section 8 certificates and vouchers) is only now being explored. As of 1989, the latest year for which data are available, roughly 240,000 elderly-headed households were participating in the certificate and voucher programs, representing 22.5 percent of all participants. A recent analysis suggests that the elderly who use these forms of tenant-based assistance experience a lower incidence of physical housing deficiencies and affordability problems compared to similar elderly not receiving housing assistance, though there is no difference in the quality of their neighborhoods, in general, or crime, in particular (Newman and Schnare 1993).

Programs such as Section 8 certificates and vouchers underwrite a portion of the household's rent in the private market. Because the certificate or voucher does not have to be used in a particular housing development such as an apartment building occupied exclusively by the elderly, the economies of scale that make it feasible to hire a service coordinator or in-home care staff in congregate housing for the elderly do not exist. The alternative mechanism currently being tested in a HUD demonstration program is to provide the tenant with an "enriched" voucher that can be used for both rental and services costs (including the costs of a case manager who can assemble appropriate services for the client). While HUD will continue to fund 100 percent of the rental subsidy, the cost of the supportive services will be divided among HUD (40 percent), the local public housing authorities (PHAs) that administer federal housing programs (50 percent), and the service recipients (10 percent). A key question HUD and Congress hope to answer is how the matching funds required of elderly recipients affect the sustainability of the program.

Home Equity Conversion Schemes. Beyond supply-side and demand-side policies aimed at assisting low-income renters, housing legislation passed in the last decade that is directed to elderly *homeowners* is also relevant to the housing–long-term care nexus. The focus of these legislative provisions is the homeowner who wishes to remain in place but is experiencing cash flow problems. Under Home Equity Conversion Mortgage instruments (HECMs), (e.g., lines of credit, lump sum payments, reverse annuity mortgages), the elderly homeowner can continue to live in the house while drawing down on accumulated equity. Thus, HECMs allow elderly homeowners to generate cash income from their housing while retaining occupancy, and do not require repayment until some future date. Legislation passed in 1982 helped make HECMs more widely available. In 1989, HUD launched the Equity Conversion Mortgage Insurance Demonstration Program to determine the need and demand among the elderly for this housing-finance instrument and to test the effects of providing FHA insurance for HECMs on participation by both the elderly and financial institutions in the mortgage markets. This demonstration program ended in September 1995. Congress reauthorized the program in 1996 to allow conversion of up to 50,000 mortgages.

From their inception, HECM strategies have attracted attention at least partly because of their significance for concerns about the long-term care needs of the elderly (Jacobs 1985; Jacobs and Weissert 1984). For many elderly households, including those who are frail and in need of assistance, the most sizable source of accumulated wealth is the home. Yet, this wealth is illiquid and inaccessible, leaving the homeowner house rich and cash poor. HECMs allow the elderly to "liquify" their housing wealth so that they can purchase what they need, including long-term care services.

In spite of this attractive feature of HECMs, the early offerings by financial institutions during the 1980s did not attract many participants. Knowledgeable observers attribute this lack of interest to four factors: (a) the inherent complexity of the structure of most HECM schemes, which make them difficult to explain to consumers; (b) an apparently strong bequest motive among the elderly; (c) supply-side constraints such as incomplete markets for resale and securitization (Chinloy and Megbolugbe 1994); and (d) perhaps most importantly, the fact that HECMs make financial sense for only a minority of the elderly – those who own their homes, whose house value is high enough to generate a good monthly income stream, and whose current income is low. Data on the number of elderly who fit into these three categories are not readily available, but the published data that are available indicate that only about 10 percent of those who own homes worth $60,000 or more have incomes below $10,000, and about 25 percent have incomes below $20,000 (Newman 1993). Anecdotal reports suggest that interest in HECMs may have increased in the last few years. However, while Congress authorized funding for up to 25,000 insured loans through 1995 under the FHA insurance demonstration, only 5,000 loans have been written since 1989. HUD reports that applications for its FHA insurance program are "slow but steady" (Krems 1993).

2. Disabled individuals and homeless individuals

Until passage of the McKinney Act in 1987, the Section 202 housing program was the major federal source of housing assistance that specifically targeted disabled individuals as a group to be served. Yet, it appears that few of the disabled have received benefits under this program. Annual counts of persons with mental illness participating in this program, for example, are exceedingly low, reaching a high of 1,741 units in 1988 (Newman 1992). An evaluation of the program's effectiveness for persons with mental illness conducted in the early 1980s emphasized three primary problems with the program that may have contributed to the low participation rates:

- the paperwork requirements were very burdensome, particularly for the small nonprofit groups who were most likely to develop housing for severely mentally ill (SMI) individuals;
- the lag time between application for program funds and occupancy of the first unit was far too long, in some cases lasting five years or more; and
- program rules did not allow the flexibility required to develop and operate a successful housing setting for SMI persons (Macrosystems 1982; Urban Systems Research and Engineering 1983).

Partly in response to these concerns, the 1990 housing legislation redesigned the program. Known as the Section 811 program, the subsidy now takes the form of a non-interest-bearing capital advance plus contracts for rental assistance. Advances need not be repaid as long as the housing remains occupied by the very low-income population of disabled individuals for whom it was

Housing Policy and Home-Based Care   197

originally intended (e.g., those with AIDS, SMI persons) for at least 40 years.

The nonrepayment feature of the financing is clearly attractive. Among other things, it may free up the nonprofit providers to devote more of their time to on-site management and assisting tenants who need help. But from the perspective of access to home- and community-based supportive services, one aspect of the program is troubling. Because the 1990 housing legislation allows the use of federal funds to cover service coordinators in Section 202 but not in Section 811, an inequity seems to have been created. It is possible that disabled individuals who continue to live in their Section 202 units would have access to the help of a service coordinator while participants in the new 811 program would not. The rationale for this distinction was the presumption that disabled individuals would rely on state-funded services to meet their needs (Harre 1993). Although developers applying for 811 funds must demonstrate that they will provide supportive services, these services must be funded separately. This separation of housing and service funding could engender the same types of problems encountered in the original Section 202 program which, in part, motivated the 1990 provision to cover service coordinators. Furthermore, from the perspective of the allocation of federal funds, the effect is unequal treatment, with those who participate in the new Section 811 program being disadvantaged relative to comparably impaired individuals in the Section 202 program.

Congress's main response to the housing plus service needs of homeless persons, including those suffering from mental illness, HIV infection, and co-occurring substance abuse, has been the Stewart B. McKinney Homeless Assistance Act, first passed in 1987 and amended in 1988 and 1990 (see Newman 1992). Subsequently, the 1992 housing act was passed, which also contains features that are relevant to homeless persons. The key provisions in both acts are: (a) the Section 8 Moderate Rehabilitation Program for Single-Room Occupancy (SRO) settings, which subsidizes the rehabilitation of SRO units and supportive services provided on site; (b) the Supportive Housing Demonstration Program (SHDP), which is a dollar-for-dollar federal/nonfederal matching-grant program that has developed 28,000 transitional and 3,000 permanent housing units as of 1992; (c) the Supportive Housing Program, which replaced SHDP in 1992 and provides matching funds for transitional, permanent and innovative housing for the homeless as well as supportive services; (d) Projects for Assistance in Transition to Homelessness (PATH), which is a formula-matching grant to the states to provide supportive services to homeless persons who are also mentally ill; and (e) the Shelter Plus Care Program, which provides HUD rental assistance that must be matched by supportive services of equivalent value and is targeted on three groups of homeless persons: the severely mentally ill, those with chronic substance-abuse problems, and those who have AIDS. (Additional information about these programs can be found in Appendix A.)

At the time of writing, the future of these, as well as other housing programs, is uncertain. According to the Clinton administration's current plan, as outlined in "A Blueprint for Reinventing HUD," homeless assistance programs would go through two phases of consolidation. Through fiscal year 1996–7, these programs would be consolidated but kept in a separate block grant to give communities time to establish a "continuum of care." In the following fiscal year, the homeless programs block grant would be combined with programs targeted on other population groups under a broader-umbrella block grant, the Affordable Housing Fund.

3. Additional observations on financing

The recent housing programs acknowledging the "more than just housing" needs of many participants, which preceded the current "reinvention" proposals, represent exceptions – albeit significant exceptions – to the typical financing structure of low-income housing. To all intents and purposes, HUD no longer provides production subsidies for the construction or substantial rehabilitation of multifamily structures (which, as noted earlier, did not consider home-based care). As a result, developers must piece together bits of financing from multiple sources that in many instances do not even include the mainstream programs just reviewed. Reliance on six or more different capital financing sources is not uncommon (Sandorf 1991). Presumably, because of the added effort required, this retail approach to capital financing may provide little leeway for also raising funds for on-site supportive services such as home-based care. Unfortunately, we can't look at past experience to judge whether generating funding for home-based services would be more likely under the kind of production-subsidy programs that existed 10 or more years ago. At that time, there was far less sensitivity to the service needs of vulnerable tenant groups and, therefore, little attention to, or documentation about, funding services in project-based subsidized housing. The one clear exception is the Section 202 program, which unarguably has succeeded in increasing the supply of service-enriched quality housing to frail and disabled low-income groups.

Housing Policy and Home-Based Care

At the more affluent end of the income spectrum, the private sector has targeted senior citizens as a market for "purpose built" projects that fall into three broad categories: independent living, assisted living, and life care. Independent-living developments are aimed at healthy, active individuals who are primarily seeking reduced home-maintenance burdens, opportunities for social interaction, and the convenience of on-site services such as meals, recreation, and housekeeping. Assisted living caters to a more frail, less independent elderly population. On-site services may range from meals and housekeeping to assistance with Activities of Daily Living and Instrumental Activities of Daily Living, such as bathing, dressing and taking medications. Life-care communities combine features of each of the first two setting types and often add a third, namely, a nursing home either located on the same campus or nearby (Newman and Scanlon 1989). While the comprehensiveness of services varies across these three settings, the financing principle is the same: residents pay for the services they receive either through the endowment payment they made upon moving in, through their monthly rental or maintenance fee, or on a fee-for-service basis. Industry experts have not yet observed any effects of long-term care insurance on these markets.

Regulations and Statutes

Housing statutes and their regulatory interpretation set the boundaries of housing policy including, importantly, the boundaries of the "allowable." The size and physical configuration of dwellings, the adequacy and condition of the housing unit and surrounding neighborhood, and the ability of individuals with varying degrees of functional impairment to reside in housing units located in the community are just some examples of the direct and indirect ways in which housing laws and regulations determine whether those in need have access to home-based care and whether its provision is feasible.

1. Housing quality standards

All housing units must comply with a mix of construction and maintenance standards, commonly called "codes," that are related to the physical condition of the building and dwelling unit. From a societal perspective, "codes represent the level of conditions which the public and their representatives consider to be economically, socially, and politically necessary, as well as acceptable and feasible at the time of their adoption" (American Public Health Association 1971). These standards, however, should not be viewed as immutable; new knowledge, demographic shifts, or changing perceptions of desirable housing conditions require that codes be subject to continuous reevaluation.

Building and other *construction codes* are enforced primarily through a system of permits, which are granted after plans and detailed specifications for the physical structure have been submitted to, and evaluated by, the relevant local government review board. These government agencies hold the power to issue, or withhold, the required permits (American Public Health Association 1971). By contrast, *housing codes* establish minimum standards essential to make dwellings safe, sanitary, and fit for human habitation by governing the physical condition of the property, its maintenance, utilities, and occupancy (American Public Health Association, 1971). Although the specific content of codes is left to the discretion of each locality, most rely on a similar set that typically covers minimum room square footage by function, natural light and air, and the state of repair of electrical, heating, and plumbing systems.

Knowledgeable observers suggest that while building and construction codes are generally well enforced, housing codes are not. In the face of major budget constraints, many cities have had to make deep cuts in services, including code enforcement. Baltimore, for example, has adopted the strategy of inspecting a portion of its multifamily housing stock each year on a rotating basis, and inspecting single-family homes on an "as need" basis only, primarily in response to complaints from occupants and neighbors. Because the modal housing structure type in Baltimore is the rowhouse, this policy means that most dwellings in the city are never inspected for code compliance. Furthermore, follow-up with property owners who have received code citations to ensure that proper repairs have been made is also viewed as inadequate (Masters Program in Policy Studies 1992). One by-product of a spotty housing-code compliance and enforcement system in many cities is its effect on home-care workers, as noted by Scharer et al. (1990): "Unsafe housing is a major problem that confronts providers of home-care services."

The federally assisted housing inventory of more than four million rental housing units is governed by a somewhat different system of housing standards and enforcement. All housing units in the assisted inventory must meet a set of housing quality standards, or HQS, which is similar in content to housing codes. The HQS covers both maintenance and structural attributes including peeling paint, malfunctioning heating, presence of rodents, and absence of complete plumbing. Within the last decade, PHAs have been given the option of substituting their local housing codes for the HUD HQS, but they are not allowed to rely on their locality's mechanism for code enforcement. Instead, every unit in the subsidized inventory must be inspected once a year by a trained HUD housing inspector. A schedule of reinspections is established for units that fail. Despite these requirements, studies conducted by the HUD Office of the Inspector General have found a substantial error rate in the application of the HQS, the most worrisome of which is what statisticians refer to as Type I errors; that is, dwelling units that are deemed physically adequate when they actually are not (*Housing and Development Reporter* 1989).

Housing codes, the HQS, and their enforcement are likely to have indirect effects on the delivery of home-based care. Several plausible scenarios of how this may occur were advanced at the outset of this chapter. Inadequate codes, or more importantly, inadequate enforcement of existing codes, may perpetuate substandard housing, thereby obstructing or preventing home-based care from being delivered. Individuals in need of home-based care services may, in turn, be denied access to these services (Scharer et al. 1990).

2. Neighborhood conditions

Unlike housing codes, which pertain to dwelling units in both the private and assisted inventory, explicit site and neighborhood standards apply to the assisted stock only and, within the assisted stock, to units receiving project-based assistance only. The main instruments for neighborhood standards in the private market are a combination of local zoning regulations and law enforcement which, by and large, fall outside the boundaries of housing policy, per se. The assisted stock is, of course, subject to these same mechanisms, but also must meet additional requirements such as the following:

- "The neighborhood must not be one which is seriously detrimental to family life or in which substandard dwellings or other undesirable elements predominate, unless there is actively in progress a concerted program to remedy the undesirable conditions";
- "The housing must be accessible to social, recreational, educational, commercial, and health facilities and services, and other municipal facilities and services that are at least equivalent to

those typically found in neighborhoods consisting largely of unassisted, standard housing of similar market rents." (Code of Federal Regulations 1990)

Both of these standards have clear applicability to the delivery of home-based care. The first, which may also fall within the jurisdiction of local zoning regulations and law enforcement, attempts to address neighborhood conditions, such as lack of safety, which can deter providers of home-based care services. According to Scharer et al. (1990), some providers have arranged for escorts from security services to accompany home-care workers visiting unsafe neighborhoods. Maintaining 24-hour, on-call services is much more difficult under these circumstances. And, as noted previously, residents living in these areas who need in-home care may be denied access to needed services. The second standard raises the issue of accessibility to health facilities and services including community-based services.

It is not possible to assess how well zoning regulations and local law enforcement promote and preserve safety in the tens of thousands of neighborhoods across the nation. This is a question best addressed by each locality. But recent research raises concerns about how well some assisted-housing programs meet their site and neighborhood standards. Newman and Schnare (1993) found that households with children living in public housing gave low ratings to the quality of their neighborhoods, and 37 percent reported crime to be a significant problem in their neighborhoods. However, residence in public housing was not significantly associated with low neighborhood ratings for other households, namely, the elderly and other nonelderly individuals without children the majority of whom are disabled; the fractions of each group reporting crime to be a problem were 10 percent and 11 percent, respectively. Because most individuals in the latter two groups reside in separate public housing developments that are explicitly targeted on the elderly and handicapped, there may be a dichotomy in the way site and neighborhood standards are applied to public housing for different household types.

3. Legislative and regulatory changes

Over the nearly 60-year history of national housing policy, legislative and regulatory changes have either facilitated, or obstructed, the linkage between housing and home-based care. Examples of the facilitation of linkage were provided in the previous section and include several new provisions enabled by the 1990 housing act, the

Housing Policy and Home-Based Care

Housing and Community Development Act of 1992, and the McKinney Act. By and large, these programs represent serious efforts to support this linkage. But examples of obstacles to linkage also exist. Perhaps the most dramatic recent case is demonstrated by the 1981 changes in regulations governing the Section 202 program.

In an effort to reduce the production levels and costs of the Section 202 program, the Reagan administration introduced a number of cost-containment requirements. These included: (a) devoting 25 percent of units in each project to efficiencies; (b) limiting unit sizes to 415 square feet for efficiencies; (c) limiting the total cost of space not attributable to dwelling use to 10 percent of total project cost; and (d) restricting amenities and design features.

An analysis of the impact of these measures concluded that they may have undermined the "ability of Section 202 projects to meet the special needs of elderly tenants," including the frail elderly who are a key target group for the program (Turner 1985). As alluded to earlier, it is hard to imagine that an efficiency unit of 415 square feet could accommodate a caregiver who may be required to stay overnight, and it may even raise logistical problems for daily home-based care visits. Limitations on common areas also raise serious concerns. Turner found that in the sample of HUD field offices she studied, these restrictions had the effect of eliminating congregate dining rooms altogether. Here, again, eliminating the option of congregate meals would appear to disadvantage the very target group of frail elderly who were the intended beneficiaries of the program. Indeed, the 1981 cost-containment regulations may have discouraged frail elderly from applying to the program in the short run, and required Section 202 residents who became frail to move out over the longer run. If that move was to a nursing home, the attempt to save money was clearly ill-conceived.

4. Residency Requirements

Historically, another way in which housing policy has indirectly affected the demand for, and utilization of, home-based care is through tenant admission and retention policies. If housing developments are able to exclude individuals with disabilities or to ask tenants to leave if they become disabled, the contours of the market for home- and community-based care will obviously be affected. One possible outcome is that more individuals in need of care will either move in with relatives or move to a setting that offers more intensive services than required. Although, as described in the next section, the Fair Housing Amendments Act and the Americans with Disabilities Act are designed to attenuate these effects, such effects have not been eliminated entirely.

Research on admission and retention policies in housing for the elderly suggests that such policies are generally ad hoc and inconsistent (Bernstein 1982). In a study of 116 HUD-subsidized housing projects for the elderly, Bernstein found that nearly equal proportions could be characterized as having policies that were "strict" and "not strict". Most developments accepted the reality of sensory changes, onset of chronic conditions, and mobility problems among many of their elderly tenants who age in place. Property owners and managers were also amenable to having these problems addressed through linkages with home- and community-based services such as home-delivered meals, housekeeping and visiting nurses. On the other hand, certain health conditions raised more problems for admission and retention partly, according to Bernstein, because these impairments are "the least amenable to help via traditional community services" (p. 312). Included here are serious emotional and mental problems, substance abuse, accident proneness, and reclusive behavior. One of the basic goals of recent fair-housing and disability-rights legislation is to take all feasible steps to accommodate individuals with a broader range of disabling conditions, including some of those just noted, in housing in the community.

5. The Fair Housing Amendments Act of 1988 and the Americans with Disabilities Act of 1990

The Fair Housing Amendments Act of 1988 (FHAA) and the Americans with Disabilities Act of 1990 (ADA) are two significant pieces of legislation for individuals with functional impairments and disabilities, including the frail elderly, and persons with mental or physical handicaps. Although the ADA addresses a far broader scope of civil rights issues beyond housing alone, the housing provisions of both the ADA and the FHAA supplement and reinforce each other (Milstein and Hitov 1993). Both are also strongly supportive of a linkage between housing and home-based care.

Until passage of these statutes, physically or mentally impaired individuals were excluded from explicit coverage by the housing discrimination provisions of the Civil Rights Act of 1968, which pertain to the sale or rental of a dwelling. As a result, landlords, owners, and management companies could use subjective and ad hoc criteria to reject applications from impaired individuals for renting or purchasing property or, in the case of rental dwellings, for renewing leases. The FHAA and ADA now prohibit such exclusion or lease termination. The only health-related basis for exclusion

Housing Policy and Home-Based Care   205

is the determination that the prospective buyers or tenants will pose a direct threat to the health and safety of others. This determination is to be based solely on the applicant's past behavior as a housing resident; landlords and sellers cannot probe into underlying medical conditions, and cannot ask different questions of a person perceived as having a disability. Thus, in the case of an elderly tenant applicant in the early stages of Alzheimer's disease, for example, landlords cannot speculate about possible future problems as a basis for denying tenancy. However, landlords are allowed to ask whether the tenant applicant qualifies for a dwelling that is only available to the handicapped. This type of inquiry is allowed because it appears to be the only way to determine whether the tenant is eligible for special government housing programs for the handicapped (Newman and Mezrich forthcoming).

A second key way in which these statutes support the linkage between housing and home-based care is by requiring owners to make reasonable modifications and accommodations that will enable a handicapped or impaired individual to live in the dwelling. Under the FHAA, "modifications" can include not only the individual's own dwelling but also common interior or exterior areas. Examples cited in the FHAA regulations include installation of grab bars in the bathroom, which may also require the installation of proper wall reinforcements, and the widening of passage doorways into, and within, the dwelling. "Accommodations" pertain mainly to adjustments in rules, policies, practices or services. Examples of accommodations include allowing a blind individual with a seeing eye dog to live in a building that doesn't allow pets, and assigning a parking space adjacent to the main entrance, to a mobility-impaired tenant in a building that does not assign parking spaces for other tenants. The ADA takes the modifications and accommodations provisions even further. In cases where undue financial and administrative burdens would exempt the owner from having to make the dwelling structurally accessible as required by the FHAA, the ADA regulations suggest additional alternatives that may achieve accessibility including assigning aides to tenants, and arranging for home visits (Milstein and Hitov 1993). Thus, the FHAA and ADA have both indirect and direct effects on home-based care. The indirect effects are connoted by provisions which enable disabled individuals to reside in housing in the community at large, thereby creating or sustaining the market for home- and community-based care. The direct effects are embodied in the ADA regulations which specifically cite home-based care as an approach to meet the needs of impaired residents.

Coordination

The feasibility of home-based care is arguably greater if housing and health policymakers, as well as those in the front lines of housing and health-service delivery, coordinate their efforts (see Pynoos 1990; Redfoot and Sloan 1991). This is particularly likely to be the case in assisted projects housing large numbers of individuals with home-based care needs. However, by and large, formal and informal signals from both the housing and health sectors have discouraged cooperation and coordination.

On a structural level, the design and funding of housing and health legislation and the implementation of housing and health programs are the responsibility of different congressional or legislative committees and governmental agencies. One observer believes that the current system compartmentalizes specific parts of underlying problems, making it almost impossible to fashion an integrated and coherent response (Walker 1990). Furthermore, local agencies vested with administrative and fiscal oversight of housing and health policy have inconsistent geographic boundaries. Health matters typically fall within the jurisdiction of single agencies within the state and local governments. While all states have a state housing agency, the primary focus of these departments has traditionally been *state* housing programs; federal housing programs are largely controlled by local public housing authorities that operate quite independently of state and local government (COSCDA and APWA 1993). Substantively, health and housing professionals and policymakers have different orientations and types of expertise. It is rare to find individuals knowledgeable in both areas, as the scarce research on housing and home-based care reviewed at the outset of this chapter demonstrates.

Funding is also a barrier to cooperation for at least three reasons. First, as noted earlier, health and housing programs differ in the time commitments of funding streams; housing programs offer multiyear commitments, while health programs represent annual appropriations. Additionally, a significant share of health programs are entitlements for all who are income eligible; housing assistance is not an entitlement. Instead, it is allocated first, to specially designated preference groups such as the homeless, and second, on a first-come first-served basis to other income-eligible households. One result of the different eligibility rules for housing and health programs is that many more income-eligible households do not receive housing assistance than do receive it. Finally, during times of fiscal austerity, all levels of government are typically less willing to launch new initiatives such as those required to foster co-ordination. Some observers have correlated the budget pressures of the last decade with the hardening of agency boundaries and a particularly vigorous effort to protect turf (COSCDA and APWA 1993). Agencies may also be prohibited by regulations from using program funding to underwrite coordination activities.

Despite these barriers, the catalyst of homelessness has resulted in a number of steps toward coordination in the last decade. Among the more important initiatives introduced during this time were: (a) a Memorandum of Understanding between HUD and HHS, which reduced bureaucratic red tape preventing staff from the two agencies from working together; (b) the federal Interagency Task Force on Homelessness, emulated by numerous task forces in many states; (c) passage of the McKinney Act, the 1990 National Affordable Housing Act, and the Housing and Community Development Act of 1992, each of which enable housing programs that *require* coordination with partners from other fields including, prominently, health and human-services experts. For example, every state must submit a Comprehensive Housing Affordability Strategy (CHAS) in order to be eligible for funding from most housing and community-development programs. Because the CHAS requires information on a broad range of topics pertaining to living conditions, poverty, and quality of life, preparing the CHAS required interagency collaboration. Another example is the Shelter Plus Care Program discussed earlier. In this competitive grant program, significantly higher points are awarded to applicants who have developed their plans in coordination with other agencies serving homeless people, and to applications that include *commitments* to provide supportive services.

Some private foundations have also been catalysts for co-ordinating programs and funding to assist the homeless. In the 1980s, for example, the Robert Wood Johnson Foundation launched two demonstration programs – the Program on Chronic Mental Illness, and the Homeless Families Program. In both cases, a Memorandum of Understanding was developed between the public housing authority and the service agencies and, with funding from HUD, Section 8 certificates were provided to individuals linked to supportive services, primarily case management.

Another population group that has generated coordination between housing and health services is the frail elderly. The Congregate Housing Services Program and the service coordinator subsidies for Section 202 and public housing for the elderly have already been discussed. Another clear example is the Supportive Services in Senior Housing demonstration program mentioned earlier that is funded by the Robert Wood Johnson Foundation. A key component of this demonstration has been for state housing finance agencies (HFA) ". . . to build and institutionalize a service responsibility within the HFA" (Feder et al. 1992). Under the demonstration, participating housing developments for the elderly have hired service coordinators using funds from the operating budgets or reserves of the individual developments and from the HFA.

Whether these initial steps toward coordination will have lasting positive impacts on recipients depends on one's interpretation. A pessimistic view would emphasize that, upon closer examination, many of the housing programs that have been initiated place less emphasis on coordination than on the housing system expanding its boundaries to also address the service needs of its clientele. From a broad policy perspective, having the housing system take on the added responsibility of the supportive-service system does little to improve efficiency. But the newness of recognizing a broader set of needs and of attempts to meet them suggest a wholly different and more optimistic interpretation. Just as the needs to be met by the health system and housing system have changed over time, so, too, must the strategies to respond to these needs. Both systems are at an early stage of exploring and testing strategies. Informal arrangements constitute one possible approach; another is to broaden the mission of each system and attempt to build more formal bridges between them. As a first step, for example, the housing and health systems need to become better acquainted with each other and more aware of the ways in which the interrelationship between health and housing can affect their clientele. One way to accomplish these objectives is through statewide or local task forces that include members of both systems who are developing strategies to address a shared problem such as homelessness or the lack of sufficient, affordable, service-enriched housing. Such strategies have the advantage of providing each system with a much better understanding of the other's mission and expertise. Whether the ultimate outcome will be true coordination and cooperation only time will tell.

Conclusions

A key message in the foregoing review is that, particularly over the past five years, housing policy in the US has taken a number of significant steps toward accommodating the special needs of some population groups, including the need for home-based assistance. Some prominent examples include the Shelter Plus Care Program, which requires sponsors to match the housing subsidies they receive from HUD with services of equal value; the Section 202 program for the elderly, and public housing for the elderly, which allow use of a portion of HUD funding to hire a service coordinator; and the combination of the Fair Housing Amendments Act and the Americans with Disabilities Act, which require that landlords make reasonable modifications and accommodations so that persons with disabilities may live in housing units in the community. Taken together, this body of policy suggests a broadened definition of the fundamental goals of housing policy as stated in the 1949 housing act: "a decent home and suitable living environment."

Most of these programs are now in flux. The Clinton administration has proposed to consolidate most of the major housing programs into three block grants. A number of programs for the elderly, the disabled, the homeless, and the general population of income-eligible households would be folded into a single Affordable Housing Fund. Because the proposal does not place priority on assisting particular target groups, some observers believe that localities may be inclined to use the funds for "historically favored" populations such as the elderly and the working poor at the expense of the homeless, persons with disabilities, and welfare recipients (*Housing and Development Reporter* 1994).

Yet, even before the Administration proposed to radically alter HUD housing-assistance programs, some questioned whether the strides that had been made at HUD set a trend for the future or were an idiosyncratic blip. In his review of the 1990 housing act, Pynoos (1992) described the alignment of research, policy, and politics which allowed the act to pass as "akin to a total eclipse of the sun." Furthermore, the fact that housing programs are not entitlements means that most of the initiatives reviewed will affect only a small fraction of those in need. Thus, a major challenge for future policies is closing the many gaps that remain. Among the most important gaps are those pertaining to the physical adequacy and safety of housing units and neighborhoods. Focusing on these two fundamental objectives has the dual advantage of affecting the greatest number of households while not relying solely on the vagaries of Congressional actions regarding HUD programs.

While virtually all communities across the nation have adopted a set of local housing codes that are designed to assure the adequacy and safety of dwelling units in each jurisdiction, the existence of these codes is of little consequence if they are not vigorously and comprehensively enforced. To the extent that the main deterrent to enforcement is lack of resources, the solution is straightforward though, in times of fiscal restraint, politically unpopular. One approach is to increase the amount of money each community receives under the Community Development Block Grant with the hope that these resources would be spent on code enforcement. Some communities, however, may require additional encouragement to target resources in this way. In these instances, a special code-enforcement program may be required, similar to the concentrated code-enforcement programs that existed in the early 1970s.

Although communities also have local law-enforcement systems in place to address the most troubling neighborhood problem – safety – experience to date suggests that the nature and extent of the problem makes it very difficult to deal with in many localities. Here, too, insufficient resources are likely to play a role and are a prime target of President Clinton's proposed Anti-Crime Bill, which would support 50,000 additional police officers around the country. But an even more fundamental problem is uncertainty regarding the most effective strategies for preventing neighborhood crime. A number of approaches are being tried such as voluntary neighborhood watch teams and the reintroduction of community policing and neighborhood beat patrols. Incentives for continuous experimentation with multiple approaches are warranted.

Another important gap is not in policies or programs but in knowledge. Little systematic research has been done on the relationship between housing and neighborhood conditions, and home-based care. As a result, we lack objective information about specific environmental features that affect home-based care access, delivery, quality, and cost. It is unfortunate that past evaluations of home-based care initiatives, including numerous demonstrations conducted in the 1970s as well as the major Channeling demonstration, did not address housing issues. Any future demonstrations should not repeat this mistake. The idea of adding a housing supplement to ongoing data collections relevant to health and long-term care, such as the National Health Interview Survey and the National Long-Term Care Survey, should also be explored (Newman forthcoming). And ongoing programs may be ripe for careful evaluations of the role of housing. Beyond offering a better understanding of the role of housing in home-based care, such studies can provide hard evidence on what works, for whom, and under what circumstances – precisely the type of information that is now lacking for informed policy decisions.

The value of solid research notwithstanding, Redfoot and Sloan point out in their legislative history of the Congregate Housing Services Program that research and logic may ultimately have little to do with the successful passage of a program because of "powerful jurisdictional and institutional barriers" (Redfoot and Sloan 1991). This brings us to the final gap – the lack of a well-developed, formal system that fosters ongoing coordination between the housing and health policy and practice arenas. Here, again, a number of strides have recently been made to forge connections between these systems. What is now needed is an overarching policy framework that ties the two systems together, where appropriate, to ensure that *both* the housing and home-based care needs of the individual are being met. There are various approaches to achieving this coordinated system. A radical approach would be to build a new integrated system essentially from the ground up. A more modest, and realistic, approach would be to reshape the existing collection of programs into a more coherent and effective system. The core objective of this reshaping would be to remove the legal and institutional barriers that have kept the two systems apart.

While a detailed analysis of alternative models of coordination is beyond the scope of this chapter, recent work on the human-resource investment system (e.g., job training, welfare-to-work) suggest several strategies (e.g., Employment and Training Administration 1991; National Governors' Association 1993). Among "top down" strategies that are either encouraged or imposed by the federal or state government are: (a) requiring each state to create an integrated plan that establishes goals, objective, and outcome expectations for each of the programs in the coordinated system; (b) ensuring that innovators will not be worse off for attempting to coordinate; (c) increasing flexibility in using funds to coordinate; (d) developing and requiring all programs to use uniform terms and definitions; and (e) standardizing the fiscal and administrative procedures across programs. "Bottom up" strategies that are locally developed include: (a) special boards to oversee all relevant programs at the local level and to approve or disapprove local plans for federal and state funds (similar to the CHAS for housing and community development subsidies); (b) "one stop shopping," where individuals in need of either housing assistance, home-based care assistance, or some combination of the two would face a single point of entry, eligibility determination, assessment, referral, and perhaps service delivery; (c) integrated management-information systems; and (d) co-location of staff from the different systems in the same building.

The informal efforts to coordinate the housing and health systems that have occurred in a number of communities, even in an environment where neither system has encouraged it, have required two characteristics – flexibility and a willingness to change – on the part of each system. It is perhaps these same characteristics that will ultimately determine the success of efforts to formalize coordination and ensure its continuity.

Note

This chapter was originally prepared for the Visiting Nurse Service of New York and Milbank Memorial Fund project, "Home-based Care for a New Century." The author gratefully acknowledges the helpful assistance of Eugene Fogel, David Harre, Pauline Magette, and Jean Whaley at the US Department of Housing and Urban Development, Burt Barnow, Anne Hendrick, and Sally Katz at Johns Hopkins, Jack Kerry of The Kerry Company, and the anonymous reviewers. A slightly different version of this chapter is published in *The Milbank Quarterly*, Vol. 73, No. 3, 1995.

References

American Public Health Association. 1971. *Housing: Basic Health Principles and Recommended Ordinance*. Washington, D.C.

Berkeley Planning Associates. 1985. *Evaluation of Coordinated Community-Oriented Long-Term Care Demonstration Projects: Final Report*. Berkeley, CA.

Bernstein, J. 1982. Who Leaves – Who Stays: Residency Policy in Housing for the Elderly. *The Gerontologist* 22(3): 305–13.

Casey, C. 1992. *Characteristics of HUD-Assisted Renters and Their Units in 1989*. Washington, D.C.: US Department of Housing and Urban Development, Office of Policy Development and Research.

Chinloy, P., and I. Megbolugbe. 1994. Reverse Mortgages: Contracting and Crossover Risk. *AREUEA Journal* 22(2): 367–86.

Code of Federal Regulations. 1990. 24 CFR Ch. VIII, Sections 880.206, 885.730.

COSCDA (Council of State Community Development Agencies) and APWA (American Public Welfare Association). 1993. *Excerpts from Interim Final Report to the Ford Foundation on Implementing Housing and Human Service Collaboration*. Washington, D.C.

Employment and Training Administration. 1991. *An Assessment of the JTPA Role in State and Local Coordination Activities*. Washington, D.C.: US Department of Labor.

Eustis, et al. 1993. Home Care Quality and the Home Care Worker: Beyond

Quality Assurance as Usual. *The Gerontologist.*
Feder, J., et al. 1992. Supportive Services in Senior Housing: Preliminary Evidence on Feasibility and Impact. *Generations* Spring: 61–2.
Harre, D. 1993.Personal communication, Office of Elderly Housing, HUD, August 4.
Housing and Development Reporter. 1994. Tenants would Fare Poorly under Block Grants, NHLP Says. 22(36): 552–3.
Housing and Development Reporter. 1989. Problems in Single Family, Voucher, Other Programs Noted in OIG Report. 17(6): 114.
Jacobs, B. 1985. A Note on Recent Analyses of the Potential for Using Home Equity to Help Finance Long-Term Care for the Elderly. Rochester, NY: University of Rochester Public Policy Analysis Program, Discussion Paper No. 8503.
Jacobs, B. and W. Weissert. 1984. Home Equity Financing of Long-Term Care for the Elderly. Rochester, NY: University of Rochester Public Policy Analysis Program, Discussion Paper No. 8401.
Krems, S. 1993. Personal communication, Office of Single-Family Housing, HUD, August 6.
Macrosystems, Inc. 1982. *Exploratory Evaluation of the HUD–HHS Demonstration Program for Deinstitutionalization of the Chronically Mentally Ill: Final Report.* Washington, D.C.
Masters Program in Policy Studies. 1992. Housing Problems Facing Baltimore. Baltimore, MD: Johns Hopkins University Institute for Policy Studies.
Mathematica Policy Research, Inc. 1987. *The Evaluation of the National Long-Term Care Demonstration: Final Report.* Princeton, NJ.
Milstein, B., and S. Hitov. 1993. Housing and the ADA. In *Implementing the Americans with Disabilities Act: Rights and Responsibilities of All Americans,* ed. L. Gostin and H. Beyers, 137–53. Baltimore, MD: Paul H. Brookes Publishing Co.
Mindel, C., et al. 1986. Informal and Formal Social Support Systems of Black and White Rural Elderly: A Comparative Cost Approach. *The Gerontologist* 26(3): 279–85.
National Governors' Association. 1993. *Bringing Down the Barriers.* Washington, D.C.: National Governors' Association.
Newman, S. 1985. Housing and Long-Term Care: The Suitability of the Elderly's Housing to the Provision of In-Home Services. *The Gerontologist* 25(1): 35–40.
Newman, S. 1992. *The Severely Mentally Ill Homeless: Housing Needs and Housing Policy.* Baltimore, MD: Johns Hopkins University Institute for Policy Studies, Occasional Paper No. 12.
Newman, S. 1993. Comment on 'Long-Term Care Reform and the Role of Housing Finance'. *Housing Policy Debate* 4(4): 551–64.
Newman, S. Forthcoming. The Effects of Supports on Sustaining Older Disabled Persons in the Community. Washington, D.C.: American Association of Retired Persons, Public Policy Institute. Issue Brief.

Newman, S., and M. Mezrich. Forthcoming. Implications of the 1988 Fair Housing Act for the Frail Elderly. *Staying Put: Adapting the Places Instead of the People*, ed. S. Lansperry and J. Hyde. Amityville, NY: Baywood Publishing Co.

Newman, S., and W. Scanlon. 1989. Delivery of Long-Term Care Services: New Developments in Nursing Homes and Housing. Paper prepared for UCLA–FHP Foundation meeting, "The Economics and Politics of Long-Term Care," Irvine, CA, October 11–13, 1989.

Newman, S., and A. Schnare. 1993. Last in Line: Housing Assistance for Households with Children. *Housing Policy Debate*, 4(3): 417–55.

Newman, S., et al. 1994. The Effects of Independent Living on Persons with Chronic Mental Illnesses: an Assessment of the Section 8 Certificate Program Component of the Program on Chronic Mental Illness. *Milbank Quarterly* 72(1): 171–98.

Newman, S., et al. 1990. Overwhelming Odds: Caregiving and the Risk of Institutionalization. *Journal of Gerontology* 45(5): S173–83.

Noelker, L. 1982. The Impact of Environmental Problems on Caring for Impaired Elders in a Home Setting. Paper presented at the 35th Annual Gerontological Society Meetings, November.

Noelker, L., and D. Bass. 1989. Home Care for Elderly Persons: Linkage between Formal and Informal Caregivers. *Journal of Gerontology* 44(2): S63–70.

Pynoos, J. 1992. Linking Federally Assisted Housing with Services for Frail Older Persons. *Journal of Aging and Social Policy* 4:157–77.

Pynoos, J. 1990. Public Policy and Aging in Place: Identifying the Problems and Potential Solutions. In *Aging in Place: Supporting the Frail Elderly in Residential Environments*, ed. D. Tilson, 167–208. Glenview, IL: Scott, Foresman.

Pynoos, J., et al. 1987. Home Modifications: Improvements that Extend Independence. In *Housing the Aged: Design Directives and Policy Considerations*, ed. V. Regnier and J. Pynoos, 277–304. New York: Elsevier.

Redfoot, D., and K. Sloan. 1991. Realities of Political Decision-Making on Congregate Housing. In *Congregate Housing for the Elderly: Theoretical, Policy, and Programmatic Perspectives*, ed. L. Kaye and A. Monk, 99–110. New York: The Haworth Press.

Sandorf, J. 1991. Supported Housing Alternatives Project: Final Report and Program Recommendations. New York.

Sangl, G. 1983. The Family Support System of the Elderly. In *Long-Term Care*, ed. R. Voegel and H. Palmer, 306–7. Washington, D.C.: HCFA.

Scharer, L., et al. 1990. Lack of Housing and its Impact on Human Health: A Service Perspective. *Bulletin of the New York Academy of Medicine* 66(5): 515–25.

Steinfeld, E. 1975. *Barrier-Free Design for the Elderly and the Disabled*. Syracuse, NY: Syracuse University.

Struyk, R., and H. Katsura. 1988. *Aging at Home: How the Elderly Adjust Their*

Housing Consumption without Moving. New York: The Haworth Press.
Struyk, R., and J.P. Zais. 1982. *Providing Special Dwelling Features for the Elderly with Health and Mobility Problems.* Washington, D.C.: The Urban Institute.
Sussman, M. 1979. *Social and Economic Supports and Family Environments for the Elderly.* AOA Grant Report No. 90-A-316(03), January.
Tennstedt, S., and J. McKinlay. 1987. Frail Older People Reliant on Formal Services: Comparison With Those Receiving Informal Care. Presented at the 40th Annual Meeting of the Gerontological Society of America, Washington, D.C., November.
Thomas, S. 1983. The Significance of Housing as a Resource. In *Long-Term Care*, ed. R. Voegel and H. Palmer, 391–414. Washington, D.C.: HCFA.
Turner, M. 1985. Building Housing for the Low-Income Elderly: Cost Containment in the Section 202 Program. *The Gerontologist* 25(3): 271–7.
US Department of Housing and Urban Development 1993. *HUD 1994 Budget: Summary Document.* Washington, D.C.
Urban Systems Research and Engineering. 1983. *Standards and Criteria for Housing for the CMI in the Section 202/8 Direct Loan Program. Final Report.* Cambridge, MA.
Walker, B. 1990. Housing and Health. *Bulletin of the New York Academy of Medicine* 66(5): 382–90.
Wan, T. 1987. Functionally Disabled Elderly: Health Status, Social Support, and Use of Health Services. *Research on Aging* 9(1): 61–79.
Weicher, J. 1980. *Housing: Federal Policies and Programs.* Washington, D.C.: American Enterprise Institute, Studies in Economic Policy.
Whaley, J. 1993. Personal communication. Office of Special Needs Assistance, HUD, August 4.

Appendix: Table A Key Features of Housing Policies and Programs Relevant to Home- and Community-Based Care

Program	Target Group(s)	Key Features	Estimated Number of Participants	Status
1. Section 202 Program for the Elderly (and Handicapped)	• Persons 62 years of age or older • Persons with mental or physical handicaps eligible until 1990 passage of Section 811 (see below)	• Subsidy for property development and operating costs • Barrier-free design • Provision of common rooms • Use of 15% of subsidy for service coordinator	286,172 units as of 1991	Ongoing
2. Congregate Housing Services Program	• Frail persons 62 years of age or older	• Subsidy for tenant rents and on-site services	@ 1,800	Ongoing
3. Public Housing	• Families • Persons 62 years or older • Single disabled persons	• Government underwrites full construction costs • Formula-driven subsidy for operating costs • Subsidized rents	@ 517,000 elderly and handicapped @ 843,000 families	Essentially no new public housing development but subsidies ongoing to existing properties
4. Section 8 New Construction; Section 8 Substantial Rehabilitation; Section 236; Section 221(d)3	• Families • Persons 62 years of age or older • Single disabled persons	• Deep subsidies for property development that have the effect of lowering rents	@ 660,000	Program discontinued but subsidies ongoing for length of contract
5. Section 8 Certificates and Vouchers	• Families • Persons 62 years of age or older • Single disabled persons	• Rental subsidy that limits tenant rent to 30% of income • Dwelling must meet housing quality standards • Subsidy amount limited by fair market rent ceiling • Units rented from private market	@ 243,800 elderly and handicapped @ 816,200 families	Ongoing; certificates and vouchers combined into one program
6. HOPE for Elderly Independence	• Frail persons 62 years of age or older	• Subsidy for both rent and services • Rental subsidy similar to Section 8 certificates and vouchers	@ 1,447	5-year demonstration program (1993–1998)

Program	Target Group(s)	Key Features	Estimated Number of Participants	Status
7. Reverse Annuity Mortgages	• Homeowners 62 years of age or older	• Allows homeowners to cash out the value of their house while retaining occupancy • FHA Insurance	@ 5,000 (FHA Insurance Program)	Ongoing
8. Section 811 Housing for Persons with Disabilities Program	• Persons < 62 years old with mental or physical disabilities	• Subsidy for property development and operating costs	@ 4,000 as of 1992	Ongoing
9. Section 8 Moderate Rehabilitation Program for SROs	• Homeless persons	• Subsidy for rehabilitation of property, tenant rents and supportive services	@ 7,900 as of 1992	Ongoing
10. Supportive Housing Demonstration Program	• Homeless persons	• Transitional housing with limit of 24 months on length of stay • Permanent housing • Nonfederal match required	• @ 28,500 as of 1992 • @ 3,300 as of 1992	Program discontinued but subsidies ongoing for length of subsidy term
11. Supportive Housing Program	• Homeless persons	• Transitional housing • Permanent housing • Innovative housing • Supportive services	Awards not made yet	Ongoing
12. Projects for Assistance in Transition from Homeless Program (PATH)	• Persons who are homeless and severely mentally ill • Substance abusers eligible	• Formula matching grant to states • Subsidies for supportive services and housing services	All states; no estimate available on persons served	Ongoing
13. Shelter Plus Care	• Persons who are homeless and mentally ill, substance abusers, and those who have AIDS	• Tenant-based assistance like Section 8 certificate or voucher • Sponsor-based assistance which reduces tenant units • SRO moderate rehabilitation subsidy which reduces tenant rents • Project-based rental assistance which reduces tenant rents	@ 2,300 as of 1992	Ongoing

Program	Target Group(s)	Key Features	Estimated Number of Participants	Status
14. Housing Quality Standards	• Building, construction and housing codes apply to full housing stock • HUD housing quality standards apply to assisted stock	State of repair of electrical, heating, and plumbing systems, and interior and exterior of dwelling	NA	Ongoing
15. Site and Neighborhood Standards	• Zoning regulations and local law enforcement apply to most neighborhoods • HUD standards apply to supply-side subsidized stock	• Regulates land use mix, noxious uses, safety • Avoidance of areas with concentrated poverty; promotes accessibility to services and resources	NA	Ongoing
16. Fair Housing Amendments Act of 1988; Americans with Disabilities Act of 1990	• All residents including those with functional impairments and disabilities	• Real estate transactions cannot inquire about health status • Landlords required to make reasonable modifications and accommodations to enable residency by disabled persons	NA	Ongoing

Notes:
[a] All target groups must meet income-eligibility guidelines. The current criticism is an income ≤ 50% of area median income.
[b] Number of elderly and handicapped participants follows Casey's (1992) estimate of 35% of households in assisted housing falling into these groups.
NA = not applicable.

Sources: Casey (1992); Interviews with D. Harre (Office of Elderly Housing); S. Krems (Office of Single Family Housing); S. Meisel (Office of Elderly Housing); J. Whaley (Office of Special Needs Assistance) of the US Department of Housing and Urban Development; J. Dawkins (Office of Demonstration Programs) of the US Center for Mental Health Services.

10

Care at Home for Children with Chronic Illness: Program and Policy Implications
James M. Perrin, Ute Thyen, and Sheila Bloom

Background

Child health care has experienced a considerable shift of interest during the past two decades. Following major advances in treating acute health conditions and a broad decline in most childhood infectious illnesses, the relatively smaller number of children with chronic disease have drawn more attention. Many of these conditions would have led to death in childhood a generation ago. With advances in medical care, however, almost all children, even with physiologically severe illnesses, now survive to young adulthood or beyond (Gortmaker and Sappenfield 1984). Many surviving children and adolescents face secondary consequences of their health condition, disabilities interfering with mobility, educational attainment, self care, or other functions. Furthermore, children and adolescents with chronic health conditions face greater risks of significant behavioral and psychological problems than do children without apparent illness (Cadman et al. 1987). Much of this secondary disability can be prevented or ameliorated through effective comprehensive programs, and the majority of young people with chronic illnesses and disability can become functioning members of society, holding jobs and participating in community and family life. Program and policy goals have shifted from combatting mortality to maximizing the functioning of young people with chronic illnesses.

Many individually rare diseases affect children, with at least 2–4 percent of children having moderate to severe chronic physical conditions (Newacheck and Taylor 1992). Thus, more than a million children in the United States have severe chronic illnesses that may significantly change their daily activities, their school performance, or their psychosocial functioning as they develop (Hobbs, Perrin, and Ireys 1985). Although children assisted in a major way by technologies (such as respirators or special feeding equipment) have been the focus of most public discussion of home care for children, the spectrum of conditions covers a continuum of children from the relatively small number with major technology assistance (less than 100,000 nationwide) (US Congress 1987) to the much larger number with relatively less severe chronic conditions, such as hemophilia, severe asthma, diabetes, and arthritis.

Many individual diseases are so rare that the child will be a single case in the community. At times, the diagnosis is difficult to establish and definitive knowledge about the prognosis for the individual child is lacking. Treatment cures few of these conditions, although most children and adolescents survive to adulthood. Technologies are used to replace or assist one or more bodily functions. Oxygen supplementation, tracheostomy, or mechanical ventilation aid breathing; dialysis replaces kidney function; intravenous or tube feeding maintains proper nutrition; intravenous medication or chemotherapy fight infections or malignancy or replace deficient proteins (e.g., immunoglobulins or clotting factor). Initially developed and administered in hospitals, mainly large tertiary-care centers, these technologies previously required children with severe chronic disease to have prolonged or frequent hospitalizations. These hospital stays markedly limited participation in normal family, school, or community activities. Technological advances have allowed the transfer of care for children assisted by technology from hospitals back to families and communities and have resulted in improved survival of these children (Pope and Tarlov 1991; Perrin, Shayne, and Bloom 1993).

Other conditions, requiring less complex assistive technologies, have also depended much less on inpatient care as a result of improved and more available medical care. Although rates of asthma have increased in the past decade (Weitzman et al. 1992), improved treatments allow the large majority of children with asthma to receive almost all care in home or community settings. home care for children with hemophilia, using replacement clotting factors administered at home, has markedly decreased the need for hospital care (Smith and Levine 1984). Increasing use of home and community care has greatly changed the roles of households in caring for children with complex long-term conditions; the activities and responsibilities of hospitals, home-care agencies, and other health providers; and the response of communities to young people with health disabilities.

Five additional key factors have supported the growth in home and community care for children with chronic illnesses. First, growing consumerism in health care, along with increasing family involvement and commitment to care for their children at home with appropriate community support, has led to much pressure to have children with long-term illnesses cared for at home. This change partly reflects greater interest among many families in maintaining responsibility for the care of their own members. It also reflects a changing view of disability, as codified in the Americans with Disabilities Act, civil rights legislation that strongly supports the integration of people with disabilities into community life (West 1991).

The second consideration supporting the transfer from hospital to home and community care has been the increasing awareness on the part of pediatricians, child psychologists, and other child-care specialists of the negative impact of long-term hospitalization on the psychosocial development of children, along with convincing evidence of improved prognosis for these children when cared for in a family and community environment. Long-term hospitalization prevents many opportunities for socialization of children and for learning that follows from exploration of the environment. Even short-term hospitalizations, if frequent enough, can interfere with many childhood activities and diminish interactions with other children.

A third key factor has been the great increase in costs for long-term hospital care, coupled with evidence of the cost effectiveness of using home and community care in many circumstances. Thus, many public and private insurers have developed programs that encourage use of home and community care rather than hospital care for many of their more expensive clients. From the point of view of parents, however, this phenomenon, while supported enthusiastically, has been a mixed blessing. On the one hand, it allows them to care for their child at home rather than in hospital;

on the other hand, many of the costs previously paid for at hospitals are now shifted to the family, increasing their financial burdens.

Fourth, child health providers, especially pediatricians, have developed increasing capability and interest in caring for children with special needs in home and community settings (Green 1983). Several states have developed regionalized programs of care for children with special health-care needs that encourage them to receive more care at the community level and that help their community physician provide much ongoing medical care. In Iowa, for example, the care of children with malignancies was decentralized from the university medical center to the community through a shared management program, with resulting decreased cost, increased patient satisfaction, and increased participation of the child in school and community life (Kisker et al. 1980).

Finally, as a practical matter, medically complex children who no longer need the acute care available at a hospital have no choice but to go home. For these children, there are few skilled care facilities or other institutions that are staffed to provide the level of care that they need. Moreover, the few institutions that do exist are regionalized and not necessarily located near families. Few parents will authorize an institutional placement that will effectively separate them, physically and emotionally, from their children.

Meeting the Needs of Families

Families now provide care at home for most childhood chronic conditions, relying on hospitals only for acute, life-threatening complications of the disease or for review by specialists. Providing that care typically requires a broad array of multidisciplinary services that may vary substantially according to the health condition and needs of the children and their families. Most families require services well beyond traditional medical and nursing care.

Replacing hospital care with home care offers advantages to families, hospitals, and insurers. Children and families are reunited in the caring environment of the home. Hospitals can reduce financial losses incurred when providing lengthy, costly care to children with complex health disorders whose care is inadequately financed. Insurers save money because they usually pay less for home care than hospital care. Nonetheless, home care may not provide overall savings. High quality home care is very expensive, and much expense is borne by families who give up jobs or reduce work hours to care for their children and then provide that care without compensation. Hospital costs may decrease, but reductions are achieved by shifting much of the burden of expense from the hospital to the family.

Hospitals routinely provide many specialized services. When these services (and their costs) are transferred to households and communities, families face significant new direct and indirect costs. Fragmentation of the health-care system, financing problems, lack of community resources, and lack of qualified and experienced personnel make the transition from hospital to home difficult for many families involved (American Academy of Pediatrics 1986).

Costs and utilization

The costs of caring for children with complex medical conditions in the home and community are high. Utilization of services far exceeds that of most other children, and the costs of services are often much higher than the costs of health services that children without apparent illness receive. Smyth-Staruch and colleagues (1984), for example, found health service utilization among children with cystic fibrosis, cerebral palsy, myelodysplasia, or multiple handicaps much higher than that of a comparison group. Chronically ill children made much greater use of all services except dental care; they had 2.7 times as many doctors' visits, 14.5 times as many hospital days, and 240 times as many physical therapy visits. An analysis of the 1980 National Medical Care Utilization and Expenditure Survey (NMCUES) compared health service use by children under 21 with limitations in activity (play, school, or work depending on age) with use by those without limitations (Newacheck and McManus 1988). Children with activity limitations used health services more than twice as often as did their peers without limitations. Increased use of health services leads to higher costs for insurers and families and increases the amount of uncompensated care for children without insurance or other resources. The costs of care for children with chronic conditions are substantially greater than costs incurred by able-bodied children. Families with children with one of ten long-term health conditions estimated the medical and non-medical expenses incurred by their children during 1987 (General Accounting Office 1989); 34 percent reported total expenses less than $250 per month ($3,000 per year), while 66 percent reported monthly expenses above this level. Other studies document the increased use of services and higher costs among children with long-term illnesses, although they also document that (even among children with serious medical conditions) a relatively small percentage uses a very large amount of total expenditures. For example, Newacheck and McManus demonstrated that the top 10 percent of children accounted for 65 percent of all charges; the top 25 percent incurred 87 percent of total charges.

Health-care costs reflect only a small portion of the total extra costs incurred by families with children with complex medical conditions. Health-care costs include hospital or physician services, medications, and specialized therapies, but this accounting leaves out transportation for doctors' visits and hospital stays, increased electric bills for powering necessary equipment, or home modifications to prepare the home and a room for the child.

Caring for a chronically ill child at home imposes costs not faced by most other families. Families have increased telephone bills; higher utility bills for heating, air conditioning, or operating supportive equipment; expenditures for extra clothing or special furnishings; a second car; home modifications; higher costs for specially trained babysitters; and special diets. These costs, rarely paid by insurance, represent a special burden for families because they must be paid out-of-pocket (usually at the time they are incurred), because they strain already thin budgets, and because they are regular expenses that families can expect to incur on an ongoing basis.

Opportunity costs are rarely documented but wreak havoc with family finances and undermine parental self-esteem. Opportunity costs include employment forgone so that a parent can stay home to provide care, raises that are refused to enable a family to continue eligibility for benefits tied to family income, and job transfers or promotions that are turned down to prevent the family from losing insurance coverage, or to keep the child near familiar, established services. The opportunity costs borne by families of children with complex chronic conditions combined with the out-of-pocket costs that they incur in the care of their children impose a substantial added financial burden on young families. At a time when the peers of the parents are becoming more secure financially and can begin to save for a home, education, or other family needs, parents of most children with complex conditions still struggle to make ends meet.

Using the 1972 National Health Interview Survey, Salkever (1982) studied the effect of a disabled child in the family on the mother's participation in the workforce. He found that in white, two-parent families, mothers with a disabled child worked outside the home about 10 percent less than mothers without disabled children. A similar study compared workforce participation of mothers of children with specific chronic illnesses (cystic fibrosis, cerebral palsy, myelodysplasia, and multiple physical handicaps) with that of mothers of children with no disabilities (Breslau, Salkever, Staruch 1982). Mothers of chronically ill children, especially those at low income levels, participated less in the workforce. A related study by Breslau (1983) compared time spent on household work (for example, cooking and cleaning) and child care. As compared with the control group, married mothers of chronically ill children spent nearly four additional hours per week on household work. No significant differences were found in time spent in child care. However, home therapy provided by parents required an average of 6.9 hours per week for those children for whom therapy was recommended. Families of chronically ill children also spent more time on doctors' visits than did families of able-bodied children. Those parents of chronically ill children who do participate in the labor force must also address the child's home-nursing-care needs during an acute illness or exacerbation of the chronic condition. General population estimates are that women working full time outside the home, on average, miss an additional seven work days per year due to a child's illness (Carpenter 1980). Increased school absence for chronic illness is well documented; and these school absences often result in more parental absence from work. In Scandinavian countries, parents of children with chronic conditions receive extra paid days' leave from work because those societies recognize the increased time demands of children with special health needs (personal communication, Dr. Bengt Zachau-Christiansen 1982).

Services

Organizing health and medical services around single or closely related conditions (such as muscular dystrophy or hemophilia) allows the development of a group of specialists with much sophistication regarding variations in prognosis, complications, therapies, and advances in medical care for specific rare conditions. Yet this emphasis on specialization requires that most services be highly centralized, insofar as the relatively low frequency of each individual condition means that satisfactory numbers of children with the condition can be found only when brought together in a large geographic or population area. This "categorical" or condition-based approach, although providing important benefits for children and families, requires that families travel long distances, face significant disruption of daily lives, and miss school or work in order to receive services. Families need access both to appropriate technologically sophisticated specialty services (usually in centralized tertiary-care centers) and to a broad array of services applicable to a wide variety of chronic health conditions. Services such as respite care, home nursing care, home-based therapies, and primary-care pediatrics, which all families with children with specialized health-care needs require, are best offered at the community level.

Schools are a significant source of services for children with special health needs. Important federal legislation assures access to education for children with handicapping conditions. Public Law 94-142, the Education of the Handicapped Act of 1975 (EHA), assures a free and appropriate public education in the least restrictive environment to children with handicaps. This act, renewed and expanded by Public Law 99-457 and renamed as the Individuals with Disabilities Education Act (IDEA) in 1991, mandates special education services throughout the United States.

The special services that are available under IDEA are of major importance to young people who have severe health impairments, and can make it possible for children to stay on track in school. Special transportation, physical therapy, medication administration during the school day, home or hospital instruction during an illness that prevents regular school attendance, psychological services, and modified physical education are just some of the services to which eligible youngsters may be entitled. The additional demands on school districts vary widely. Especially for small or significantly underfunded districts, financial demands can be severe and create difficult choices among competing priorities – extensive services for relatively few children or basic services for all children.

Households and stress

The stress of living with a child's severe chronic illness takes many forms. Caring for chronically ill children at home affects the functioning and activities of all family members, marital relationships, and living arrangements. Several studies indicate a high risk of increased physical and mental health problems in families, in particular, among care-taking mothers but also among children and siblings (Gortmaker et al. 1990). Many families face social isolation. Families whose children are assisted by technology depend heavily on home-based nursing services. Many families experience problems with home nurses because of a lack of privacy, minimal experience with the child's condition, and lack of staff continuity. Other children may have less need for technology, but may require frequent hospital visits, interfering with usual household activities. Communities may lack needed preventive or supportive therapies or counseling services.

Marital relations are strained by having a chronically ill child.

Care at Home for Children with Chronic Illness

Distress between parents with chronically ill children is higher than that of other families. In spite of increased distress, however, divorce rates are no higher for these families (Sabbeth and Leventhal 1984) probably reflecting relatively high rates in society in general, with childhood chronic illness having only a marginal influence.

Home and community care affects sisters and brothers. Many siblings benefit from having a brother or sister with a health impairment living at home. Older siblings can gain strength and competence from helping to provide care (Feinberg 1985). Yet, the tremendous demands on the time and energy of parents in caring for the ill child may leave little parental attention for the other children (Thorp 1987; Ruben et al. 1982). Feinberg observes, "Parents may valiantly strive to continue to attend the ballet recitals or football games of their other children. But the demands of the ill child or their own exhaustion make the continuation of these normal activities extremely difficult" (p. 38). Siblings may feel angry, jealous of the sick child, and guilty about their own good health. Unable to verbalize their feelings and fears, and affected by their parents' anxiety, they may experience emotional and behavioral difficulties.

Financing Services for Families

Despite insurance benefits or Medicaid coverage, many families face continuing financial burdens due to a lack of reimbursement for non-medical items or therapies, transportation, necessary home renovations for the child's needs, and equipment. Loss of a job (to stay home to care for the ill child) or missed career opportunities may reduce family resources.

Sources of payment for health services for children with complex medical conditions include private health insurance, public financing programs such as Medicaid and the Title V (Maternal and Child Health) program for Children with Special Health Needs, and school programs through the Education of the Handicapped Act of 1975 and its revisions. These several programs, although providing an important base of financing, leave many families without any source of payment and many more with only partial coverage.

The United States finances health care for children through a variety of unrelated programs (Perrin et al. 1994). Virtually all of the elderly in the United States have identical basic coverage for health expenses through the single federal program Medicare. In contrast, multiple sources finance children's health care, including federal–state partnerships, parents' employers (group health coverage), insurance directly purchased by the family, out-of-pocket payment, or charity care resulting from non-payment.

Private health insurance

The private health insurance system, including both commercial and Blue Cross/Blue Shield plans, pays for the majority of health care for children in the United States. In some cases, special benefits from private health insurance support home care for children with complex medical conditions, although private insurance has many limitations in meeting family needs. Even with seemingly adequate health insurance, many families with children with complex medical conditions find themselves with major financial burdens because of the limitations and terms of coverage. Specific problematic provisions include:

1 lack of coverage of pre-existing conditions;
2 deductibles, coinsurance, and stop-loss limits;
3 lifetime ceiling on benefits; and
4 depth and breadth of coverage for needed services.

Private insurance companies often deny or restrict coverage of pre-existing conditions, health conditions that were known at the time that the insurance went into effect. These limitations are particularly burdensome because they deny (or postpone) coverage to those people who most need it (those with health problems) and also make families pay large amounts out-of-pocket for needed health care while waiting for coverage. Rather than accept this risk, most families choose to forgo job transfers or other life changes that will affect insurance or coverage. Other families learn about pre-existing-condition exclusions only after making a job move, too late to avoid the loss of needed health insurance.

In recent years, the availability of employer-based health insurance coverage for children with special health needs has eroded in several ways (Rosenbaum, Hughes, and Johnson 1988). First, many employers have stopped providing health insurance for dependants or offer it only at high cost to the employee, an extra burden for young families with marginal incomes. Second, employers increasingly change the company from whom they purchase insurance, and the new insurer may apply a pre-existing-condition clause, thus removing needed coverage even when the employee has not changed jobs. Third, the move to

Care at Home for Children with Chronic Illness

Preferred Provider Organizations (PPOs) created financial barriers to the use of "non-approved" specialists, who may include the child's established, ongoing providers.

The family's out-of-pocket expenses are largely determined by the deductible, coinsurance, and stop-loss provisions of private health insurance. Although the cost to families with able-bodied children for these provisions may be substantial but not devastating, the ongoing annual burden of these expenses for a family with a medically complex child can severely undermine the family's financial stability (American Academy of Pediatrics 1987). The lifetime ceiling on benefits is a provision of health insurance that families with able-bodied children often ignore but families with children with complex medical conditions find of major concern. While people in good health may believe that $1 million of health insurance coverage more than adequately covers any medical need, families with ventilator-assisted or other medically fragile children will attest to its limitations.

Although most third-party payers provide adequate coverage for hospitalization and physician services, few insurers offer satisfactory benefits for home care. Policies that provide home-care benefits usually apply many restrictions. In most cases, coverage for home-care services is linked to recent hospitalization, services are provided in lieu of hospitalization, and the recipient of services must be at home or homebound, a limitation rarely applying to children. Implicit in these requirements is the assumption that home care costs the insurer less. In many cases, cost savings must be demonstrated for coverage of home-care services.

Many, but not all, group insurance plans provide coverage for the special home services needed by families of chronically ill children. Fox and Newacheck (1990) documented the breadth and depth of benefits provided by group insurance policies in a survey of 150 employers, of which 140 provided insurance coverage to employees. Of the 140 firms offering coverage, 122 (87 percent) provided visiting nurse benefits; 104 (74 percent) covered home health aides; 96 (69 percent) covered home-care services such as occupational, speech, physical, and respiratory therapy and social work but 75 percent of these firms limited visits. Mental health counseling was covered by 129 firms (92 percent) but 52 limited the number of sessions per year, and 34 applied other limits; and 72 firms (51 percent) offered individual benefits management. The available benefits for home-care services meet the basic needs of most families but are inadequate in scope and depth to meet the needs of a family with a child with a complex medical condition.

Other restrictions in coverage for home health-care services for children abound. Insurers may cover direct home-nursing procedures but will often not reimburse for education about illness or training family caregivers. Likewise, many insurers insist for children (as they do for adults) that a child must be at home and all services provided in the home. This requirement precludes payment by insurance for private duty nursing at school for a ventilator-assisted child who requires around-the-clock care. This requirement has been challenged through litigation in some instances, and plaintiff children's positions have been reviewed favorably by the court (*Detzel* v. *Sullivan*).

Capitated health plans

Prepaid plans (such as health maintenance organizations or independent practice associations) are conceptually attractive models for providing care and coverage to children with complex health conditions. These practices agree to provide inpatient and outpatient care and a range of additional services, in exchange for a fixed total payment (usually paid monthly). Prepaid practices therefore should have incentives to provide many services (beyond basic hospitalization and physicians' services) that families with medically complex children need – for example, preventive care, preventive mental health services, home care, and care coordination – in order to prevent costly hospitalization.

A survey of prepaid group practices by Fox and colleagues (1993) sheds some light on the adequacy of these organizations in meeting the needs of children with complex medical conditions. In general, prepaid group practices offer very good coverage for acute-care services but are less generous in their benefits for chronic care. The use of primary-care physicians as "gatekeepers" who must authorize many services restricts children's access to services such as specialty physicians, hospital outpatient departments, ancillary services (such as occupational, physical, and speech therapies), mental health services, and substance abuse treatment. Additional restrictions on the use of these benefits may be applied through limitations on the number of visits or dollar amount of services that will be covered. Home health benefits are covered by nearly all the plans surveyed, but again, access is limited by physician referral or other requirements. Case management is usually offered as a limited service but does not include the multidisciplinary, comprehensive coordination of care that families with medically complex children require (Perrin and Bloom, in press).

Restrictions on access to services must be against the clear benefits of prepaid group practice enrollment: families have low out-of-pocket expenses and excellent protection against the catastrophic cost of hospitalization. An additional benefit, not significant to most families with apparently well children but of crucial importance to families with children with complex medical conditions, is that prepaid group practices rarely exclude coverage for pre-existing conditions.

Unfortunately, there is little conclusive evidence about the actual performance of prepaid group practices in caring for children with complex medical conditions. Some families are very satisfied with the care and services they receive, having learned to "work the system" to get the most from their plans. Yet, many anecdotes from other families and from providers indicate that prepaid group practices fall short of their potential in meeting families' needs. In particular, access to specialty providers is reported to be restricted, thereby denying children access to needed services; and contrary to the results of Fox's survey, home-care benefits are said to be severely limited and inadequate to meet the needs of medically complex children at home.

Medicaid
Although states must provide a set of basic benefits for their Medicaid populations, they offer optional benefits at their discretion; and states may apply limitations to all benefits, both mandatory and optional. Depending on the states' choices regarding eligibility and benefits, the Medicaid program may be a rich resource with great depth and breadth of services or more impoverished, meeting only minimal needs for the poorest of the poor. The great interstate variation in eligibility criteria and benefits creates major inequities in the Medicaid program.

Two main factors determine eligibility for Medicaid: disability and financial status. A disabled child meeting income and disability criteria for Supplemental Security Income (SSI), the federal program of cash assistance for aged, blind, or disabled people, receives Medicaid in most states. The SSI program historically served relatively few children; in 1990, approximately 290,000 children received SSI benefits, most of whom were eligible for Medicaid (Fox and Greaney 1988). Eligibility for children had been limited by difficulty in determining the functional abilities of very young children with disabilities, accounting for additive effects of multiple handicaps, and assessing the many rare conditions that disable children. As a result of a US Supreme Court ruling in early 1990 (*Sullivan* v. *Zebley*), the Social Security Administration developed new regulations to ease the eligibility determination process for children. As of June 1994, the numbers of childhood beneficiaries had grown to almost 800,000 with expectations of well over a million child and adolescent beneficiaries ultimately, depending on the methods of implementing the new regulations (Perrin and Stein 1991). With the Medicaid eligibility that accompanies SSI enrollment in most states, SSI provides a valuable financial benefit for families.

The second main avenue for Medicaid eligibility, through enrollment in the Aid to Families with Dependent Children (AFDC) program, requires meeting family-structure guidelines and state-specific income-need standards. The optional medically needy program provides another route for Medicaid eligibility. This program provides Medicaid coverage for people who meet the "categorical" requirements for Medicaid (i.e., have family structure or disability like other AFDC recipients) and have income between the AFDC payment level on May 1, 1988, and 133 percent of the current AFDC payment set by the states. In addition, similar families whose incomes exceed this ceiling but whose medical expenses will offset the excess income are also eligible for Medicaid through the "spend down" provision. While this program offers great potential to meet the needs of children with complex medical conditions, its complex administration provides substantial barriers to enrollment.

Medicaid expansions authorized by Congress over the past several years provide coverage to all eligible children, including those with chronic illness, whose family incomes meet established standards. States must provide Medicaid coverage to pregnant women and children up to age six whose family incomes are up to 133 percent of the federal poverty level. States also have the option of raising the income level threshold for Medicaid eligibility up to 185 percent of the poverty level for pregnant women and infants up to age one. Beyond these expansions, Congress passed legislation in 1990 that requires a phase-in of Medicaid coverage for children up to age 19 whose family income is below 100% of the federal poverty level; this phase-in will be completed by October 2001 (National Governors' Association 1993).

Two Medicaid options, waiver programs and state amendments to Medicaid plans, offer additional promise for helping families care for complex chronically ill children at home. The Medicaid waiver programs began in 1982. Prior to this innovation, Medicaid would pay medical expenses while a child was in the hospital but would not continue to cover her if she returned home and had substantially lower, although still considerable, expenses.

The Medicaid waiver programs allow approved states to forgo certain Medicaid requirements (for example, income standards for eligibility, deeming rules, and freedom of choice of providers) or to provide additional benefits so long as home care is safe and costs to the Medicaid program will not increase. Section 2176 Home and Community-Based Services Waivers includes two types of programs: the "regular" waivers that permit an unlimited number of enrollees and the "model" waivers that are limited to 200 individuals. The Section 2176 waivers allow states to offer expanded services beyond the standard Medicaid benefits to targeted recipients (aged, disabled, mentally retarded, or mentally ill) to avoid more costly institutionalization. Allowed additional services provided through a waiver (beyond the state's usual Medicaid services) include case management, homemakers, home health aides, personal care services, adult day care, habilitation, respite care, private duty nursing, and home modification (Fox 1984; Hall 1990).

The Section 2176 waiver programs can improve financing and services for children with complex medical conditions. As of 1989, 36 states were approved for a total of 66 waivers that serve children. Of these 66 waivers, 42 are regular waivers and 24 are model waivers (Hall 1990). The value of the waiver to families of complex chronically ill children is substantial. Children who, in the absence of the waiver, would have stayed in hospital to remain on Medicaid now live at home with their families and still keep their coverage. Moreover, the additional services available through the waivers help families to cope long-term with the stress of a medically complex child at home.

Nevertheless, the waivers fall short of meeting the needs of many families. Model waivers are limited to 200 individuals regardless of the population of the state, so the needs of the 201st child and all subsequent children remain unmet in states where the waiver slots are filled. Under these circumstances, an additional waiver may be requested by the state. Waivers also fail to serve children whose home care is more costly to Medicaid than their hospital care. This situation can arise when a child's hospital care is paid by private insurance that will not provide home-care benefits. In such a case, Medicaid is obligated to pay nothing for hospital care so that any home-care plan that would be paid by Medicaid would not meet the cost-effectiveness requirement.

Amendments to states' Medicaid plans provide another option to serve the special needs of children with complex medical conditions. These state plan options offer states the advantage of expanding eligibility for Medicaid benefits to certain populations in the state without requiring special approvals from the Health Care Financing Administration. This mechanism to expand Medicaid eligibility is easier administratively than applying for a waiver and had been selected in 17 states as of 1989 (Hall 1990). This option for serving medically complex children is most beneficial in states that have a generous Medicaid program because the benefits are limited to those available through the regular program. Through this option, states may target Medicaid eligibility to certain needy groups without opening eligibility to a more general population.

Programs to Help Families

Key program and policy changes in the areas of home and community care for children with chronic illnesses can be, at least in part, based on evidence. There is sufficient knowledge to develop comprehensive care systems coordinating inpatient and outpatient services, including discharge and family service plans and standards of home nursing care. Rather than the characteristics of each condition, success in home care more typically reflects certain characteristics of households, the supports available to families, and the degree to which programs develop family partnerships that account for stages in family development (Perrin, Shayne, and Bloom 1993).

Furthermore, issues in financing care and assuring access to a broad array of services substantially influence outcomes. Strengthened nursing services in many hospitals and community agencies have led to improved discharge planning, better in-home care, and a broader array of outpatient services for children with chronic illnesses. There is also sufficient evidence to define elements of care coordination and to determine households most likely to benefit from these services. However, predicting which families will succeed in home care is an uncertain art; policymakers, families, and providers will benefit from more careful exploration of this question.

Care coordination activities have a long history in the human-service arena, where staff from public or private agencies have helped families determine needs and gain access to cost-effective services (Weil and Karls 1985). Care coordination was applied to children with special health-care needs over a decade ago, often with initial goals and services similar to those for other human-service clients. This service empowers families, helping them learn to manage their own care, rather than having an external agent direct services (Anderson 1985).

Care coordination or case management is an allowed additional service provided through the Medicaid waiver (beyond the state's usual Medicaid services) that helps to alleviate some of the problems that families experience as a result of having a health-impaired child at home (Hall 1990). Furthermore, it is a service increasingly offered by private insurers as a cost-saving measure. For many families, coordination of care is an additional, important family-support service with several functions.

The functions of care coordination include teaching families about their children's care, working with families to develop a plan for ongoing care, helping families access needed services (such as health care, insurance, school, social benefits, respite care, or recreation), monitoring progress and revising the care plan accordingly, and teaching families over time to advocate for themselves and to provide their own coordination (Perrin and Bloom, in press). In addition to these main functions, some care coordinators offer direct care to children. They provide this service with several goals in mind: to assess a child's current medical status, to help a family provide care, to model appropriate caregiving techniques for family members, and to provide a concrete service for families to help to build rapport with parents. Further research is needed in the evaluation of home-care services, including means to determine best personnel standards and determine outcomes.

Many other programs help families. These include programs that coordinate services from tertiary centers with those in the community (Kisker et al. 1980; Lie 1990), hospice and respite-care programs for severely ill or dying children, day-care programs for chronically ill or medically fragile children (Pierce, Lester, and Fraze 1991), and parent support groups.

Health policies regarding the care of chronically ill children must reflect changing society values. The community increasingly assumes responsibility for these children and adolescents, and there is a broad commitment to make their survival a positive experience for the family as well as the community. Ethical guidelines for home care for chronically ill children will emerge as a result of an ongoing exchange of views and debate among the involved youngsters and adolescents, their families, professionals, community groups, and policymakers, reflecting changing societal and cultural values.

Lessons from Europe

European countries have supported households with chronically ill children and adolescents in several ways. In Great Britain, for example, families with children with long-term illnesses may receive different types of financial support, including an Attendance Allowance for a dependant over two years old who requires substantial care at home, with a higher rate paid for those who need constant attendance day and night. In addition, a caretaking parent can receive an additional Invalid Care Allowance. A Mobility Allowance is a further benefit for people aged 5–80 who are unable to walk. Social service programs provide or assist with special housing, care, or education.

Once it is clear that a child has special needs, he or she is entered on a register in the district health authority. "The consultant community pediatrician assumes responsibility for monitoring the progress of all children registered, obtaining and reviewing regular reports from the various professionals involved in the child's care. The district handicap team also identifies a 'named person,' usually one of the professionals directly involved in the child's care, who acts as a contact and reference point for parents in all matters concerning the child" (Goodwin 1990).

In Norway and Sweden, most children are seen by general practitioners, but area-pediatricians, specialists working closely with family physicians in a given region, take special responsibility for children with chronic diseases and handicaps, and link the regional pediatric department with primary health care. Regular co-payments for doctor visits and medications do not apply for people with chronic conditions, who receive free care. Parents can apply for cash benefits (care allowance) if they care for a disabled child at home. Parents can take off 12 workdays per year with full compensation if the child is ill or they need to go to the doctor. Social domestic assistance provides support for housework and child care when parents or children are ill. Parents can apply for home nursing, home aid, or home-care grants (Lindstrom and Kohler 1991).

The German social system reimburses up to 25 hours per month of home nursing. If the family can manage the care on their own, they receive financial support both from the sickness funds and from the welfare system. If the family has cared for a chronically ill family member for at least 12 months, they are entitled to reimbursement for respite care for up to four weeks. Exceptions from the 25-hour monthly limit can occur (e.g., for a child discharged on a ventilator), when the sickness fund decides it will be cheaper to pay for nursing rather than intensive-care unit costs (Wysong and Abel 1990; Bundesminister für Arbeit und Soziales 1990).

Making the System Work for Children and Families

Programs and policy in the area of home and community care for children with chronic illnesses should enhance family or household functioning and ensure the best growth and development of the child in the context of severe long-term illness. As the large majority of children with severe long-term illnesses survive at least to young adulthood, and as most of these young adults are capable of employment and participation in most activities of their peers despite ongoing physical disability, policy goals should include maximizing long-term productivity and independence of children and adolescents with chronic illnesses. In the short term, goals of home care should include the integration of the child and household into the community and the maintenance of family lifestyle in the context of the child's health condition.

Principles for policy
Three main principles should guide the formulation of policy for home and community care:

(a) families must have the central role in guiding the care for their children,
(b) benefits and services must be flexible, recognizing that the needs of children and families change over time and that needs vary among families, and
(c) children with chronic illness and their families should be integrated to the maximum extent possible into their home communities and activities.

With appropriate assistance and adaptation, close to complete integration of the child and family can happen.

These principles and the previous discussion support the notion that policies and programs must view the family (and at times the community) as the unit of intervention rather than directing services primarily to the child. Services should enhance family well-being and be broad enough to include not only home-based direct care (nursing and other) but also respite services, family counseling, and educational planning. The goals of such services should include not only the optimal functioning of the child but also assisting families to cope with altered lifestyles.

Home and community services

We recommend a system of long-term care that uses a generic definition of chronic illness (Perrin et al. 1993) (rather than one based on specific diagnoses), that provides broad and comprehensive benefits, and that includes a mechanism to ensure that families gain access to the range of benefits and services appropriate to their and their child's needs. This mechanism is best based on a system of coordination of care, with the care coordinator, in collaboration with medical consultation, working with the family to assure access to appropriate services. Limiting eligibility to conditions that engender lengthy hospitalization and requiring home-care plans that are less costly than hospital-based programs (as has been done with Medicaid waiver programs) exempts most children who can benefit from home and community care. Furthermore, such rules offer potentially inflationary incentives through encouraging unnecessary hospitalization of children with chronic illnesses.

A child and adolescent long-term care plan should provide four basic groups of services:

(a) direct care services in the home based in a continuum of health and medical services,
(b) services to integrate the child into school and the community,
(c) family support services, and
(d) care coordination.

Family support services should target the whole family, including siblings and the extended family when appropriate.

Access to services should be based on a family service plan, jointly developed by the family and a coordinator of care, and outlining appropriate services in each category. Plans should be monitored and revised regularly to assure flexibility of benefits in the context of changing child and family needs, and include the child or adolescent as he or she grows older so that at adulthood decision making and central focus has transferred to him or her.

Financing and organization

To finance health services, the nation needs a system of health insurance with national standards, ensuring an adequate level of care for all children. Such a system would provide the same basic benefits to children regardless of the parents' economic status, place of residence, or employment. However, universal health insurance alone will not meet the needs of children with severe illnesses unless it includes appropriate long-term care benefits and financial support to households. The extra financial burdens their families carry merit additional benefits, such as cash payments through SSI or tax breaks. Health insurance and extra financial benefits would help offset parents' stress from economic worries and allow them to focus on their top priority – taking care of their children with special health needs. Four main financial and organizational efforts should support home and community care for children with chronic illnesses. First, most health and medical care services should be financed by universal insurance under health-care reform, as part of the acute-care benefit structure. Second, recognizing that the care for a child with severe long-term health disability creates significant financial burdens for the family, public programs should provide direct financial payments to families. (Such payments provide families with additional resources to choose those services they feel most beneficial to their well-being.) This recommendation builds on the current Supplemental Security Income program for children, but we recommend further changes in SSI so that the program enhances children's abilities rather than encourages continuing disability to maintain benefits, and so that it covers a larger number of households (with a graded benefit based on family income). Efforts must be made in the financial structure to provide these families with resources that enable them to enjoy what other families without a child with a chronic illness or disability enjoy. Families should not need to sacrifice their standard of living nor siblings face compromised futures because so much of their income must be used for this one family member.

Third, based on broad eligibility criteria noted above and on development of an appropriate specific family/household plan, children and households should have access to an additional long-term care benefit package (including respite care), supporting appropriate comprehensive services. Families with children with severe illnesses have further service needs that are unlikely to be covered by basic health insurance programs. Some needed services fall into a category of direct care services, such as in-home nursing or specialized homemaker services, respite care that is flexible (in-home, out-of-home, varying time frame, pre-scheduled, or crisis relief), and hospice care, equipment, specialized transportation, or coordination of care. Some services may be available through the "basic" insurance program, but many will require a supplemental benefit package that should be available to families whose children meet a broad and generic definition of severe chronic illness. Although these benefits could be financed in a generally available universal insurance program, they presumably will not be available to all families, but rather just to those meeting specific eligibility criteria.

Fourth, additional funds will be needed to support the development and maintenance of regional programs of care that integrate home and community care with specialty health services for children with complex medical conditions.

Among these four items, the first three will be likely to come from federal efforts. Benefits (items one and three) should be part of public or private health insurance schemes. Direct household financial support should come through social security arrangements. The fourth item, support for regionalized systems, is likely to be mediated through state Title V Maternal and Child Health programs in collaboration with specialized health centers and community service programs, or through similar ventures at the state and community level funded with public monies and carried out by private programs. Public resources must support the organization and delivery of services at the state, regional, and community level.

Note

Prepared for Milbank Memorial Fund/Visiting Nurse Service of New York Conference, Harriman NY, November 1993. This chapter reflects in part work supported by Grants MCJ 253795 and 250581 from the Maternal and Child Health Program (Title V, Social Security Act), Health Resources and Services Administration, Department of Health and Human Services. The authors thank Dr Priscilla Lincoln of the Visiting Nurse Services of New York for her review and helpful comments in the development of this chapter.

Portions of this chapter have appeared in an earlier version in J.M. Perrin, M.W. Shayne, and S.R. Bloom, *Home and Community Care for Chronically Ill Children*. Oxford University Press, New York, 1993.

References

American Academy of Pediatrics (Committee on Children with Disabilities). 1986. Transition of Severely Disabled Children from Hospital or Chronic Care Facility to the Community. *Pediatrics* 78: 531–4.

American Academy of Pediatrics. 1987. Health Care Financing for the Child with Catastrophic Costs. *Pediatrics* 80: 752–7.

Anderson, B. 1985. Parents of Children with Disabilities as Collaborators in Home Health Care. *Coalition Quarterly* 4(2 and 3): 1–18. Publication of

Federation for Children with Special Needs, 312 Stuart Street, Boston, MA02116.
Breslau, N., D.S. Salkever, and K.S. Staruch. 1982. Women's Labor Force Activity and Responsibility for Disabled Dependants. *Journal of Health, Society, Social Behaviour* 23: 169–83.
Breslau, N. 1983. Care of Disabled Children and Women's Time Use. *Medical Care* 21: 620–9.
Bundesminister für Arbeit und Soziales. 1990. *Soziale Sicherheit-Sozialgesetzbuch.* Buch No. 5: Krankenversicherung. Bonn.
Cadman, D., M. Boyle, P. Szatmari, D.R. Offord. 1987. Chronic Illness, Disability, and Mental and Social Wellbeing: Findings of the Ontario Child Health Study. *Pediatrics* 79: 805–13.
Carpenter, E. 1980. Children's Health Care and the Changing Role of Women. *Medical Care* 18(2): 1208–18.
Detzel v. Sullivan 895 F.2d 58 (2d Cir 1990).
Feinberg, E.A. 1985. Family stress in Pediatric Home Care. *Caring* 4(5): 38–44.
Fox, H. 1984. A Preliminary Analysis of Options to Improve Health Insurance Coverage for Chronically Ill and Disabled Children. Prepared for the US Department of Health and Human Services, Division of Maternal and Child Health, Habilitation Services Branch, September.
Fox, H.B., and A. Greaney. 1988. Disabled Children's Access to Supplemental Security Income and Medicaid Benefits. Prepared for the University of California at San Francisco with support from the US Department of Health and Human Services, Bureau of Maternal and Child Health and Resources Development. Fox Health Policy Consultants, Inc., December.
Fox, H.B., and P. Newacheck. 1990. Private Health Insurance of Chronically Ill Children. *Pediatrics* 85: 50–7.
Fox, H.B., et al. 1993. Health Maintenance Organizations and Children with Special Health Needs. *American Journal of Diseases of Children* 147: 546–52.
General Accounting Office. 1989. Home Care Experiences of Families with Chronically Ill Children. Gaithersburg, MD: US Government Printing Office. (Report No. GAO/HRD-89-73).
Goodwin, S. 1990. Children with Special Needs: Their Care in England and Wales. *Pediatrics* 86: 1112–16.
Gortmaker, S.L., and W. Sappenfield. 1984. Chronic Childhood Disorders: Prevalence and Impact. *Pediatric Clinics of North America* 31: 3–18.
Gortmaker, S.L., D.K. Walker, M. Weitzman, and A.M. Sobol. 1990. Chronic Conditions, Socioeconomic Risks, and Behavioral Problems in Children and Adolescents. *Pediatrics* 85: 267–76.
Green, M. 1983. Coming of Age in General Pediatrics. *Pediatrics* 72: 275.
Hall, L. 1990. Medicaid Home Care Options for Disabled Children. Washington D.C.: Health Policy Department, Human Resources Policy

Studies Division, Center for Policy Research, National Governors' Association.

Hobbs, N., J.M. Perrin, and H.T. Ireys. 1985. *Chronically Ill Children and Their Families*. San Francisco: Jossey-Bass.

Kisker, C.T., F. Strayer, K. Wong, et al. 1980. Health Outcomes of a Community-Based Therapy Program for Children with Cancer. *Pediatrics* 66: 900–6.

Lie, S.O. 1990. Children in the Norwegian Health Care System. *Pediatrics* 86: 1048–52.

Lindstrom, B., and L. Kohler. 1991. Youth, Disability and Quality of Life. *Pediatrician* 18: 121–8.

National Governors' Association. 1993. *State Coverage of Pregnant Women and Children—January 1993*. Washington, D.C.: Center for Policy Studies.

Newacheck, P., and M. McManus. 1988. Financing Health Care for Disabled Children. *Pediatrics* 81(3): 385–94.

Newacheck, P.W., and W.R. Taylor. 1992. Childhood Chronic Illness: Prevalence, Severity, and Impact. *American Journal of Public Health* 82: 364–71.

Perrin, J.M., and S.R. Bloom. In press. Coordination of Care for Households with Children with Special Health Needs. In *Maternal and Child Health Practices*, 4th edn, ed. H.M. Wallace, R.P. Nelson, and P.J. Sweeney. Oakland, CA: Third Party Publishing.

Perrin, J.M., R.S. Kahn, S.R. Bloom, et al. 1994. Health Care Reform and the Special Needs of Children. *Pediatrics* 93: 504–6.

Perrin, E.C., P. Newacheck, I.B. Pless, et al. 1993. Issues Involved in the Definition and Classification of Chronic Health Conditions. *Pediatrics* 91: 787–93.

Perrin, J.M., M.W. Shayne, and S.R. Bloom. 1993. *Home and Community Care for Chronically Ill Children*. New York: Oxford University Press,

Perrin, J.M., and R.E.K. Stein. 1991. Reinterpreting Disability: Changes in SSI for Children. *Pediatrics* 88: 1047–51.

Pierce, P.M., D.G. Lester, and D.E. Fraze. 1991. Prescribed Pediatric Extended Care: The Family Centered Health Care Alternative for Medically and Technology Dependent Children. In *The Medically Complex Child: The Transition to Home Care*, ed. N.J. Hochstadt and D.M. Yost, 177–90. Chur: Harwood Academic Publishers.

Pope, A.M., and A.R. Tarlov, eds. 1991. *Disability in America – Toward a National Agenda for Prevention*. Washington, D.C.: National Academy Press.

Rosenbaum, S., D. Hughes, and K. Johnson. 1988. Maternal and Child Health Services for Medically Indigent Children and Pregnant Women. *Medical Care* 26: 315–32.

Ruben, R.J., et al. 1982. Home Care of the Pediatric Patient with a Tracheotomy. *Annals of Otology, Rhinology and Laryngology* 91(6): 633–40.

Sabbeth, B.F., and J.M. Leventhal. 1984. Marital Adjustment to Chronic

Childhood: A Critique of the Literature. *Pediatrics* 73: 762–8.

Salkever, D. 1982. Communications: Children's Health Problems and Maternal Work Status. *Journal of Human Resources* 17(1): 94–109.

Smith, P.S., and P. Levine. 1984. The Benefits of Comprehensive Care of Hemophilia: A Five-Year Study of Outcomes. *American Journal of Public Health* 74(6): 616–17.

Smyth-Staruch, K., et al. 1984. Use of Health Services by Chronically Ill and Disabled Children. *Medical Care* 22(4): 310–28.

Thorp, E.K. 1987. Mothers Coping with Home Care of Severe Chronic Respiratory Disabled Children Requiring Medical Technology Assistance. Dissertation submitted to the faculty of the School of Education and Development, George Washington University, Washington, D.C., May 1987.

US Congress, Office of Technology Assessment. 1987. *Technology-Dependent Children: Hospital vs. Home Care.* Washington, D.C.: US Government Printing Office. (OTA-TM-H-38).

Weil, M., and J.M. Karls. 1985. Historical Origins and Recent Developments. In *Case Management in Human Service Practice*, ed. M. Weil, J.M. Karls, and Associates, 1–28. San Francisco: Jossey-Bass.

Weitzman, M., S.L. Gortmaker, A.M. Sobol, and J.M. Perrin. 1992. Recent trends in the prevalence and severity of childhood asthma. *Journal of the American Medical Association* 268: 2673–7.

West, J., ed. 1991. The Americans with Disabilities Act: From Policy to Practice. *Milbank Quarterly* 69: Supplements 1/2: 1–360.

Wysong, J.A., and T. Abel. 1990. Universal Health Insurance and High-Risk Groups in West Germany: Implications for US Health Policy. *Milbank Quarterly* 68: 527–60.

11

AIDS and Home Care: Lessons for Policy and Practice
David A. Gould

I Introduction

AIDS has challenged the American health-care system with an unparalleled suddenness and intensity, stimulating advances in biomedical knowledge and clinical practice and precipitating several radical shifts in how communities organize to advocate for and deliver health and social services. Amid the tragedy and conflict engendered by AIDS, the growth of a large and diverse system of community-care services is often heralded as a bittersweet victory won in the continuing battle against AIDS. The foundation of that system of community care is the provision of home-care services, without which many of the other community services would prove inadequate.

This chapter will examine the emergence of home-care services for persons with AIDS (PWAs),[1] with one eye focused on discerning what new challenges were encountered and the other on delineating commonalities among what are often perceived to be two distinct home-care systems serving PWAs and the elderly. Bringing these two views together should create a perspective that will help identify how policymakers seeking to reshape the home-care system can benefit from the experience gained by providing home-care services to PWAs.

A few caveats are in order before we begin our investigation. First, there is a substantial literature on AIDS and long-term care, the best of it written by Ted Benjamin, which has heavily influenced my thinking on the topic. But that literature customarily presents home care as a small part of a larger system or as a response to the demands of that system. In this chapter I will attempt to keep the spotlight on how home care works and what that tells us about the design of the larger health-care system. Second, although there is a slowly blossoming literature on home care and AIDS, I have drawn extensively on the experience, insights, and opinions of a diverse group of health-care professionals who pioneered the development of home-care services for PWAs in New York City during the past decade. Their views were gained through a series of individual interviews and panel discussions, and I have done my best to synthesize them without blurring important differences. The following analysis also was enriched by a review of the substantial body of planning documents produced by city and state agencies and several public–private collaborations.

A final note: although AIDS is a problem of national scope, my observations are largely confined to the experience gained in New York City. Although my perspective is admittedly parochial, Dr. Nicholas Rango, the late director of the New York State AIDS Institute, often reminded us that New York is home to the three population groups separately affected in other urban areas: gay men, injection drug users (IDUs), and women and their children. In this respect, New York is not so much exceptional as it is a microcosm of AIDS in America.

II AIDS in New York City: Dimensions and Trends

The following figures briefly present some basic data about the incidence and growth of AIDS in New York City. To no one's surprise, AIDS is not equally prevalent in all of New York's communities, whether these are defined by geography or population group. The concentration of AIDS in several neighborhoods follows a pattern that roughly parallels its spread from a disease found predominantly among gay men living in Greenwich Village and Chelsea/Clinton to one that has ravaged the communities of Harlem, the South Bronx, and Central Brooklyn (table 11.1).

AIDS and Home Care 247

Table 11.1 Aids in New York City neighborhoods

	AIDS Rate		Adult	Homicide Rate	Percent of Population	
	Per 100,000 Population 1992	Percent Change 8/88-12/92	AIDS Cases 1992	Per 100,000 Population 1990	White Non-Hispanic 1990	Medicaid Eligible 1992
Chelsea-Clinton	2632.0	119.6	3240	7.6	67.5	17.2
Greenwich Village-Soho	2262.0	142.6	1847	5.9	69.7	7.4
East Harlem	1411.6	150.0	1672	58.8	5.9	45.5
Upper West Side	1386.2	142.2	3076	12.9	66.7	10.8
Gramercy Park-Murray Hill	1328.6	134.9	1594	4.0	81.3	4.1
Union Square-Lower East Side	1290.7	134.3	2521	23.4	45.5	23.7
Central Harlem-Morningside Hghts	1163.1	243.3	2192	71.3	7.9	45.3
High Bridge-Morrisania	1090.2	217.7	1810	74.7	2.1	50.8
Hunts Point-Mott Haven	1076.5	182.4	1147	99.6	1.4	61.5
Crotona-Tremont	946.4	207.9	1540	96.6	3.5	54.8
Lower Manhattan	810.4	124.1	218	17.7	66.9	16.5
Downtown-Heights-Slope	770.9	175.7	1643	23.0	45.7	20.0
Bedford/Stuyvesant-Crown Hghts	689.7	315.3	3122	61.2	4.4	35.4
Greenpoint-Williamsburg	590.3	270.7	1401	32.9	33.7	40.6
Fordham-Bronx Park	556.6	226.0	1352	43.0	24.1	33.8
Jamaica	498.6	191.0	1237	29.7	13.9	19.7
Upper East Side	489.9	97.8	993	3.5	87.0	3.3
East New York	485.3	256.7	858	59.7	10.9	37.2
Pelham-Throgs Neck	466.0	250.3	1210	28.9	38.5	19.8
Washington Heights-Inwood	462.2	191.1	916	54.6	18.3	38.7
West Queens	412.3	163.0	1593	22.7	33.5	14.8
Stapleton-St. George	394.0	268.0	379	11.1	67.7	16.1
Sunset Park	387.6	196.4	371	23.8	32.1	29.1
East Flatbush-Flatbush	371.5	190.0	1197	26.9	28.4	18.6
Port Richmond	330.9	187.9	148	15.5	64.1	16.6
Northeast Bronx	319.9	219.9	539	24.3	32.4	14.3
Rockaway	305.1	458.1	307	17.2	44.0	28.2
Long Island City-Astoria	299.6	305.2	571	8.2	57.3	12.7
Southwest Queens	239.6	222.9	527	9.9	56.6	12.3
Kingsbridge-Riverdale	238.7	135.6	199	19.4	62.3	12.2
Coney Island-Sheepshead Bay	206.8	230.9	544	13.0	73.9	18.7
Bensonhurst-Bay Ridge	201.8	193.0	356	8.3	84.6	9.6
Southeast Queens	198.6	150.0	377	13.7	33.0	9.6
Ridgewood-Forest Hills	179.4	255.6	385	5.4	76.6	9.6
Borough Park	178.4	209.9	372	7.1	73.1	19.1
Canarsie-Flatlands	170.5	219.6	264	18.8	68.4	10.0
South Beach-Tottenville	142.2	438.7	218	6.1	91.0	4.8
Fresh Meadows	125.2	218.2	104	11.8	67.9	7.0
Flushing Clearview	122.6	218.6	290	8.8	61.4	7.5
Bayside-Little Neck	111.2	268.8	87	3.7	76.9	3.5
Willowbrook	107.3	360.0	91	6.3	83.9	6.0
BRONX	655.4	NA	7797	51.2	24.2	33.3
BROOKLYN	440.2	NA	10128	30.3	42.0	24.5
MANHATTAN	1237.9	NA	18269	26.4	51.3	21.2
QUEENS	281.2	NA	5478	14.5	48.4	12.8
STATEN ISLAND	220.6	NA	836	8.7	79.7	9.6
NEW YORK CITY	582.7	NA	42508	27.6	44.6	21.4

Sources: Health Systems Agency; New York City Department of Health, Office of AIDS Surveillance.

Here we find almost all PWAs to be persons of color and, on average, to be more economically and socially disadvantaged. Substance abuse, especially with injection drugs, is the predominant vector of infection in these communities, but carries with it a secondary stream of infection: female partners of IDUs and their children (figure 11.1).

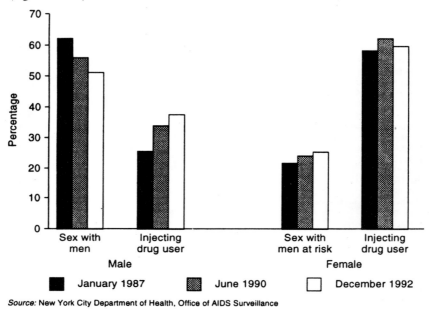

Figure 11.1 AIDS in New York City by sex and selected risk factors

While it is crude generalization, the perception of a movement of AIDS from a largely white, middle-class, gay community to a set of low-income, socially marginalized communities devastated by a host of social ills including crime, unemployment, substandard housing, and rampant drug abuse guides much of this chapter's analysis. This generalization does not mean that AIDS has left the gay community, which continues to account for almost half of all cases and is home to a large number of HIV-infected but as yet symptom-free men. Nor does it mean to imply that AIDS is found only in these neighborhoods of highest incidence. But the generalization does help focus on the emergent need to bring home-care services to at least two differently populated and organized communities.

From the very outset, the city agency with lead responsibility for providing home and community services to PWAs, the Human

Resources Administration (HRA), understood that the crisis called for something other than business as usual. HRA anticipated an explosive demand for an unprecedentedly complex array of income supports, housing, and social and legal services, in addition to intensive home-care services. The agency also appreciated the unpredictability of the disease, recognizing that a PWA's clinical status and consequent need for in-home services were likely to change quickly. This called for the capability to adapt the plan of in-home services just as quickly, a managerial responsiveness not found in HRA's large Medicaid personal-care program. It was also evident that the intensity of care and risks associated with delivering it would require a rate of payment significantly higher than provided to the city's personal-care program or the local certified home health agencies.

HRA's response was, given its bureaucratic culture, unorthodox. While it created a new Division of AIDS Services (DAS) to provide comprehensive case-management services, it also tested a new approach to delivering home-care services to PWAs. A limited special program conducted with the Red Cross in 1984 proved inadequate and led the next year to a prime contract with the Visiting Nurse Service of New York (VNSNY) to coordinate and manage the provision of all home-care services to all Medicaid-eligible persons with HIV disease and AIDS in New York City. Significantly, no other agency seriously bid on the contract. (Concerns with being stigmatized as an AIDS agency and the need to function in all parts of the city are said to have curbed the interest of other agencies.)

HRA's contract with VNSNY incorporated two special features, each essential to the nurturing of the fledgling care system. First, it conveyed extra financing through the personal-care services rate to meet the extraordinary costs of staff recruitment, training, and support. Second, it authorized VNSNY to independently adapt the plan of in-home services according to its professional judgment. Under the contract, VNSNY could, for example, change the frequency of nursing visits or hours of personal-care services as it saw fit, informing the HRA medical review unit of the change and seeking its retroactive approval. This type of professional latitude was not found in HRA's personal-care program, as it more typified the management style of the certified home health agency. The change was a significant policy departure for HRA. At the same time, HRA required VNSNY to work with DAS case workers to devise an initial plan of care, which required the approval of a separate medical review staff before initiating services. This scheme of collaboration mixed with a hearty dose of utilization review suggests the limits of HRA's willingness to redefine its organizational ethos.

III The Home-Care Caseload: More and Less

The prime contract with VNSNY represented a creative response to a service crisis that threatened to grow exponentially in both size and complexity. And, as the caseload numbers in table 11.2 indicate, growth has been an abiding theme. For example, in the three years from December 1989 to December 1992 the DAS caseload more than tripled in size, while the numbers receiving home-care services only doubled. The proportion of DAS cases receiving home care declined from 12.6 percent to 7.8 percent. The growth in the average number of PWAs served by the VNSNY's Medicaid AIDS Project also follows a similar trend.

Table 11.2 Selected services for PWAs, 1989–1992

	HRA, Division of AIDS Services		VNSNY Medicaid AIDS Project	PWAs in Hospital
	Active	Home	Average monthly census	One-Day census
December 1989	3,515	444	387	1,981
December 1990	5,869	769	606	2,209
December 1991	9,028	695	735	2,244
December 1992	11,788	914	713	2,444

Sources: Greater New York Hospital Association; New York City Human Resources Administration, Division of AIDS Services; Visiting Nurse Service of New York.

While changing definitions of eligibility for services provide an occasionally slippery statistical slope for fine-grained analyses, these few numbers point to a trend surprising to most observers of the service response to AIDS in New York City. Simply put, projected demand for home-care services has far exceeded expressed demand. While this holds for most services, the dramatic growth anticipated in home care – largely driven by the need to shorten exceedingly long, expensive, and inappropriate hospital stays – has not been fully realized. To illustrate, the demand level projected by the report of the Health Systems Agency/New York City AIDS Task Force for 1989, a caseload of 1,670 PWAs, has not been approached even four years later.

AIDS and Home Care 251

While it is easy to second-guess such projections and exhort today's experts to refine our system models, it may be more instructive for the purposes of this chapter to explore why demand for home-care services has fallen short of expectations. Doing so will tease out some of the problems of service delivery which are important for both understanding the past and planning for the future.

Clearly much of the shortfall can be attributed to a slowed growth in hospital admissions for HIV-related diseases and AIDS and the expansion of residential health-care services for PWAs. With fewer episodes of acute care and more institutional care alternatives, demand for home-care services would necessarily slacken. Beyond these powerful system influences, however, we should examine how the special constraints and requirements of home care for different sub-groups of PWAs have further slowed the growth of the service system.

It is important to recognize that available service data are incomplete and, at times, inconsistent. Some PWAs undoubtedly receive home-care services unrecorded by various governmental and provider information systems: the care is purchased privately (and often off-the-books) or is provided solely by family and friends. These numbers are small, however, and probably declining given the movement of the epidemic toward lower-income populations.

A more significant issue is the marked deterioration of the DAS case-management function since its creation by HRA in 1986. After a brief administrative honeymoon, DAS quickly succumbed to what might be called regression to bureaucratic mediocrity: significant turnover among the case-work staff generated hard-to-fill vacancies and eventual replacements with less ardor and competence. Caseload ratios increased dramatically, leading to significant delays of several months in intake and assessment during the past three years. Thwarted by the reemergence of bureaucratic behaviors, some PWAs have reportedly given up their efforts to secure services while others have literally died waiting. Similarly frustrated, hospital discharge planners are reportedly circumventing the DAS approval process for home-care services by referring cases directly to agencies.

If the system has grown less able to respond quickly to the care needs of PWAs, it is also important to grapple with aversion of other PWAs to the notion of receiving home-care services. For reasons we will explore more fully later in this chapter, an unknown but not negligible number of PWAs reject home-care services, equating them with defeat and imminent death. This attitude, which often blends a steely drive for autonomy and self-reliance with blinding denial, simply cannot permit the intrusion of home care. The broad rejection of hospice care by most PWAs reflects the starkest statement of this assessment and motivation, which applies as well to home-care services.

The youth of most PWAs, the sudden onset of their illness, and expectations of a quick and complete recovery of functional capabilities also reinforce latent denial of the need for home-care services. Some analysts argue that in this regard PWAs are fundamentally different from elderly persons whose chronic health conditions have prepared them to accept and even seek service. But the well-known hesitancy of many elderly persons to accept in-home care suggests that we may be observing a threshold barrier common to both populations, but one which looms higher for PWAs.

For some PWAs home care is an intrusion unwelcome for quite different reasons. Substance-abusing PWAs, most typically IDUs, cannot tolerate the constant surveillance that accompanies the provision of home-care services. Whether they are dealing or just using drugs, these PWAs have a need for privacy that generally overwhelms the desire for services.

Substance-abusing PWAs are not alone in confronting home care's intrusion on their privacy. Other PWAs live in such fear of stigmatization and social abandonment by family, friends, or neighbors that they conceal, as best they can, the nature if not the fact of their illness. In this regard, home-care services represent a threat. The regular arrival and departure of nurses and aides, together with the delivery of equipment and supplies, signal a serious health problem which can trigger a sequence of socially explosive disclosures. Professionals report of parking their automobiles several blocks from the PWA's residence, of not having sickroom supplies delivered directly to the PWA's residence, and similarly crafted evasions which speak to the profound fear of stigmatization. And while we might hope that with the knowledge and familiarity that come with the passage of time irrational fears of AIDS might abate, it is likely that the movement of the epidemic from the gay communities to the more recently affected low-income communities has negated such a change. Increasing numbers of PWAs live in neighborhoods whose social, cultural, and religious mores are aggressively hostile to the behaviors associated with the spread of AIDS. This observation does not minimize the continuing, hard-fought battle waged in the gay community against employment and housing discrimination triggered by AIDS; but instead it underscores the sad truth that the same battles must be fought again and again.

If social stigmatization can thwart or distort the demand for home-care services, some analysts believe that many PWAs living in minority, low-income neighborhoods (where the epidemic is spreading most rapidly) are culturally less well prepared to seek and receive services. A variety of factors are at play, including suspicion of government, a belief that family should look after its own, poor self-esteem, and a long established tradition of being the givers, not the receivers, of service. Other analysts, however, observe a general familiarity and comfort with entitlements in these very same neighborhoods. When coupled with the often manipulative behavior of persons with addiction histories, it is easy to depict an alternative scenario of heavy service utilization. While the accurate measurement of the respective influence of cultural background and individual personality traits on service demand requires a substantial research program, it may be true that for some minority of cases a basic appetite for service overwhelms otherwise powerful cultural inhibitions.

While cultural expectations may well have a net effect of suppressing demand for home-care services, two other factors of life in low-income communities also play significant but not well-documented roles in shaping demand. First is the simple fact that without housing, a PWA cannot receive home-care services. To the extent that PWAs are homeless (and all studies find a proportion to be so), they are excluded from home care. More difficult to measure is the number of PWAs who live in housing that is so substandard as to be unserviceable. This may mean single rooms without refrigerators, dependable electricity, telephones, private toilets, or adequate physical space to accommodate a personal-care worker or needed equipment. Housing of this sort cannot support a home-care plan. Residences where crime is so rampant that agencies cannot send in professional or paraprofessional staff also cannot be serviced. The prevalence of shockingly poor housing in most low-income neighborhoods has in all likelihood reduced the demand for service.

Even when adequate housing is available, it is valuable to remember that, as the saying goes, a house is not a home, which is required for home care. Without the dependable support of family, friends, or caring neighbors, home care is often not a viable service option. Consequently the availability of these informal caregivers – most commonly found in stable environments – has become an increasing concern to agencies charged with providing home care to more socially isolated or marginal persons.

In conclusion, this brief review of the obstacles impeding the delivery of home-care services to PWAs is indeed sobering; at the same time, it is important to recognize what has been achieved against significant odds in New York City in the past decade. But if we are to learn how to better deliver more accessible and appropriate services with greater efficiency and effectiveness, we need to design and execute rigorous, longitudinal, person-based research. While we look forward to the products of this research, our analysis to date has identified three core themes which are integral to home-care services for PWAs:

1 home-care personnel, especially nurses and paraprofessional aides;
2 the caregiving environment, including PWA attitudes and the role of informal supports provided by family and friends; and
3 the administrative and regulatory structure guiding service provision.

A fuller examination of these themes, drawing on the experience gained to date in providing home-care services to PWAs, will allow us to speculate on the direction of several important trends. By relating that experience to other populations served by the home-care system – especially the dependent elderly – we will try to extract several generalizable lessons of encouragement and caution.

IV Staffing the System

Among the various types of health-care services perhaps none is so dependent on personnel as home care. It was therefore a grave concern in the early years of the epidemic that rampant fear of AIDS – grounded in a poor understanding of the risks of transmission for health-care workers and played out in a generally tight labor market – would cripple the creation of AIDS health services. Fearing the absence of adequate staffing, some health planners floated concepts of a dedicated AIDS corps, lauded the ethos of the plague doctors, and budgeted hefty salary increases and service bonuses.

Much to the surprise of most observers, securing adequate staffing for a burgeoning AIDS services network never proved to be a broad or irreversible problem. To be sure, there have been spot shortages in particular institutions, agencies, or neighborhoods, but not the industry-wide problem anticipated by so many.

The reasons for this unexpected outcome are, in retrospect, not so surprising. The ready supply of home-care nurses – right in the midst of the ballyhooed nursing shortage – speaks to two important factors. First, nurses quickly incorporated the facts about transmission and risk, and their knowledge of infectious diseases overcame fear and anxiety. Second, home-care nursing for PWAs presented an unusually challenging opportunity to use and hone their genuine capacity for caring, and their clinical and management skills. For many nurses, care of PWAs perfectly captured their motivation for choosing nursing as a profession.

Personal care workers (aides and attendants) were also feared to be in short supply. Several agencies fielded special recruitment and training programs which offered extra incentives and resources to prospective staff. Although few of these programs were rigorously assessed, they appeared to be well received and of high quality, and their efforts undoubtedly lessened some worker fears. But a more negative phenomenon probably accounts for the relatively ready supply of personal care workers since the late 1980s – a sour economy. The recession effectively limited the job options available to these paraprofessionals, yielding the twin effect of reducing departure from the existing workforce and bringing to it an increasing flow of eager and otherwise thwarted applicants.

Because of these professional and social trends the home-care services system for PWAs has had an adequate supply of personnel. Accordingly, the focus of attention shifted to how to better train and support these staff. The perception that AIDS presented complex and dynamic clinical issues and that professional caregivers were at greater risk of "burnout" stimulated the creation of special training and support services. While the reasons are diverse, and change with time and place, nursing administrators commonly identify three special sources of additional stress: the disease's complexity in terms of its clinical manifestations and psychosocial effects; the imminence of patient death; and the fact that most of these terminally ill patients are relatively young and of the same generation as their formal caregivers. Caring for PWAs appears to be harder on the mind and the spirit.

Most home-care agencies have enhanced their orientation and in-service training resources and enriched their supervisory capacities to meet these additional demands. By most accounts their efforts have been well received and workforce skills have risen to the desired level.

The agencies' efforts to address the psychological and emotional toll exacted by caring for PWAs, however, have yielded more mixed results and some interesting lessons. The creation of caregiver support groups has by and large proven to be poorly received. The activities fit neither the schedule nor preferences of home-care nurses, among whom there appears to be a reluctance to admit a need for help. Consequently, they appear to fare better with individually tailored programs of counseling and respite. Good, supportive supervision seems to be adequate to the task, and, resources permitting, a feature of competent agency management.

Anticipation of professional burnout encouraged the VNSNY to carefully consider how it would deploy its nursing staff to cover a growing PWA caseload. Rather than create a dedicated AIDS services unit, which might have had advantages in terms of targeting educational resources and refining clinical expertise, VNSNY decided to maintain nursing caseloads that mixed PWAs with other types of patients. As a result, it established some capacity for "structured respite," enabling nursing staff to step out of the especially intensive, emotionally draining PWA service environment.

Other agencies have pursued a dedicated AIDS service strategy out of both necessity and choice. Some agencies have been established only to meet the needs of PWAs and have no access to mixed caseloads. Others, motivated in part by a concern with building clinical expertise and managing competition between AIDS and other types of cases for nursing attention, have opted for special units. They, too, have had success in meeting the support needs of their nurses and report low levels of turnover together with continuing high rates of personal satisfaction and commitment.

Discussions with nursing administrators suggest that nursing care for PWAs accentuates many of the characteristics of care for geriatric patients: death is more imminent; crisis management more common; services more complex; and plans of care more fluid. While not discounting the demands of geriatric home care, the VNSNY clearly sees it as a respite from the emotional toll exacted by PWA care.

Looking to the future demands on nursing and paraprofessional staff, two phenomena – one new and one renewed – loom large on the horizon. Each threatens to further distinguish care for PWAs from care for the dependent elderly. First, the new. AIDS is becoming more of a chronic disease as we learn how to reduce the frequency or intensity of opportunistic diseases and related medical complications. Many of these treatments are delivered by infusion, bringing to increasing numbers of homes a comparatively complex technology. Substandard housing and undependable informal supports will undermine the viability of this type of home care or place greater burdens on home-care staff at greater cost to the system. As infusion technology is introduced into high-risk environments, it will demand more sophisticated decision making from nurses and attentive, supportive care from paraprofessionals. Given the direction of the epidemic in terms of the persons affected and the neighborhoods in which they live, we can only expect an escalation in the challenges home-care personnel confront.

If infusion technology poses new challenges, the resurgence of tuberculosis (TB) represents an insidiously renewed threat to sustaining a committed, competent workforce. Infectious-disease experts, who dealt well with exaggerated fears of accidental HIV transmission, find the threat posed by TB more difficult to address. A significant number of all PWAs will have active TB, which after proper treatment for a considerable time will not be infectious. But the corridor for error in either diagnosis or treatment is wide, potentially exposing home-care staff to real risks of infection, which take on a heightened significance in light of the spread of multiple drug resistant (MDR) TB. These risks are greatest for aides who often spend long hours with PWAs in close quarters.

Home-care agencies, supported by government, will have to institute aggressive TB screening and educational campaigns to bring a greater measure of security to their staffs. Failure to act, coupled with a few well-publicized mini-epidemics of TB (such as those that have already coursed through several prisons and hospitals), could grievously undermine the confidence and commitment of the home-care workforce.

V Informal Supports

Without informal supports – the direct caregiving, management assistance, and environmental support provided by family and friends – home care becomes increasingly difficult and expensive to deliver. Not only does it become necessary to purchase more formal services, the home-care plan also becomes more tenuously grounded, more unstable. A shortage of information and support resources in the home heightens the risk of inattention and inaction in response to the inevitable but unpredictable crisis. The rich literature detailing the importance of informal supports to the viability and quality of home-care services informed the early development of home care for PWAs; the varied experience of the past decade has further enriched our understanding.

It is all too easy to drift from helpful generalizations to extreme, misleading stereotypes. Therefore, we must carefully appraise two common images: the community of empowered, mutually supporting gay PWAs and the Hobbesian world of the socially outcast, drug-abusing PWA. Behind most stereotypes lies some reality – and these are no exception – but a closer examination reveals more ambiguous patterns offering both hope and concern.

The first model AIDS service system emerged in San Francisco in the early 1980s, grounded on the voluntary efforts of family, friends, and community. The self-help ethos, driven by necessity and sociopolitical preference, manifested itself in New York as well, perhaps most visibly and productively in the form of the Gay Men's Health Crisis. As members of New York's gay community centered in Greenwich Village and Chelsea Clinton advocated with unprecedented fervor and effectiveness for prevention, health care, social services, and the like, it was only natural that their supportive caregiving for ill partners and friends would become an expected and common feature of the home-care system. Home-care professionals are quick to praise this mutual support, on which so much home care depends, but they also remind us that all is not what we might wish.

Various stresses and obstacles undermine the informal support system that has served so many gay PWAs so well. Professionals have observed that as the city's DAS caseworkers – for all the criticism leveled against them – implement publicly financed service plans, it becomes more difficult to keep in place direct care given by family and friends. (This phenomenon of formal services substituting for, rather than complementing, informal services is a feature of the geriatric home-care system as well, but hard evidence documenting its prevalence and pattern is lacking.)

Looking not to the system's issues but to the psycho-dynamics of caregiving, professionals also note a pattern of frequent and accelerated burnout among many caregivers. Seeing too much of themselves and their futures in the illness of their friends, some caregivers flee from the caregiving role in a form of self-defense. For others, the physical and time demands of caregiving may gradually outstrip their personal resources, particularly if they themselves are ill.

While the predominant patterns of informal caregiving in the gay community remain positive but subject to deterioration, the picture that surfaces in low-income, minority neighborhoods where drug abuse is the most significant vector of infection is not as bleak as first anticipated. For one thing, a significant portion of the PWAs in these neighborhoods are women and their children who are able to marshall an extensive array of family supports. Many of these women have been responsible for heading their households for some time. However, for some women their relatively stable family and community roles ironically can constitute a serious obstacle to receiving informal support. According to some reports, the stigma of AIDS remains so potent that some women fear disclosure if they seek aid and choose instead to struggle without help to avoid the risk of familial and social ostracism.

Analyzing the informal supports available to male PWAs, who often are active drug users, poses an even more difficult challenge. Some, to be sure, are social isolates: homeless, without family or friends able to offer assistance. By all reports, however, most drug-abusing PWAs have more extensive supports than originally anticipated. What has been difficult for home-care agencies to identify and assess is the quality, reliability, and durability of these supports. The personal and social disorganization of many PWAs, their impulsive behavior, their manipulative yet often charming ways, do not drive away all family supports. The cultural imperative to look after one's own remains powerful in most communities, and, despite their often anti-social behavior, most of these PWAs have access to various sources of informal support.

With experience, home-care agencies have grown more accustomed to dealing with unorthodox patterns of support, and remain impressed with how families in crisis can cobble together some imaginative care plans. What has proven especially difficult for the agencies is the issue of predictability. Given the complexity of care to be provided at home and the volatility of the PWA's clinical status, can a comprehensive plan of care prove viable if the informal supports so integral to the plan are not truly reliable? And what risks are run in the event that the PWA rejects informal aid or that its provision, initially made in a period of short-term crisis, is not extended over time? The assessment of these risks and benefits seriously challenges the skills of home-care nurses with unprecedented complexity and consequences.

The fragility of informal support systems for PWAs is, according to the reports of professionals, more pronounced than is found in families caring for dependent elderly. And, referring again to the basic distinction between gay, middle-class PWAs and largely minority, low-income, drug-abusing PWAs, we find greater fragility in the informal supports available to the latter.

Several factors account for these differences. As compared to the elderly, the clinical status of PWAs is perceived as more demanding and distressing. Not only do caregivers have to deal with clinical manifestations of the disease that are more physically demanding, but the clinical status is more likely to change dramatically and suddenly. Clinical volatility poses a significant added burden as it plays havoc with predictable expectations of the PWA's needs, and such predictability is important to informal caregivers, as it enables them to define their role and activities.

Concomitant with changing clinical status are variable psychosocial conditions. The unsurprising prevalence of anger among PWAs about their illness takes a special toll. To it we must add a powerful desire for independence, for maintaining self-mastery, and for engaging in as social a life as possible. As a result of these needs – coupled with often astounding improvements and declines in clinical status – informal supports for PWAs carry especially heavy responsibilities and are often the only object available for a range of extreme emotions and behaviors. Similarly, the effect of dementia among PWAs on their informal caregivers reportedly takes a different and more demanding course. Largely because of their relative youth and anger, dementia in PWAs can lead to more frequent and more physical behavior changes, which further jeopardize the viability of informal supports.

These clinical and psychosocial factors suggest how difficult it will prove to be to sustain informal supports in the home-care plans of PWAs. The intensity of these factors challenges the commitment and capabilities of family and friends in ways different from the challenge presented to caregivers of dependent elderly. Moreover, these caregiving demands are being made in what are increasingly more trying and unsupportive environments. As more PWAs are found in socially disadvantaged, low-income neighborhoods, caregivers must function in the midst of marginal housing and without benefit of deep social and financial resources. Living so close to the edge, the caregiving role of family can be overwhelmed by a significant change in either the PWA's condition or the social environment they share. It is no comfort, therefore, to hear of case conferences with families struggling under these circumstances in which, in the words of one nurse, "AIDS never comes up," because the families are buffeted by such competing social needs as housing, crime, employment, or welfare.

Home-care agencies, working in tandem with government and community-based service organizations running the gamut from churches to self-help groups of PWAs, must directly address the problem of precarious and deteriorating informal supports. Devising programs to encourage, reward, and give respite to caregiving family and friends should be central to this effort, and the lessons learned from the design of similar programs for family caregivers of the dependent elderly should be instructive. At the same time, it is important to remember that elder care tends to demand long-term commitment to less intense situations. While care for PWAs is no longer quite so short-term and crisis-oriented, we have seen that its demands are qualitatively different and will not be well-served by a cookie-cutter replication of existing programs.

A second theme which requires careful attention involves the assessment, conducted largely by nurses, of the appropriateness and viability of family supports. This assessment process engages two difficult tasks. First, nurses need to understand and translate the value of supports being offered in different cultures and social environments. This diagnostic exercise brings true meaning to the concept that home-care professionals are guests in the homes of the people they serve and they need to understand the mores and behaviors of those homes. The second and no less difficult task requires the nurse to work with her professional colleagues and her patient and family to define and apply the concept of acceptable risk. Although easy to state, this process involves a consideration of not only professional obligations but also the interests of PWAs and their families, which of course are not always identical or compatible. As home-care services become more technologically complex and managerially demanding, and as they are provided in more socially marginal settings, it becomes increasingly important that we devise a decision-making process that satisfactorily integrates and balances the needs and preferences of PWAs, families, and health-care professionals.

VI Shaping a System

The enormous supply of formal and informal caregiving resources for PWAs is directed and supported by what we commonly call the "system," a word that implies more structure and consistency than reality would justify. The following observations do not attempt to fully define what services an ideal system might comprise or how they would be organized. Our goal is more modest: to examine a series of issues about the structure, delivery, and staffing of home-care services for PWAs that testify to newly gained strengths and reveal potential faults. From this brief examination we will identify several lessons of value to the broader home-care and health-care system.

Planning for Care

The process of designing and implementing care plans for PWAs is subject to two problems familiar to analysts of services for the dependent elderly: inadequate hospital discharge planning and a deliberately segmented government structure for need assessment and service approval. In both respects, the experience of PWAs seeking home care underscores the limitations of familiar policies and programs.

Hospital discharge planners working with PWAs are not quite so constrained by time, because hospital stays for AIDS patients in New York continue to be paid through a per diem rate. But the product – the service plan – is limited by the availability of so few choices of post-hospital care services and the practical difficulties of accurately assessing in the hospital what the needs, preferences, and resources of PWAs and their families will be after the hospitalization. The range of services has broadened in recent years with the creation of additional institutional resources, several day-treatment programs, and an AIDS-specific certified home health agency. But service choices remain limited; and, as we have seen, the potential for bringing home care into an increasing number of PWA homes is challenged by unfavorable housing and family environments. What is more, the resurgence of TB – a real threat to both formal and family caregivers – threatens to overwhelm hard-pressed planning and service resources.

Compounding the problems of discharge planning is the frustration of PWAs and health-care professionals with the HRA "two-step": need assessment, service planning, and case management by DAS and service authorization by the separate Bureau of Medical Review. Familiar arguments about the need to separate client advocacy from service authorization from service provision rule the day and compel PWAs (and dependent elderly persons alike) to negotiate a fragmented care system. The fragmentation leads to extensive delays and continuing difficulties with co-ordinating services.

These system deficiencies – and the design of suitable alternatives – have long been debated by students of home-care and long-term care services. The recent national debate centering on managed care has taken the issues into the context of the health-care system most broadly defined. The experience of PWAs, with their fast growing numbers, complex care needs, and uncertain home environments, casts these familiar issues into stark relief. Regrettably, that experience has not yet surfaced significant innovations that could advance progress toward a more streamlined, responsive system for planning care.

Managing care
Home care for PWAs has always been distinguished by an appreciation of its special intensity, complexity, and volatility. As we have seen, HRA concluded that the unpredictability of change in the clinical status of PWAs and the speed at which care services had to be deployed called for an unorthodox approach to care management. VNSNY nurses were empowered to independently alter service plans, and by all reports their ability to do so has been critically important to the success of the program. What is more, agency changes have seldom met with retroactive disapproval from HRA.

As care in the home is likely to become more complex with the expanded role of infusion technology and a greater diversity of drug therapies, it is especially important to preserve the professional discretion of home-care nurses. Their ability to assess, educate, monitor, and make swift resource-allocation decisions will become even more pivotal in the delivery of home-care services to PWAs. While nurses continue to play so important a role, it is fair to ask what role physicians should play.

Since the first years of the epidemic, a small number of physicians have occupied prominent positions in the struggle to understand the disease, devise appropriate interventions, and advocate for necessary financing and supportive public policies. But when it comes to home-care services, the report card is not so positive. Nursing administrators and others perceive a system in which physicians are noticeable by their absence, a pattern which holds equally true for the provision of home care to the dependent elderly.

The most fundamental criticism of physicians is that they do not understand home care – what it can do and for whom – and that as home-care services expand so does the gap between their hospital-based practices and the full range of needs of their patients. As physicians become more involved with and knowledgeable about home care, critics also argue that they will bring some sorely needed strengths to home care. Continued advances in the use of increasingly complex drug therapies will depend in part on physicians' ability to monitor patient status, adjust dosages, and manage symptoms. Much of this work would be done in collaborative partnership with nurses, which speaks to the desire for another profound change: physicians must become more active care leaders but as integral players on a necessarily multidisciplinary team. If they remain uninformed, unengaged, and unsupportive, it will be difficult to expand and improve the quality of home-care services.

Advocates for greater physician involvement also point out that home care could better understand and respond to physician needs. For example, rather than require a physician to deal with a different nurse for each patient receiving home care – a logistical and communications nightmare – a liaison or coordinating nurse could greatly improve the management of care and more productively engage physicians.

The management of home-care services for PWAs has shown real promise in the work accomplished by nurses and in the expanded role physicians could play. While the care of dependent elderly persons may not typically demand such intensive care-management resources, patterns of care needs suggest that elder care is moving in the direction of PWA care: sicker individuals, more complex interventions, and more uncertain informal supports. Consequently, it would be in the interests of public funders and regulators to test the utility of empowering home-care agencies with greater responsibility for the type of independent care management that has worked so well with the PWA caseload. The proven ability of government to define and monitor this authority constitutes a solid platform from which it could be extended more broadly in the home-care system.

Looking beyond the management of in-home services to the management of all needed supports – housing, income, legal services, and the like – we find the PWA experience with what is called case management less encouraging. It is critical to recall that home care is, or should be, one of an array of complementary community-care services. The division of responsibility between DAS and the home-care agency (which can be further compounded by the involvement of a variety of service agencies each of which may perceive a role for itself in the overall management of the case) has seriously inhibited the development of a comprehensive, coordinating mechanism. The complexity of PWA care needs heightens the demand for a responsive, comprehensive management capacity.

Again, we find a comparable, though less universal and intense, need among geriatric home-care clients. Recent analyses of how well complementary services are utilized to effectively support increasingly frail and dependent persons underscore both the potential value and regrettable absence of an effective management resource. While not all elderly persons may need case management to the extent PWAs do, we should aggressively experiment with different strategies to create genuine case management. Failure to do so will force the system to blindly demand more of in-home services, which in turn will escalate their costs while undermining their safety and viability.

Thinking about care

Although often shunted to the periphery of the debate over national health-care policy, home care – and more specifically home care for PWAs – offers several important lessons about the likely direction and limitations of the reform impulse.

More intriguing than shifts in approaches to structuring and financing PWA health-care services is the admittedly incomplete and still elusive reappraisal of what used to be called patients. Many PWAs are anything but: they do not, as the dictionary definition would have it, endure their condition with calmness; nor do they acceptingly await the outcome of a fatal disease. These PWAs shed some revealing light on a key actor in the promised world of managed care and managed competition – the consumer, informed and deliberate as well as anomic and recalcitrant.

The activism of some PWAs, many of them gay men conditioned to wage battle by a long struggle for civil rights and protection against discrimination, has reaped several stunning victories. The modification of sacrosanct policies governing the testing and distribution of new pharmaceuticals and alternative treatments testifies to the power of their impassioned, well-organized activism. For these PWAs, AIDS as a personal or community challenge became a defining crisis. Many took charge of their own care, selecting and setting the pace of treatment. Often knowing as much as their physicians (or at least believing they did), these PWAs represent a type of informed, empowered consumer unlike anything conjured up in Jackson Hole.

The experience of these medico-social PWA activists also surfaced a theme that courses unevenly through much of the debate over health-care reform: a sharply ambivalent attitude toward physicians and corporate health care. The traditional respect for physicians as a professional elite, once so typical of elderly patients, is not common among PWAs. To be sure, a PWA's own physician may be lauded, but it seems that individual experiences do not translate into general appraisals.

Increasing hostility toward physicians is intimately entwined with antagonism toward what is perceived to be a prosperous lifestyle. Growth in personal incomes, much like the hefty profit margins of pharmaceutical companies, leaves a bitter taste in a community marked by deterioration and death, and does little to sustain traditional attitudes grounded in the concepts of physician service and patient deference. As the receipt of health-care services becomes so deeply etched by economics, roles and expected behaviors must change: a world of physicians and patients is being replaced by a marketplace of providers and consumers.

For the other albeit stereotypical PWA – the personally and socially disorganized individual often living with the consequences of a history of substance abuse in a low-income, minority neighborhood – AIDS has evoked a response that also jeopardizes visions of a world of informed, managed health care. These PWAs also are not reverential, or even deferential, toward physicians and the health-care system. They are, too often, non-compliant with medical instructions, but for reasons more typically associated with indifference than self-conscious, organized militancy.

For many of these PWAs (and their families) AIDS is not the defining issue it has become in many parts of the gay community. It is but another in a litany of social woes, having to compete for attention and limited resources. Adhering to medication regimens, for example, in the face of poverty, homelessness, continuing substance abuse, and the like is no easy matter, as documented by recent studies of the completion of TB treatment. While their environmental circumstances make it difficult for some socially disadvantaged PWAs to successfully act the role of compliant patient, for others personality is a major obstacle to care. The often demanding and manipulative behaviors described by many professionals defy notions of a patient's calm endurance. Rather than follow a steady course, many PWAs exhibit mercurial swings of heavy service utilization and abrupt disengagement from the system.

These PWAs – whose behaviors and motivation are far more complex than the preceding discussion conveys – pose a different sort of challenge to health-care reform premised on the concept of the informed choices made by responsible consumers. We have already seen a bold policy initiative for childhood immunizations run headlong into the reality that real access involves more than adequate financing and infrastructure for service delivery. Drawing on the past decade's experience, students of home care for PWAs would have quickly cautioned the Clinton administration that prospective consumers have to both share a belief in the value of the proffered service and live in circumstances that are, at minimum, not hostile to its provision. Unless these necessary conditions are satisfied, expectations for the full participation of either traditional patients or more futuristic consumers in the health-care system will not be realized. Systemic reform will be at best grossly incomplete, leaving many of the most vulnerable only tangentially engaged and served by the health-care system.

In conclusion, the PWAs' experiences with home care, and the health-care system more generally, suggest that we must thoughtfully reappraise definitions of patient and consumer behavior. As we have seen, home-care services must be reorganized to better satisfy what are increasingly divergent perceptions of need and the social contexts in which they are to be provided. The campaign for national health-care reform – so heavily grounded on the principle of informed consumerism and appropriately directed to bringing marginalized populations into a mainstream health-care system – has much to learn from what should be a period of bold experimentation in the design of home-care services for PWAs.

Note

1   In this chapter the term PWA comprises both persons with HIV-related illness as well as persons living with CDC-defined AIDS.

12

Home Care for Persons with Serious Mental Illnesses

Allan V. Horwitz and Susan Reinhard

Introduction

Despite the many deficiencies of state hospitals, these institutions historically provided people with serious mental illnesses a panoply of benefits including shelter, food, medical care, and social interaction. However, for the past several decades policy has emphasized the benefits of living in the community and the detriments of hospital life for people with serious mental illnesses (Grob 1991). The impact of this deinstitutionalization policy has been dramatic: between 1955 and 1992 the number of patient residents in state and county mental institutions dropped from 550,000 to under 100,000 (Center for Mental Health Services 1992). Yet, systems to replace services previously found within state institutions have not yet been developed to any great extent for the growing numbers of people with serious mental illnesses in the community. There is no consistent and integrated home-care policy in the United States to deal with this group. Policies of home care must be considered within the context of providing a range of integrated services to people with serious mental illnesses who will live in the community for most of their lifetimes and require at most only short and intermittent institutional stays.

The provision of home care for seriously mentally ill people involves a number of complex issues. The concept of "home care" itself is inherently problematic for the majority of the seriously mentally ill. Because few people with serious mental illnesses spend extended periods of time within institutions, this population is no longer homogenous in regard to their places of residence. Instead, persons with persistent mental illness fall within at least three residential categories.

One group – estimated to encompass between one- and two-thirds of persons with serious mental illnesses – live with family members, usually parents (Goldman 1982). However, the ability of parents to provide long-term care is limited by age and disability. Further, clients, family caretakers, and professionals agree that family homes do not provide the best long-run living arrangements for consumers. A second group resides in residential treatment facilities provided by state, non-profit, and private for-profit organizations. These include board and care facilities, group homes, halfway houses, mental institutions, and supervised apartments. Residential alternatives to inpatient institutions currently house only a small proportion of persons with serious mental illnesses (Randolph, Ridgway, and Carling 1991). Finally, one highly publicized group – the homeless mentally ill – has no consistent place of lodging at all. Although estimates of the number of homeless mentally ill vary tremendously, they form a substantial group (Bachrach 1992). Housing is clearly the most pressing priority for the homeless mentally ill (Adams 1993; Milstray 1993). None of these three groups has homes in the traditional sense of owning or renting their own dwellings. The vast range and diversity of living situations makes any single definition of "home" problematic for this population.

We define home care as services that promote the use of regular housing stock, consumer choice in living arrangements, a separation of treatment and residence, permanency in housing, and flexible supports delivered in natural living environments (e.g. Test and Stein 1980; Bond et al. 1988; Bond et al. 1989; Taube, Goldman, and Salkever 1990; Carling 1993). One essential element of home care is that clients live in normal community housing rather than in institutions or in residential treatment facilities. Because few clients with serious mental illnesses live in their own homes, the *provision* of a "home" is usually an aspect of home care. Further, in home care, service delivery is organized around the client's own environment. Health-care providers reach out to clients rather than expect clients to go to mental health facilities for essential services.

Home Care for Persons with Serious Mental Illnesses

Evidence (outlined below) has accumulated that programs promoting service provision in clients' own homes lead to higher rates of community tenure, less use of inpatient facilities, and higher perceived quality of life than other modes of service delivery. Although many persons with serious mental illnesses still require long-term care, this care no longer need be synonymous with custodial or residential care. Instead, long-term care can provide continuous management of disabilities that promotes independent community living consistent with client choices and goals (Mechanic 1993). The challenge for policymakers is to implement home care in a mental health-service environment in which budgets are still disproportionately oriented toward institutional care and services are still too fragmented to provide optimal benefits to the seriously mentally ill population.

Home care is the policy most consistent with the philosophy of individual autonomy and choice that underlies contemporary policies toward disabled populations. Although there have been numerous critiques of many aspects of deinstitutionalization and community care (e.g. Lamb 1988; Johnson 1990; Lamb 1993), it is highly unlikely that trends away from institutional care will be reversed in the foreseeable future. Legal mandates forbidding involuntary commitments except under tightly defined circumstances, the desires of people with serious mental illnesses to live in the community, the shift in policymaking toward community treatment, and a social environment favorable toward personal liberty and hostile toward institutional care, ensure that most people with serious mental illnesses will spend most of their time in the community. The challenge is to develop policies that maximize the well-being and liberties of afflicted individuals, support their familial caregivers, and replace services that institutions previously provided in the most cost-effective ways possible.

Components of Home Care

There is broad agreement among experts that, aside from a small proportion of seriously mentally ill people who need extended periods of hospitalization, home care is both a feasible and an essential component of optimal mental health treatment (Mechanic 1986; Morrissey and Levine 1987; Goering et al. 1988; Lamb 1988; Seling and Johnson 1990; Torrey 1990; Thompson, Griffith, and Leaf 1990; Mechanic 1991). There is less consensus, however, on exactly what aspects of home care are most essential. Services that are provided within the home include therapeutic, social, coping, problem-solving, medication management, family education, and physical health interventions (Ritchie and Lusky 1987; Holt 1989; Brooker and Butterworth 1993; Duffy, Miller, and Parlocha 1993). Because systematic delivery of home-care services has been limited largely to model programs and to a few states, conclusive evidence on the particular components of successful home care does not exist. Aspects of effective home care include:

- Integration into a total service-delivery package that includes clinical, psychosocial, vocational, social, welfare, and physical health services (Morrissey and Levine 1987; Borland, McRae, and Lycan 1989; Kanter 1989; Thobaben 1989; Witheridge 1989; Taube et al. 1990; Bachrach 1989).
- Responsibility for clients on a long-term, not episodic, basis (Mechanic 1986; Kanter 1989; Morse et al. 1992). The persistent nature of major mental illnesses and the resulting impact on many aspects of social functioning mandate continuous rather than sporadic service provision.
- A stable funding component (Torrey 1990; Mechanic 1991). The fragmentation of funding for mental health services must be overcome and home care encompassed within permissible service delivery by major funding sources such as Medicaid and Medicare.
- Utilization of a multidisciplinary team, not an individual case manager (Holt 1989; Newton and Brauer 1989; Taube et al. 1990; Stein 1992).
- Flexible provision that varies by individualized client needs (Morrissey and Levine 1987; Kanter 1989; Brown et al 1991; England and Cole 1992). Services are not pre-packaged but change according to the social, psychological, and situational circumstances of clients.
- Stability of residence (Bond et al. 1989). An essential precondition of home care is that clients can count on a stable and secure place to live. The provision of housing is the most essential aspect of home care for the homeless mentally ill.
- Provision for social control of disruptive behaviors including programs of aggressive medication maintenance (Falloon et al. 1985; Lamb 1988). Because disruptive symptoms present a genuine threat to the possibility of successful community living, effective home-care programs will embody strategies of symptom management.

Home Care for Persons with Serious Mental Illnesses

- Integration of clients, professionals, families, and others (e.g. landlords, employers, roommates, etc.) in the natural living environment (Grella and Grusky 1989; Bernheim 1990; Taube et al. 1990; Brooker and Butterworth 1991; Mills and Hansen 1991; Carpentier et al. 1992; McFarlane, Stastny, and Deakins 1992). Home care recognizes the importance of significant others in community maintenance and brings them into treatment planning.
- Home care ideally involves clients living independently from their families. Most clients, families, and mental health professionals agree that community living outside of family homes is the preferred arrangement (Ridgway and Zipple 1990).
- When it is not possible for clients to reside independently, home care for persons living with families should include family support services including information about medication management and psycho-education (Brooker et al. 1992; McFarlane et al. 1992).

Evidence

A number of studies concur on outcomes consistently associated with successful home care and outcomes that are more variable across studies (Test and Stein 1980; Witheridge and Dincin 1985; Bond et al. 1988; Borland et al. 1989; Torrey 1990; Olfson 1990; Taube et al. 1990; Brown et al. 1991; Stein 1992; Burns 1993). Here, we only outline these conclusions. First, there is considerable evidence that clients in home-care programs have fewer episodes and shorter periods of hospitalization than those who do not receive these services. Second, participants in home-care programs consistently achieve longer tenure of independent life in the community than non-participants. Third, clients in home-care programs perceive a better quality of life. Finally, most authorities agree that effective home care can be provided at no more, although usually at no less, cost than institutional treatment (Weisbrod, Test, and Stein 1980; Bond et al. 1988; Taube et al. 1990; Halvorson 1992). In general the cost savings from lower hospitalization rates are offset by additional costs of providing community services.

Beyond the demonstrated decrease in hospitalization, increase in community tenure, and enhanced levels of consumer satisfaction, the benefits of home care have not been conclusively demonstrated.

There is considerable debate over whether home care raises client functioning, enhances employment status, ensures better medication compliance, and reduces symptoms (Lehman, Possidente, and Hawker 1986; Goering et al. 1988; Stein and Test 1980; Morse et al. 1992) or has little effect on these outcomes (Bond et al. 1988; Borland, McRae, and Lycan 1989; Olfson 1990; Taube et al. 1990; Burns 1993). Further, comparisons of home care and institutionalized groups sometimes do not fully control for differences in levels of disability. In addition, most studies that compare the costs of home care with those of other forms of care might underestimate the true costs of home-care services because they do not fully cost all community services (Wolff and Helminiak 1993). Finally, a major unresolved issue is exactly what aspects of home care account for its presumed effectiveness (Olfson 1990; Taube et al. 1990). Although a number of issues remain unresolved, the proven benefits of these programs as well as the values home care promotes warrant further efforts to diffuse these programs throughout the mental health-service system.

Special Populations

Because the seriously mentally ill are not one group but many subgroups with different problems, degrees of disability, and needs, the effective provision of home care must vary by several factors (Mechanic 1986). Those who exhibit symptoms involving acting out, violent and self-destructive behaviors, and drug abuse provide the most difficulties in arranging for home care and need more highly structured residential environments (Shanks 1989; Lamb and Lamb 1990). Aggressive social-control measures, including proactive medication management, might be necessary for maintaining this group in the community.

Clients of different ages seem to benefit from different sorts of home care. Home care for children and younger adolescents can usually be delivered in the family home (Halvorson 1992; England and Cole 1992). Services for youths should be aimed at bolstering and enhancing family support systems. Older adolescents and young adults with schizophrenia may desire independent living arrangements yet need structured residential care that includes external controls (Lamb 1988; Birmingham, MacLeod, and Farthing 1990). Home care for this group will ideally be outside the family home and recognize the fragile coexistence of desires for independence with

Home Care for Persons with Serious Mental Illnesses   275

intense dependency needs. Particular efforts at outreach must be made for the elderly, who rarely seek mental health care on their own initiative (Kruse and Wood 1989; Morgan and Weiman 1990). For the elderly, the involvement of primary health-care providers is a crucial aspect of home care in order to locate individuals in serious need of mental health services and to provide for extensive physical, as well as mental, health services (Buckwalter and Light 1989). Women may be especially concerned with home-care issues concerning children and safety (Goering et al. 1990). Providing home care to homeless mentally ill populations also presents special problems and issues including unusually stressful environments, high residential mobility, and value differences with professionals (Linn, Gelberg, and Leake 1990; Lamb and Lamb 1990; Goering et al. 1990; Bachrach 1992; Morse et al. 1992).

Implementation

The implementation of home-care policies can only be considered within the broader context of the overall mental health-care system. We believe that the major problem of this system lies in the lack of integration and fragmentation of services and funding. The most urgent needs are to establish mechanisms that provide home care within an integrated system of mental health services. Fundamental changes are required in the mental health-care system to establish home care as a component of an integrated system of care. Although some new funding would be necessary during the implementation stages, once operational, a system oriented toward home care need not require more funding than the current system. Rather, home care could be implemented through redirecting existing monies within the mental health system and capitalizing on existing federal programs. The most important changes that are needed must occur in four areas: housing, system integration, funding, and mental health professional education.

Housing

The most fundamental problem of home-care programs for persons with serious mental illnesses is that their clients are not likely to have homes. Unlike many other disabled populations, most of the seriously mentally ill do not own or rent their own homes. Therefore, these programs cannot consist solely of services brought to the home but must begin with the provision of an adequate residential setting itself.

Stable residences are an essential precondition for the provision of home care. However, a shortage of housing in communities is perhaps the most serious gap in most mental health systems (Carling 1993). The amount of low-cost public housing fell dramatically during the 1980s. The lack of adequate housing is a problem common to all economically disadvantaged groups, including the seriously mentally ill. The definition of who ought to provide housing for the seriously mentally ill is often not clear. Mental health agencies define housing as outside of their responsibilities. Public housing agencies, in turn, consider housing for the mentally ill as an issue the mental health system ought to handle. The result is that housing needs of the mentally ill are often ignored.

No single housing initiative will address the needs and preferences of consumers and families (Morrissey and Levine 1987; Tanzman 1993). The ideal system would include a range of supervised and supported housing settings that are part of an integrated service system (Lamb 1988; Bachrach 1989). Many experts now advocate a supported or normal housing model that is characterized by permanent residence in regular, scattered site, community housing (Cohen and Somers 1990; Knisley and Fleming 1993). The supported housing paradigm matches supports to the client rather than the house. Hence, the client can remain in one place while the intensity of services changes as the needs of the client change. Case-management teams deliver many services in clients' natural living environments; clients may seek other services in community facilities. However, residence and treatment are geographically separate. An additional benefit of supported housing is that it does not face the same degree of neighborhood opposition that hampers the implementation of group homes and other residential facilities. The National Association of State Mental Health Program Directors has issued a national policy statement urging states to move toward this sort of supported-housing (Livingston and Srebnick 1991).

The prospect of increased use of a supported housing model raises several policy issues:

- The provision of housing must be seen as a central aspect of the mental health-service system; when this is not feasible localities should consider the development of a specialized agency to

manage housing for persons with serious mental illnesses (Knisley and Fleming 1993).
- Collaborative efforts between federal, state, and local authorities and between the public and private sectors are necessary to develop new sources of housing or to capitalize on sources such as Housing and Urban Development (HUD) Section 8 housing (Carling 1990; Knisley and Fleming 1993). An important example is the five-year national demonstration program to provide Access to Community Care and Effective Services and Supports (ACCESS). Developed in cooperation with the Departments of HUD, Veterans Affairs, Labor, Education, and Agriculture, ACCESS creates incentives to integrate housing, treatment, and supportive services (Adams 1993).
- Unless developed as part of an integrated service system or under the aegis of a central mental health authority, scattered housing can reinforce the fragmentation of service delivery.
- Housing initiatives should be developed in tandem with integrated programs of case management discussed below. Otherwise, they may lack the necessary degree of structure and supervision that are found in more programmatic settings.
- Supported housing programs must be combined with non-residential programmatic activities to combat the possible loneliness, isolation, and lack of structured daily activities that might accompany community living (Hatfield 1993).
- More data are needed about what types of persons with serious mental illnesses require what types of housing situations and, in particular, which clients will need more structured residential settings (McCarthy and Nelson 1991).

System Integration

A central problem in delivering services to persons with serious mental illnesses is that different components of service packages — monetary assistance, housing, therapy, medication management, rehabilitation, health care, etc. — stem from different systems that are not themselves integrated with one another (Mechanic 1991). An additional complication is that different regulations and bureaucracies are attached to each separate component. Because home care is delivered outside of traditional mental health settings, it potentially can reinforce the fragmentation of this system. Therefore, it is critical that home care be incorporated within an integrated package of service delivery. There are several levels of system integration that can promote home care.

Case management
Case management has become an integral part of service delivery to persons with serious mental illnesses. An efficient system of case management can promote community living through helping consumers access and negotiate services within the mental health system. To maximize effectiveness, however, case managers should be more than links or brokers on behalf of the seriously mentally ill. Rather, they should be an integral part of the delivery system (Mechanic 1991). Ideally, a team of professionals would have long-term responsibility and authority for a caseload of between ten and twenty individuals (Taube et al. 1990; Stein 1992). Multidisciplinary continuous-care teams would provide, not just arrange, assertive outreach and direct care in natural living environments seven days a week (Kanter 1989; Thompson, Griffith, and Leaf 1990; Burns and Raftery 1991; Stein 1992).

Policies toward case management should emphasize:

- A continuous-care model that delivers services in a natural environment (Stein 1992).
- Care to a defined group of individuals rather than services to a catchment area (Mechanic 1992).
- Services provided by a team rather than a person; teams lend more stability and continuity because turnover is less problematic and problem-solving abilities are richer.
- Seven day, 24-hour availability of services optimizes crisis management and the ability of clients to remain in a community (Stein 1992).

PACT (Program in Assertive Community Treatment)
PACT is a further promising development in service integration. It uses, but goes beyond, continuous case management in providing an integrated range of services to clients in their natural living environments. This model of home care, developed in Madison, Wisconsin, is now widely used in five states (Delaware, Michigan, Ohio, Rhode Island, and Wisconsin) and 20 additional states have some PACT teams. In the PACT model, community-based teams provide a wide range of mental health, psychosocial, rehabilitation, and health-care services. This team is available seven days a week for 24 hours a day on a long-term basis. Services are provided in the

natural living environment of the client so the client need not seek help in an office- or clinic-based setting. PACT is also marked by an aggressive approach to medication compliance and social control to improve the quality of life of clients and their families.

We believe the principles of PACT can be one prominent model of home-care services for a number of reasons:

- PACT emphasizes independent living in normal housing.
- Home care is one component of an integrated system of mental health services.
- The recent diffusion of PACT across the country indicates the enthusiasm for this model within the public mental health system.
- Carefully controlled studies indicate several benefits of PACT compared to alternatives (less hospitalization, longer tenure in the community, higher perceived quality of life); in no area do PACT clients fare worse than those in alternative programs (client functioning, symptom reduction, medication compliance, employment status).
- Cost-effectiveness studies indicate that PACT programs are not more costly than institutional alternatives.
- The principles underlying PACT are flexible and easily modifiable to suit local environments.
- Because PACT is based on non-dogmatic principles it can be combined with other types of model programs (e.g. Fountain House; Fairweather Lodges).
- The flexible roles of providers, lack of distance between clients and providers, and emphasis on treatment in natural living environments render PACT suitable for populations such as younger clients, urban minorities, and dually-diagnosed individuals that are most difficult to serve through traditional treatment programs.
- Research has been an integral part of the development of PACT programs and has led to significant changes in these programs.

For all these reasons we feel that the expansion of PACT programs is warranted. Using a request for proposal (RFP) strategy, state governments could create financial incentives to replicate PACT. Further, policymakers should press for funding changes (discussed below) that will allow for more ample and stable funding for these programs. It is particularly important to test the effectiveness of these programs in urban areas, with minority populations, and with persons with co-morbid substance-abuse disorders (Burns 1993).

Mental health authorities

Mental health authorities are another option that can promote the integration of the mental health system. They are the central feature of the nine-city RWJ demonstration project. These agencies integrate the various agencies that service persons with serious mental illnesses into a single, local mental health authority (Goldman et al. 1994; Morrissey et al. 1993). They have responsibility for the entire mental health budget, all clinical mental health services (inpatient, outpatient, home care), and the administration of the mental health system in a defined area. The promise of mental health authorities is that they can integrate funding streams, direct resources to housing, and provide a variety of services in a flexible manner. Evidence from the RWJ demonstration project indicates that most demonstration sites successfully created local mental health authorities, although they were less successful in reorganizing community support systems (Morrissey et al. 1993). Because legislative changes are sometimes needed to create mental health authorities and because of the opposition from current mental health agencies, the political and administrative difficulties of implementing such far-reaching changes should not be underestimated. At the state level, the leadership, cooperation and commitment of governors, legislators, mental health-agency officials, and mental health advocates are crucial in creating these authorities.

Funding

A stable funding stream will be the essential underpinning for the expansion and diffusion of home-care policies. In an era of fiscal stringency, policymakers must capitalize on currently available resources. The major financial problems of implementing home care lie in the continued targeting of existing resources toward institutional rather than community-based care and in the restrictions on home care in the Medicaid and Medicare programs.

Funding for home-care programs requires negotiating the complicated maze of various funding streams available for certain types of home care. At present, the nation's mental health-care system is an uncoordinated mix of programs that cost $23.3 billion, with 70 percent of these costs financed through the public sector (Redick et al. 1992). State governments bear the greatest burden. Including their share of Medicaid, states account for about 45 percent of funding for treatment for persons with mental illnesses. About 60 percent of these funds are spent on inpatient care in state mental hospitals, with 21 percent spent on ambulatory care, and 8 percent on residential programs (Lutterman and Hollen 1992). The federal government accounts for about 18 percent of total treatment costs, including the federal share of Medicaid, Medicare, VA, and block grants, with local governments responsible for 7 percent of the total costs (Redick et al. 1992).

One obstacle toward implementing home-care policies is that, despite the dramatic decline in the actual use of state mental institutions, a disproportionate amount of public funding continues to support these institutions. In 1980, for example, 43 percent of direct costs for mental health care was spent in state mental hospitals and nursing homes that cared for only 7 percent of the nation's seriously mentally ill population (Sharfstein, Stoline, and Goldman 1993). Most of the remaining money goes to psychiatric treatment in general hospitals, community mental health centers, other outpatient care, and residential treatment facilities. The fraction spent on home care is so small that "home care" (or some synonym) does not even appear in data analyses of public expenditures.

Some inpatient facilities will continue to be necessary to provide intermittent stays for the most intractable cases of serious mental illness. However, as long as adequate community-based programs are available, there are no therapeutic reasons for maintaining extensive state hospital systems. To change the skewed funding ratio toward community care, state policymakers have to face the political challenge of closing, not merely downsizing, psychiatric hospitals. While this is a challenge that requires the courage and commitment of elected officials, it has been done in some states (Ohio is a notable example). One way of managing this challenge is to work with public employee unions to retrain their members as providers in natural living environments. New funding for home-care services can be captured from funds saved from current state hospital budgets. Mobilization of support from consumer, family, and professional advocacy groups is essential in redirecting funds and strengthening the infrastructure for community living.

Policymakers must also advocate changes in the Medicaid program. This program, administered by states but jointly funded by state and federal governments, accounts for 13 percent of public dollars spent on mental health care (Redick et al. 1992). There is substantial state-by-state variation in Medicaid eligibility and benefits (Lesseig 1987). This program has a built-in bias toward certain types of institutional care. Its coverage is limited to specific service incidents in health facilities (on-site, episodic care) rather than continuous supportive services for people living in the community. Although several important components of community-based care, including home care, case management and psychosocial rehabilitation, are optional under Medicaid, the majority of states have chosen to exclude them from Medicaid coverage. Further, reimbursable case management is limited to a "targeted" model that includes linking and monitoring functions but excludes direct provision of services and crisis intervention (Taube, Goldman, and Salkever 1990). Medicaid's restriction regarding on-site provision of clinical services prevents reimbursement for mobile clinic programs that are a central feature of assertive case management provided in the natural living environment of clients.

Medicare is a second federal program that might offer some opportunities for capturing funding for home care with appropriate changes in regulations. About 7 percent of Medicare dollars are spent on mental health care (Redick et al. 1992) to cover acute illness and the medical (but not the social) management of chronic illness. Possible beneficiaries include mentally ill persons over 65 and those of any age who have received SSDI for at least two years. Although in-home skilled mental health services have been reimbursed by Medicare since 1979 (Pelletier 1988), home-care eligibility is restricted to persons who are homebound (Trimbath and Brestensky 1990), a definition diametrically opposed to the implementation of home care for persons with serious mental illnesses. As with all Medicare-reimbursed home care, care is short-term in nature (Harper 1989).

We advocate the following changes in existing public funding:

- States should consider global budgeting for mental health to provide mental health systems the flexibility to allocate and shift funding to various types of mental health care (including home care). In global budgeting systems, the funding unit (county, municipality, etc.) receives a single budget for mental health and is able to choose how to allocate this budget across different types of care. Wisconsin, for example, gives each county a global budget that allows them to coordinate home-care programs with outpatient and inpatient facilities.
- States should continue to enroll all eligible persons with serious mental illnesses into the SSI program to access Medicaid (Taube, Goldman, and Salkever 1990; Koyanagi and Goldman 1991).
- All states should take advantage of options to provide home care, case management, and psychosocial rehabilitation under Medicaid.

Home Care for Persons with Serious Mental Illnesses 283

- The definitions of home care, case management, and psychosocial rehabilitation should be expanded to encompass services of proven effectiveness for persons with serious mental illnesses.
- Restrictions on eligible types of case management should be removed. Targeted case management that is directly involved in service provision and crisis intervention should be reimbursed under Medicaid (Taube, Goldman, and Salkever 1990).
- Financial barriers to providing clinical services outside the traditional clinic model should be reduced. Medicaid should fund mobile clinic programs that provide outreach care to persons in their natural living environments.
- Structure reimbursement to change patterns for service delivery (Mechanic 1991). For example, states should create inducements for Medicaid providers to link inpatients to outpatient care, including home care.
- Eliminate the Medicare homebound status requirement for home-care eligibility for the seriously mentally ill and provide for more long-term follow-up.
- Parents are currently the primary caregivers for the majority of people with serious mental illnesses. A crisis in caregiving will arise upon the death or disability of parental caregivers. To enhance the long-term welfare of clients, families should be allowed to set up trusts for SSI recipients (Koyanagi and Goldman 1991).
- Focus cost-containment efforts on inappropriate institutional care, not on benefits for community providers (Taube, Goldman, and Salkever 1990).
- Integrate funding streams so that they follow clients through different types of programs, including home care.
- The capitation approach is one mechanism to integrate funding and place providers at risk for costs exceeding a pre-paid amount for each enrolled client (Hadley, Schinner, and Kinosian 1989; Taube, Goldman, and Salkever 1990; Mechanic 1991; Mechanic and Rochefort 1992). Capitation systems have a built-in incentive for using home care, to the extent that it is a cost-effective mode of service delivery.
- Managed competition might provide opportunities to promote home care. Incentives in such a system should be geared to establishing community-based services for persons in their natural living environments.

Education

Home care requires a reorientation in the socialization, training, and professional rewards of mental health professionals. The mental health professions are currently oriented to office-based practices with persons who do not have serious mental illnesses. Professional training is not oriented toward working with clients and families in their own territories and home care is not a highly esteemed activity among most professionals. Policymakers have limited ability to control the various mental health disciplines. There are, however, several incentives for professionals that could promote home-care oriented service-delivery systems (Lefley, Bernheim, and Goldman 1989). Perhaps the most effective way policymakers can change the orientation of mental health professionals is through changes in the types of disorders reimbursable with public monies. If third-party payers would provide more generous payments for the treatment of serious mental illnesses (or require smaller co-payments for these illnesses), a shift toward the treatment of these illnesses would naturally occur. To the extent that home care is seen as the optimal form of treatment, the new interest in treating the seriously mentally ill could be channeled into home-care programs. Shifts in reimbursement policies, discussed above, would naturally result in some reorientation of professional education from episodic, on-site treatment to community treatment and to emphasize the social as well as the physical and psychological aspects of rehabilitation (Witheridge 1989; Gerace et al. 1990).

Obstacles

Although there are many reasons why home care should be a central policy in the mental health system, there are also numerous obstacles to its widespread implementation. These include problems in providing adequate housing, the lack of system integration in providing services to people with serious mental illnesses, the structure of reimbursement for mental health services, few incentives for mental health professionals to provide home care, little commitment on the part of elected officials, and the opposition of various groups that continue to benefit from an institutionally oriented system.

Home Care for Persons with Serious Mental Illnesses

A number of these obstacles have been addressed but warrant further emphasis:

1 Home care depends on the availability of suitable housing in the community. The lack of affordable and suitable housing in many communities hinders the possibility of providing care in stable living environments. Even when such housing exists, community opposition and stigmatizing attitudes toward the seriously mentally ill can be a barrier to establishing home care (Alisky and Iczkowski 1990).

2 Effective home care requires an integration of housing, social, therapeutic, social welfare, and habilitative services. In most communities, however, services are fragmented across a variety of uncoordinated systems. Implementation of home-care programs must occur as part of broader efforts to coordinate and integrate mental health services (Stein and Diamond 1985; Mechanic 1986). Further, the lack of integration of home care into centralized service-delivery systems has prevented the development of standards and regulations for appropriate care in the home. The delineation of what types of providers, facilities, and services are necessary and effective is necessary for the widespread adoption of home care.

3 Home care requires a stable and adequate funding base. However, budgetary, as well as programmatic, fragmentation of mental health services has accompanied deinstitutionalization (Scallett 1990; Torrey 1990; Mechanic 1991). Some funding streams restrict provision of non-institutional services. Others will only pay for certain types of home services that involve acute care rather than long-term management. Different incentives exist at different levels (e.g. local, state, federal) that lead to service delivery that can shift costs to other levels rather than to better service provision (Taube, Goldman, and Salkever 1990). While some funding for home care can be accomplished through optimal use of entitlement programs, diversion of funds from institutional to community-based care is a logical policy option. However, several interest groups associated with maintaining the service-delivery status quo (e.g. public employee unions, state hospital administrators, some state legislators, and local officials) have strong incentives to oppose funding reallocation. Whenever feasible, efforts at home-care programs that involve transferring dollars from institutional funds should involve these groups, particularly public employees, in planning and implementing home-care initiatives.

4. Consumer, family, and professional choices for appropriate home care may not be congruent. Consumers typically desire maximum independence and minimal structure and supervision while families and professionals tend to prefer more structured and supervised living arrangements (Bond et al. 1989). The difficulties of balancing the liberty interests of clients with treatment and control interests should not be minimized. However, efforts to implement home care should capitalize on the current effective advocacy provided by family and consumer groups to develop coordinated home-care programs without excessive control. The active involvement of consumers and families in the design and implementation of home-care programs can promote this end.

Most important in meeting these challenges is the political will and skill of elected and appointed officials to reshape the mental health system. While the general principles behind home care should be broadly importable from model programs like PACT, the particular programs based on these principles may have to be modified to suit the local context (Bachrach 1989). Therefore, policymakers must be sensitive to the local political, economic, and organizational climate (Mechanic 1991). They need to work with policy stakeholders, such as consumers, families, professionals, and public-employee groups, to negotiate strategies to prepare clients, providers, and communities for home- and community-based care. Failure to do so will assure continued skewed funding and inadequate care for seriously mentally ill persons.

Conclusion

The last thirty years have moved mental health policy for the seriously mentally ill away from an institutionally based model. They have failed, however, to overcome the resulting fragmentation of services to develop community-based programs. While it is clear that persons with serious mental illnesses can remain in communities, using short-stay hospital care intermittently, if at all, they can do so with an adequate quality of life only when supported by an integrated range of supports. Home care will be a central component of these programs. The challenge of the next thirty years will be to integrate and deliver mental health services within the natural living environments of persons with serious mental illnesses. Effective

Home Care for Persons with Serious Mental Illnesses

home-care programs can accomplish the initially idealistic goals of community mental health to maximize the autonomy and quality of life of the mentally ill within the least possible restrictive environment.

Note
This chapter is a revised version of a paper prepared for the Milbank Memorial Fund and Visiting Nurse Service Project on Home and Community Care. We are grateful to Tom Romeo, Joan Wagnon, and Arthur Webb for their comments on that paper.

References
Adams, P. ed. 1993. Program Helps Homeless Individuals with Severe Mental Illness. *Substance Abuse and Mental Health Services Administration News* 1: 12–13.
Alisky, J.M., and K.A. Iczkowski. 1990. Barriers to Housing for Deinstitutionalized Psychiatric Patients. *Hospital and Community Psychiatry* 41: 93–5.
Bachrach, L. 1989. Case Management: Toward a Shared Definition. *Hospital and Community Psychiatry* 40: 883–4.
Bachrach, L. 1992. What We Know About Homelessness Among Mentally Ill Persons: An Analytical Review and Commentary. *Hospital and Community Psychiatry* 43: 453–64.
Bernheim, K. F. 1990. Promoting Family Involvement in Community Residences for Chronic Mentally Ill Persons. *Hospital and Community Psychiatry* 41: 668–70.
Birmingham, M., R.J. MacLeod, and F.R. Farthing. 1990. A Supported Independent Living Program for Youth. *Hospital and Community Psychiatry* 41: 924–7.
Bond, G., L. Miller, R. Krumwied, and R. Ward. 1988. Assertive Case Management in Three CMHCs: A Controlled Study. *Hospital and Community Psychiatry* 39: 411–18.
Bond, G., T. Witheridge, D. Wasner, et al. 1989. A Comparison of Two Crisis Housing Alternatives to Psychiatric Hospitalization. *Hospital and Community Psychiatry* 40: 177–83.
Borland, A., J. McRae, and D. Lycan. 1989. Outcomes of Five Years of Continuous Intensive Case Management. *Hospital and Community Psychiatry* 40: 369–76.
Brooker, C., and C. Butterworth. 1991. Working with Families Caring for a Relative with Schizophrenia: The Evolving Role of the Community Psychiatric Nurse. *International Journal of Nursing Studies* 28: 189–200.
Brooker, C., and T. Butterworth. 1993. Training in Psychosocial Intervention: The Impact on the Role of Community Psychiatric Nurses. *Journal of Advanced Nursing* 18: 583–90.
Brooker, C., N. Tarrier, C. Barrowclough, A. Butterworth, and D. Goldberg.

1992. Training Community Psychiatric Nurses for Psychosocial Intervention. *British Journal of Psychiatry* 160: 836–44.

Brown, M.A., P. Ridgway, W.A. Anthony, and E.S. Rogers. 1991. Comparison of Outcomes for Clients Seeking and Assigned to Supported Housing Services. *Hospital and Community Psychiatry* 42: 1150–3.

Buckwalter, K., and E. Light. 1989. New Directions for Psychiatric Mental Health Nurses: The Chronically Mentally Ill Elderly. *Archives of Psychiatric Nursing* 3: 53–4.

Burns, B.J. 1993. Brief Overview on the Effectiveness of Programs of Assertive Community Treatment (PACT). Durham: Duke University Medical School. Unpublished manuscript.

Burns, T., and T. Raftery. 1991. Cost of Schizophrenia in a Randomized Trial of Home-Based Treatment. *Schizophrenia Bulletin* 17: 407–10.

Carling, P. 1990. Major Mental Illness, Housing, and Supports. *American Psychologist* 45: 969–75.

Carling, P. 1993. Housing and Supports for Persons with Mental Illness: Emerging Approaches to Research and Practice. *Hospital and Community Psychiatry* 44: 439–49.

Carpentier, N., A. Lesage, J. Goulet, P. Lalonde, and M. Renaud. 1992. Burden of Care of Families Not Living with Young Schizophrenic Relatives. *Hospital and Community Psychiatry* 43: 38–43.

Center for Mental Health Services and National Institute of Mental Health. 1992. *Mental Health, United States, 1992*, ed. R.W. Manderscheid and M.A. Sonnenschein. DHHS Publ. No. (SMA)92-1942. Washington, D.C.: US Government Printing Office.

Cohen, M.D., and S. Somers. 1990. Supported Housing: Insights from the Robert Wood Johnson Foundation Program on Chronic Mental Illness. *Psychosocial Rehabilitation Journal* 13: 43–50.

Community Support Network News. 1990. Collaboration Between Public Mental Health Systems and Universities. Boston, Massachusetts: Center For Psychiatric Rehabilitation.

Dial, T., et al. 1992. Training of Mental Health Providers. In *Mental Health, United States, 1992*. R. Manderscheid and M. A. Sonnenschein, 142–62. DHHS Pub. No. (SMA)92-1942. Washington, US Government Printing Office.

Duffy, J., M. Miller, and P. Parlocha. 1993. Psychiatric Home Care. *Home Healthcare Nurse* 11: 22–8.

England, M., and R. Cole. 1992. Building Systems of Care for Youth with Serious Mental Illness. *Hospital and Community Psychiatry* 43: 630–3.

Falloon, I.R.H., J.L. Boyd, C.W. McGill, et al. 1985. Family Management in the Prevention of Morbidity of Schizophrenia: Clinical Outcome of a Two-Year Longitudinal Study. *Archives of General Psychiatry* 42: 887–96.

Gerace, L., J. Tiller, J. Anderson, L. Miller, M. Ward, and J. Munoz. 1990. Development of a Psychiatric Home Visiting Module for Student Training. *Hospital and Community Psychiatry* 41: 1015–17.

Gilman, S.R. and R.J. Diamond. 1985. Economic Analysis in Community

Treatment of the Chronically Mentally Ill. In *The Training in Living Model: A Decade of Experience*, ed. L.I. Stein and M.A. Test, 77–84. San Francisco: Jossey-Bass.

Goering, P., D. Paduchack, and J. Durbin. 1990. Housing Homeless Women: A Consumer Preference Study. *Hospital and Community Psychiatry* 41: 790–4.

Goering. P., D. Wasylenski, M. Farkas, W. Lancee, and R. Ballantyne. 1988. What Difference Does Case Management Make? *Hospital and Community Psychiatry* 39: 272–6.

Goldman, H. 1982. Mental Illness and Family Burden: A Public Health Perspective. *Hospital and Community Psychiatry* 33: 557–60.

Goldman, H., J. Morrisey, and S. Ridgely. 1994. Evaluating the Robert Wood Johnson Foundation Program on Chronic Mental Illness. *Milbank Quarterly* 72: 37–48.

Goldman, H., A. Lehman, J. Morrissey, S. Newman, R. Frank, and D. Steinwachs. 1990. Design for the National Evaluation of the Robert Wood Johnson Foundation Program on Chronic Mental Illness. *Hospital and Community Psychiatry* 41: 1217–21.

Grella, C. E., and O. Grusky. 1989. Families of the Seriously Mentally Ill and their Satisfaction with Services. *Hospital and Community Psychiatry* 40: 831–5.

Grob, G. 1991. *From Asylum to Community: Mental Health Policy in Modern America*. Princeton, NJ: Princeton University Press.

Hadley, T., A. Schinner, and M. Kinosian. 1989. Capitation Financing of Public Mental Health Services for the Chronically Mentally Ill. *Administration and Policy in Mental Health* 16: 201–12.

Halvorson, V.M. 1992. A Home-Based Family Intervention Program. *Hospital and Community Psychiatry* 43: 395–7.

Harper, M. 1989. Providing Mental Health Services in the Homes of the Elderly. *Caring* 8(6): 5–9.

Hatfield, A. 1993. A Family Perspective on Supported Housing. *Hospital and Community Psychiatry* 44: 496–7.

Holt, S. 1989. Securing the Future Through Innovation. *Caring* 8(6): 35–41.

Johnson, A.A. 1990. *Out of Bedlam: The Truth about Deinstitutionalization*. New York: Basic Books.

Kanter, J. 1989. Clinical Case Management: Definition, Principles, Components. *Hospital and Community Psychiatry* 40: 361–8.

Keck, J. 1990. Responding to Consumer Housing Preferences: The Toledo Experience. *Psychosocial Rehabilitation Journal* 13: 51–8.

Knisley, M., and M. Fleming. 1993. Implementing Supported Housing in State and Local Mental Health Systems. *Hospital and Community Psychiatry* 44: 456–60.

Koyanagi, C., and H. Goldman. 1991. The Quiet Success of the National Plan for the Chronically Mentally Ill. *Hospital and Community Psychiatry* 42: 899–905.

Kruse, E., and M. Wood. 1989. Delivering Mental Health Services in the

Home. *Caring* 8(6): 28–34.

Lamb, H.R. 1988. Deinstitutionalization at the Crossroads. *Hospital and Community Psychiatry* 39: 941–5.

Lamb, H.R. 1993. Lessons Learned from Deinstitutionalization in the US. *British Journal of Psychiatry* 162: 587–92.

Lamb, H.R., and D.M. Lamb. 1990. Factors Contributing to Homelessness Among the Chronically and Severely Mentally Ill. *Hospital and Community Psychiatry* 41: 301–5.

Lefley, H., K. Bernheim, and C. Goldman. 1989. National Forum Addresses Need to Enhance Training in Treating the Seriously Mentally Ill. *Hospital and Community Psychiatry* 40: 460–70.

Lehman, A.F., S. Possidente, and F. Hawker. 1986. The Quality of Life of Chronic Patients in a State Hospital and in Community Residences. *Hospital and Community Psychiatry* 37: 901–7.

Lesseig, D. 1987. Home Care for Psych Problems. *American Journal of Nursing* 87: 1317–20.

Linn, L.S., L. Gelberg, and B. Leake. 1990. Substance Abuse and Mental Health Status of Homeless and Domiciled Low-Income Users of a Medical Clinic. *Hospital and Community Psychiatry* 41: 306–10.

Livingston, J., and D. Srebnick. 1991. States' Strategies for Promoting Supported Housing for Persons with Psychiatric Disabilities. *Hospital and Community Psychiatry* 42: 1116–19.

Lutterman, T., and V. Hollen. 1992. Change in State Mental Health Agency Revenues and Expenditures between Fiscal Years 1981 and 1990. In *Mental Health, United States, 1992*, ed. R. Manderscheid and M.A. Sonnenschein, 163–207. DHHS Pub. No. (SMA)92-1942. Washington, US Government Printing Office.

McCarthy, J., and G. Nelson. 1991. An Evaluation of Supportive Housing for Current and Former Psychiatric Patients. *Hospital and Community Psychiatry* 42: 1254–6.

McFarlane, W.R., P. Stastny, and S. Deakins. 1992. Family-Aided Assertive Community Treatment: A Comprehensive Rehabilitation and Intensive Case Management Approach for Persons with Schizophrenic Disorders. *New Directions for Mental Health Services* 53: 43–53.

Mechanic, D. 1986. The Challenge of Chronic Mental Illness: A Retrospective and Prospective View. *Hospital and Community Psychiatry* 37: 891–6.

Mechanic, D. 1991. Strategies for Integrating Public Mental Health Services. *Hospital and Community Psychiatry* 42: 797–801.

Mechanic, D. 1992. Editorial: Managed Care for the Seriously Mentally Ill. *American Journal of Public Health* 82: 788–9.

Mechanic, D. 1993. Mental Health Services in the Context of Health Insurance Reform. *Milbank Quarterly* 71(3): 349–64.

Mechanic, D., and D. Rochefort. 1992. A Policy of Inclusion for the Mentally Ill. *Health Affairs* 11(1): 128–50.

Mills, P., and J. Hansen. 1991. Short-Term Group Interventions for

Home Care for Persons with Serious Mental Illnesses 291

Mentally Ill Adults Living in a Community Residence and their Families. *Hospital and Community Psychiatry* 42: 1144–50.

Milstray, S. ed. 1993. President Clinton Calls for a Plan to End Homelessness. *ACCESS* 5: 1.

Morgan, A., and D. Weiman. 1990. Mental Health Home Visits to Nonhomebound Elderly. *Hospital and Community Psychiatry* 41: 1339–41.

Morrissey, J., and I. Levine. 1987. Researchers Discuss Latest Findings, Examine Needs of Homeless Mentally Ill Persons. *Hospital and Community Psychiatry* 38: 811–12.

Morrissey, J., M. Calloway, W.T. Bartko, M.S. Ridgely, H.H. Goldman, and R.I. Paulson. 1993. Local Mental Health Authorities and Service System Change: Evidence from the Robert Wood Johnson Foundation Program on Chronic Mental Illness. *Milbank Quarterly* 72: 49–80.

Morse, G., R. Calsyn, F. Allen, B. Tempelhoff, and R. Smith. 1992. Experimental Comparison of the Effects of Three Treatment Programs for Homeless Mentally Ill People. *Hospital and Community Psychiatry* 43: 1005–10.

Neese-Todd, S., and J. Weinburg. 1992. Public Academic Liaison: One Clubhouse Approach to Research and Program Evaluation. *Psychosocial Rehabilitation Journal* 16: 147–61.

New Jersey Division of Mental Health and Hospitals. 1993. Community Mental Health Academic Linkage Task Force Goals. Trenton, New Jersey.

Newton, N., and W. Brauer. 1989. In-Home Mental Health Services. *Caring* 8(6): 16–19.

Olfson, M. 1990. Assertive Community Treatment: An Evaluation of the Experimental Evidence. *Hospital and Community Psychiatry* 41: 634–41.

Pelletier, L. 1988. Psychiatric Home Care. *Journal of Psychosocial Nursing* 26(3): 22–7.

Randolph, F., P. Ridgway, and P. Carling. 1991. Residential Programs for Persons with Severe Mental Illnesses: A Nationwide Survey of State-Affiliated Agencies. *Hospital and Community Psychiatry* 42: 1111–15.

Redick, R., M. Witkin, J. Atay, and R. Manderscheid. 1992. Specialty Mental Health System Characteristics. In *Mental Health, United States, 1992*, ed. R. Manderscheid and M. A. Sonnenschein, 1–141. DHHS Pub. No. (SMA)92-1942. Washington, D.C.: US Government Printing Office.

Ridgway, P., and A. Zipple. 1990. The Paradigm Shift in Residential Services: From the Linear Continuum to Supported Housing Approaches. *Psychosocial Rehabilitation Journal* 13(4): 11–31.

Ritchie, F., and K. Lusky. 1987. Psychiatric Home Health Nursing: A New Role in Community Mental Health. *Community Mental Health Journal* 23: 229–35.

Scallet, L. J. 1990. Paying for Public Mental Health Care: Crucial Questions. *Health Affairs* 9(1): 117–24.

Seling, M., and G. Johnson. 1990. A Bridge to the Community for Extended-Care State Hospital Patients. *Hospital and Community Psychiatry* 41: 180–3.

Shanks, J. 1989. Mental Illness Services in Britain: Counting the Costs, Weighing the Benefits. *Hospital and Community Psychiatry* 40: 878–9.

Sharfstein, S., A. Stoline, and H. Goldman. 1993. Psychiatric Care and Health Insurance Reform. *American Journal of Psychiatry* 150: 7–18.

Soreff, S. 1983. New Directions and Added Dimensions in Home Psychiatric Treatment. *American Journal of Psychiatry* 140: 1213–16.

Stein, L. 1992. On the Abolishment of the Case Manager. *Health Affairs* 11(3): 172–7.

Stein, L., and R. Diamond. 1985. A Program for Difficult-to-Treat Patients. *New Directions for Mental Health Services* 26: 29–39.

Stein, L., and M.A. Test. 1980. Alternatives to Mental Hospital Treatment, I: Conceptual Model, Treatment Program, and Clinical Evaluation. *Archives of General Psychiatry* 37: 392–7.

Tanzman, B. 1993. An Overview of Surveys of Mental Health Consumers' Preferences for Housing and Support Services. *Hospital and Community Psychiatry* 44: 450–45.

Taube, C., H. Goldman, and D. Salkever. 1990. Medicaid Coverage for Mental Illness: Balancing Access and Costs. *Health Affairs* 9(1): 5–18.

Taube, C., L. Morlock, B. Burns, and A. Santos. 1990. New Directions in Research on Assertive Community Treatment. *Hospital and Community Psychiatry* 41: 642–7.

Test, M.A., and L. Stein. 1980. Alternatives to Mental Hospital Treatment, III: The Social Cost. *Archives of General Psychiatry* 37: 409–12.

Thobaben, M. 1989. Developing a Psychiatric Nursing Home Health Service. *Caring* 8(6): 10–14.

Thompson, K., E. Griffith, and P. Leaf. 1990. A Historical Review of the Madison Model of Community Care. *Hospital and Community Psychiatry* 41: 625–33.

Torrey, E.F. 1990. Economic Barriers to Widespread Implementation of Model Programs for the Seriously Mentally Ill. *Hospital and Community Psychiatry* 41: 526–31.

Trimbath, M., and J. Brestensky. 1990. The Role of the Mental Health Nurse in Home Health Care. *Journal of Home Health Care Practice* 2(3): 1–8.

Weisbrod, B., M.A. Test, and L. Stein. 1980. Alternatives to Mental Hospital Treatment, II: Economic Benefit-Cost Analysis. *Archives of General Psychiatry* 37: 400–5.

Witheridge, T. 1989. The Assertive Community Treatment Worker: An Emerging Role and its Implications for Professional Training. *Hospital and Community Psychiatry* 40: 620–4.

Witheridge, T.F., and J. Dincin. 1985. The Bridge: An Assertive Outreach Program in an Urban Setting. *New Directions for Mental Health Services* 26: 65–76.

Wolff, N., and T.W. Helminiak. 1993. The Anatomy of Cost Estimates: The Other Outcome. *Advances in Health Economics and Health Services Research* 14: 159–80.

Index

AAPCC methodology, 110-11
Abel, T., 237
access, concerns over, 7
Access to Community Care and Effective Services and Supports (ACCESS), 277
ACR methodology, 110-11
acute care health insurance, 148
acute care home health service
  costs of, 137, 145
  as distinct from long-term care, 136
  integration with long-term care services, 72-9, 89-92, 108, 111-14, 124, 129
  InterStudy project (1988), 106
  projected cuts in, 178
Adams, P., 270, 277
adult day-care centers, 161
adult foster-care homes, 27, 30, 35
Agency for Health Care Policy Research (AHCPR), 146
agency theory, 122-5, 128
aging interest groups, 56-8
Aid to Families with Dependent Children (AFDC), 232
AIDS patients, 245-67
  care management, 263-5
  care planning, 262-3
  case management, 249, 251, 264
  Community Medical Alliance, 79
  demand for home-care services, 250-4
  growth in numbers of, 53
  housing policy, 197, 198, 253
  informal support for, 253, 257-61
  integrated care programs, 90, 92
  in New York City, 246-50, 258
  staffing issues, 254-7
  structure of service provision, 261-7
AIDS Services, Division of, 249-50, 251, 262, 264
Alexander, J.A., 18
Alisky, J.M., 285
Alliance for Aging Research, 176
Alzheimers Association, 56-7
Alzheimer's disease, 161
American Academy of Pediatrics, 223
American Association of Retired Persons, 56-7, 58, 73
American Federation of State, County and Municipal Employees (AFSCME), 160
American Nurses Association, 37
American Physical Therapy Association, 161
American Public Health Association, 189, 200
American Public Welfare Association, 206, 207
Americans with Disabilities Act (ADA), 37-8, 59, 90, 203-5, 209, 221
Anderson, B., 235
Ansello, E., 83
Applebaum, R.A., 31
Arizona Department of Economic Security, 76
Arizona Health Care Cost Containment System (AHCCCS), 76-7, 89
Arizona Long-Term Care System (ALTCS), 76-7, 89
Arkansas, 81
arthritis, 220
asset protection, 144, 147

294 Index

assisted living centers, 2, 27–9, 30, 42–3, 199
   financing of, 43–4
   Medicaid waiver program, 33–4
   nurse delegation, 35, 36
   requirements for, 37–8
   state government policy, 38–40
asthma, 220–1

Bachrach, L., 270, 272, 275, 276, 286
Baker, M.O., 36, 37
Baltimore, 200
Barnow, B., 156, 162, 163, 164, 165
Bass, D.M., 85, 185
Batavia, A.I., 44
Bayer, E., 156, 165, 167
Benjamin, A.E., 3, 64, 66
   benefits for the elderly, 56
   case management, 175
   competition for clients, 11
   concept of home, 29
   historical context, 48
   managed care systems, 99
   Medicare, 164
Benjamin, Ted, 246
Bergthold, L.A., 6, 9, 11
Berkeley Planning Associates, 185
Bernheim, K.F., 273, 284
Bernstein, J., 204
Binney, Elizabeth A., 2–3, 15
Binney, L., 158
Binstock, Robert H., 58, 65
Birmingham, M., 274
Bishop, C., 9, 10, 170, 171, 173, 174, 175, 183n
Bloom, Sheila, 3–4, 220, 230, 234, 235
Blue Cross/Blue Shield plans, 228
board-and-care homes, 27, 29, 30, 38–40, 42, 270
Bond, G., 270, 272, 273, 274, 286
Borland, A., 272, 273, 274
Boston, 79
Bradley, V.J., 88
Brannon, D., 172
Brauer, W., 272
Breslau, N., 225
Brestensky, J., 282
Brody, Kathleen K., 3
Brooker, C., 272, 273
Brookings–ICF Long-Term Care Financing Model, 63
Brown, Lawrence, 49, 51, 56, 58, 62, 64
Brown, M.A., 272, 273
Buckwalter, K., 275
building codes, 200
Bundesminister für Arbeit und Soziales, 237
Burbridge, L., 160, 161
Bureau of Labor Statistics, 157, 158-9, 167–9, 171, 182n
Bureau of Medical Review, 262
Bureau of the Census, 12
bureaucratization, 14

Burner, S.T., 155, 158
Burns, B.J., 273, 279
Burns, T., 278
Burton, J.R., 43
Bush, George, 48
Butterworth, C., 272, 273
Button, James W., 56

Cadman, D., 219
California, 95, 160
California In-Home Supportive Services (IHHS) program, 176, 177
California Multipurpose Senior Services Project, 86
California SCAN, 73, 112
Canada, 27
Canalis, D.M., 17
Cantor, M., 160, 162
Caplan, A.L., 30
care management, 148
   elderly, 264
   persons with AIDS, 263–5
Carling, P., 270, 276, 277
Carpenter, E., 225
Carpentier, N., 273
Carrell, D.S., 16
case management, 123–4, 175–6
   chronically ill children, 230, 235
   elderly, 264–5
   mentally ill, 277, 278, 282, 283
   persons with AIDS, 249, 251, 264
Casey, C., 194
Center for Mental Health Services, 269
cerebral palsy, 90, 223
chain systems, 7, 157, 158, 171
chemically dependent, 84
Chichen, E., 160, 162
childhood immunization policy, 266
children
   lead-based paint, 190
   mentally ill, 274
   special health needs of, 53, 56
   see also chronically ill children
Chinloy, P., 195
Christianson, J.B., 86
chronic illnesses
   future of nursing homes, 43
   integrated care, 79
   objective conditions of, 50, 52–3, 65
   out-of-pocket expenses, 137
   public attitude to, 50, 54–6, 65
Chronic Mental Illness Program, 207
chronically ill children, 219–40
   capitated health plans, 230–1
   care co-ordination, 234–5, 238
   case management, 230, 235
   costs of caring for, 223–5
   European practice, 236–7
   family needs, 222–7
   financial aspects, 227–34, 238–40
   Medicaid, 227, 231–4, 235

Index 295

policy goals, 237–40
private health insurance, 227, 228–30
service requirements of, 225–6
stress in the home, 226–7
utilization of services, 223-5
Civil Rights Act (1968), 204
claims review mechanisms, 175
Clare, F.L., 161
class divisions, 15
Clauser, S., 175
Clinton, Bill, 17, 25, 47, 51, 57, 72, 149, 210
Code of Federal Regulations, 201–2
Cohen, M.D., 276
Cole, R., 272, 274
Colorado, 35
Committee on a National Agenda for the Prevention of Disabilities, 116–17
Committee on Ways and Means, 161
commodification, 15–16
Commonwealth Fund, 173, 176
Community Assisted Independent Living (CAIL), 82
Community Development Block Grant, 210
Community Medical Alliance (CMA), 79, 90, 91–2
competition
for clients, 11, 14
promotion of, 6
Comprehensive Assessment, Care Planning and Care Management (CAPM) programs, 82, 83, 93
Comprehensive Housing Affordability Survey (CHAS), 207
Congregate Housing Services Program (CHSP), 193, 211
Consortium of Citizens with Disabilities (CCD), 57, 83, 93
construction codes, 200
consumer-driven service models, 173, 176–7
consumer groups *see* interest groups
Continuing Care Retirement Communities, 2, 34, 139, 140
"Contract with America", 178
corporate retiree programs, 72–3
cost-containment, 2, 10–12, 146–8
housing policy, 203
labor market, 156, 161–2, 174, 178
cost-effectiveness, 31–4
costs, 137–8, 150
acute care, 137, 145
chronically ill children, 223–5
family caregivers, 141, 145
hospitals, 171, 172, 221–2
impact of employee practices on, 169–72
mentally ill, 273, 274
nursing homes, 52, 54, 137, 146–7, 150
Council of State Community Development Agencies, 206, 207
Cowan, C., 158
Cready, C.M., 31
Crown, W., 160, 162, 165, 182n

culture of caring, 15–16
Current Population Survey (CPS), 159, 160, 182n
cystic fibrosis, 223

day-care programs, 235
De Lissovoy, G., 13
Deakins, S., 273
death, 122, 125
DeJong, G., 44
Delaware, 81–2, 278
dementia sufferers, 37, 260
demographics, 12, 52
deregulation policy, 6
Detzel v. Sullivan, 230
developmentally disabled *see* mentally retarded
diabetes, 220
diagnostically related groups (DRGs), 72, 107
Diamond, R., 285
Dincin, J., 273
disability groups, 59, 93, 173
disabled
Community Medical Alliance, 79, 90, 91–2
difficulty in identifying programs, 79
housing, 186, 190, 196–8, 204–5, 209
integrated care, 72, 81–2, 83–4, 89–92, 93–4
Medicare eligibility, 6
personal assistant services, 25
see also chronic illnesses; chronically ill children; mentally ill; young disabled
disease prevention programs, 161
divorce, 136, 227
Dole, Bob, 57
Donham, C., 158
Donovan, R., 160, 162
Doty, P., 86, 87
drug abuse *see* substance abuse
Duffy, J., 272
durable medical equipment (DME) companies, 13, 17, 182n

Eckert, J.K., 38
Edelman, P., 85, 86
Education of the Handicapped Act (EHA) (1975), 226, 227
effectiveness, 123, 127, 128–9
efficiency, 123, 124, 127, 128
elder foster-care programs, 161
elderly
aging interest groups, 56–8, 93, 173
care management, 264
case management, 264–5
demand for home-care services, 252
growth in numbers living alone, 137
growth in numbers needing care, 136
housing, 186, 187–8, 192–6, 199, 203, 204, 207–8, 209

296 Index

increased home health care utilization, 9
informal care of, 84–5, 259, 261
integrated care, 72, 73–8, 80–1, 83–4, 89–90, 93–4
and labor demand, 161
long-term care expenses, 53
long-term care insurance, 140, 141
and Medicare, 26, 100, 227
Medicare HMO risk demonstrations, 112
meeting demands of, 66–7
mentally ill, 275
out-of-pocket costs, 137
PACE, 1, 33, 75–6, 89–90, 175
population growth of, 12, 52, 161
public attitudes to, 54, 56
SHMOs, 72–5, 76, 89–90, 112, 114
state integrated care programs, 76–8, 80–1, 83–4, 93–4
Elderplan, 73, 112
Ellison, M., 89
Employee Benefit Research Institute, 140
employees *see* home-health aides; homemakers; licensed practical nurses; occupational therapists; physical therapists; registered nurses
employer-based health insurance, 228–9
employers *see* home health agencies (HHAs)
Employment and Training Administration, 211
England, M., 272, 274
Equity Conversion Mortgage Insurance Demonstration Program, 195
Estes, Carrol L., 2–3, 158, 171
access to care, 7
competition for clients, 11
future implications, 16
HHAs adaptability to change, 11–12
industry transformation, 14
lack of constraints on market entry, 17
market growth, 6, 7, 9
"niche" providers, 13
social and supportive services, 15
sources of payment, 11
uncertified agencies, 8
Europe, 27, 236–7
Eustis, N., 83, 156, 165, 172, 187
Evashwick, C.J., 43
expenditure, 141–3, 146, 158
growth of, 1, 10, 137, 142, 155
Extended Care Facility, 102–4, 109

Fair Housing Act (FHA), 37–8, 196
Fair Housing Amendment Act, 203, 204–5, 209
Falik, M., 26
Falloon, I.R.H., 272
Families USA, 52, 56–7, 58, 142
family caregivers, 150
chronically ill children, 221, 222–35
effects of housing, 187, 188
financial burdens of, 227–34, 239
limits on ability to provide care, 161
mentally ill, 270, 273, 274
needs of, 222–7
programs available, 234–5
stress, 226–7
training of, 117
see also informal caregivers
Farmers Home Administration (FmHA), 193
Farthing, F.R., 274
Feder, Judy, 43, 137, 208
feedback, 123, 124, 127, 128
Feinberg, E.A., 227
Feldman, Penny Hollander, 3, 156, 162, 166
home-health aides, 160
independent providers, 159, 177
labor shortages, 165
labor unions, 60
Feustle, J.A., 13
finance, 43–4, 135–41
chronically ill children, 227–34, 238–40
current arrangements, 141–4
housing policy, 191–9, 206–7
integrated care, 72–3
mentally ill, 272, 280–3, 285
public finance expansion, 144–9
reform of, 150–2
FIND/SVP, 10
Fischer, L., 156, 165, 172
Five-Hospital Program Community Care Project, 86
Fleming, M., 276, 277
Florida Frail Elderly Option, 77
for-profit agencies, 1, 6–8, 14, 157, 158, 159
Ford Foundation, 166
Fox, H.B., 229, 230, 231, 233
Fox, P.D., 107
Fraze, D.E., 235
Friedland, Robert B., 3, 156, 166, 167
Friedlob, A., 32
Friedman, B., 18
Fullerton, H., 161

Gabel, John, 137
Gallup poll (1993), 140–1, 152n
gay men, 246, 248, 252, 258, 265
Gay Men's Health Crisis, 258
Gelberg, L., 275
geographic mobility, 136–7
Gephant, Richard A., 62
Georgia, 89
Gerace, L., 284
Germany, 236–7
Gifford, B.D., 18
Gilbert, N., 162
Ginsburg, S., 26
Glendenning, C., 88
Goering, P., 271, 274, 275
Goldberg, S.C., 15, 16
Goldman, C., 284
Goldman, H., 270, 280, 281, 282, 283, 285
Goodwin, S., 236

Gortmaker, S.L., 219, 226
Gould, David A., 4
government agencies, 8
government policies
　impact on labor market, 156, 158, 163–4, 177–8
　on nursing home care, 146
　see also health-care reforms
governmental structure, 50, 61–3, 66
Greaney, A., 231
Great Britain, 236
Green, M., 222
Green, V.L., 121
Greenberg, George D., 62, 64
Greenlick, Merwyn R., 3, 103
Grella, C.E., 273
Griffith, E., 271, 278
Grob, G., 269
Group Health, Inc., 110, 112
group insurance plans, 229
group residential settings *see* adult foster-care homes; assisted living centers; board-and-care homes
Grusky, O., 273
Guterman, S., 9

Hadley, T., 283
halfway houses, 270
Hall, L., 233, 234, 235
Halvorson, V.M., 274
Hanley, R., 85, 86
Hansen, J., 273
Harper, M., 282
Harre, D., 197
Harrigan, M., 31
Harrington, Charlene, 63, 74
Harris, Katherine M., 52
Harrison, S.C., 9
Hatfield, A., 277
Hawes, C., 27
Hawker, F., 274
Health and Human Services, Department of, 90, 92, 95, 207
Health Care Financing Administration (HCFA), 105, 161, 170–1
　cost-containment strategies, 10
　HMOs, 110–11
　Medicare examination, 44
　Minnesota LTCOP, 77, 78
　SHMOs, 73
　state Medicaid plans, 234
Health Care Financing Review, 172
health-care reforms, 17–18, 25, 51, 89, 122, 129
　high-tech home care, 13
　persons with AIDS, 265–7
　task force, 47, 63, 66, 93–4, 95
Health Insurance Association of America, 140
Health Maintenance Organizations, 1, 99–118

Index   297

　early research, 100–5
　expansion of services, 107
　integration of acute and long-term care services, 108, 111–14
　integration of population based models, 107–11
　InterStudy Project (1988), 105–7, 110
　and Medicare, 100, 104, 105–7, 108–9, 110, 112
　personnel policy, 114–18
health promotion programs, 161
Health Security Act, 25, 27, 72, 94
Helbing, C., 10
Heller School of Brandeis University, 112
Helminiak, T.W., 274
hemophilia, 220, 221
Henry J. Kaiser Family Foundation, 151
Heumann, J.E., 26
Hitov, S., 204, 205
HIV infection *see* AIDS patients
Hobbs, N., 220
Hofland, Brian F., 59, 83
Hollen, V., 281
Holt, S., 272
home, concept of, 29
home-care model, 29–31
home-care reform
　demand structure, 50, 56–61, 65–6
　governmental structure, 50, 61–3, 66
　objective conditions, 50, 52–3, 65
　policy context, 49–50, 51–2, 64–5
　public attitudes and values, 50, 54–6, 65, 150–2
　technology, 50, 63–4
home-care restructuring, 5–18
Home Equity Conversion Mortgages (HCCMs), 195–6
home health agencies (HHAs), 157–9, 182–3n
　adaptation to change, 11–12
　authorization of, 5–6
　employee earnings, 167–9
　growth of, 6–9
　impact of employment practices, 169–72
　transformation of, 14
　visit costs, 173
home-health aides, 102–4, 115, 116, 158, 159–60
　CHR demonstration program, 112
　growth of, 155, 161
　persons with AIDS, 254–7
　quality of work life, 162, 165–7
　wages, 169, 170
　workweek, 182n
Homeless Families Program, 207
homeless persons, 207, 209
　mentally ill, 197–8, 270, 272, 275
　persons with AIDS, 197, 198, 253
homemakers, 115, 158, 159
Horwitz, Allan V., 4
hospices, 8, 17, 235, 252

298   Index

hospital-based agencies, 8, 157, 158, 159, 182–3n
hospitals, 1, 49
  chronically ill children, 220–3
  cost containment pressures, 161–2
  cost increases, 171, 172, 221–2
  discharge planning of persons with AIDS, 262
  discrimination process, 37
  employee earnings, 167–9
  expansion of influence, 114–15
  impact on labor market, 161
  integrated state programs, 82
  Kaiser Permanente Portland Study, 102, 103
  mentally ill, 269, 273, 281
  use-reduction goals, 122, 123–4
  workweek, 159, 182n
housing, 185–212
  and the disabled, 186, 190, 196–8, 204–5, 209
  and the elderly, 186, 187–8, 192–6, 199, 203, 204, 207–8, 209
  finance, 191–9, 206–7
  and health issues, 189–90, 206–8, 211–12
  legislative and regulatory changes, 202–3
  mentally ill, 188, 196–8, 270, 272, 275–7, 285
  neighborhood conditions, 201–2, 209–10
  persons with AIDS, 197, 198, 253
  quality standards, 199–201, 209–10
  regulations and statutes, 199–205
  research evidence, 187–9
  residency requirements, 203–4
  Section 202 program, 186, 192, 193, 196, 197, 198, 203, 209
Housing Act (1949), 209
Housing Act (1990), 202, 209
housing allowance, 147
Housing and Community Development Act (1992), 203, 207
Housing and Development Reporter, 201, 209
Housing and Urban Development (HUD), 192, 193, 194–5, 209
  FHA insurance programs, 196
  and HHS, 207
  homeless, 198, 207
  housing quality standards, 201
  mentally ill, 277
  production subsidies, 198
housing codes, 200–1, 210
housing finance agencies, (HFAs), 206
Hudson, Robert, 64
Hughes, D., 228
Hughes, S., 8, 86
Human Resources Administration (HRA), 248–50, 251, 262, 263
Hurtado, A., 103

Iczkowski, K.A., 285
Illinois, 81, 86

Illston, L.H., 33
implementation problems, 122–6, 129
incentive structure, 123–5, 127–8, 129
income protection, 147
income tax, 151
independent living developments, 199
independent providers (IPs), 157–8, 159, 160, 173, 176–7, 183n
Individuals with Disabilities Education Act (IDEA) (1991), 226
informal caregivers, 15, 84–9, 94–5
  cost estimate of, 141, 145
  diminishing role in future, 136
  elderly, 84–5, 259, 261
  persons with AIDS, 253, 257–61
  see also family caregivers
infusion therapy, 13, 256–7, 263
injection drug users (IDUs), 246, 248, 252
Institute for Health and Aging, 8
Institute of Medicine, 117
institutional care *see* hospitals; nursing homes
insurance, 138–41
  chronically ill children, 222, 238–40
integration
  acute and long-term care services, 72–9, 89–92, 108, 111–14, 124, 129
  administration/funding of state programs, 79–83, 92–3
  chronically ill children, 237
  disabled, 72, 81–2, 83–4, 89–92, 93–4
  for diverse long-term care populations, 83–4, 93–4
  elderly, 72, 73–8, 80–1, 83–4, 89–90, 93–4
  of formal and informal care, 84–9, 94–5
  mentally ill, 84, 272, 273, 275, 277–80, 285
  mentally retarded, 72, 76–7, 83, 84, 94
  persons with AIDs, 90, 92
Interagency Task Force on Homelessness, 207
interest groups, 39–40, 65–6, 83–4
  disabled, 59, 93, 173
  elderly, 56–8, 93, 173
  mentally ill, 285
  mentally retarded, 59
  young people with disabilities, 58, 59, 93
Intergovernmental Health Policy Project (IHPP), 79
InterStudy Project (1988), 105–7, 110
Iowa, 222
Ireys, H.T., 220
Irvin, K., 76, 77

Jacobs, B., 195
Jamieson, A., 27
Johnson, A.A., 271
Johnson, G., 271
Johnson, K., 228
Jones, P.A., 17, 155, 165
Justice, D., 80, 81, 82, 86

Index

Kaiser Permanente Center for Health Research (CHR), 100–1, 112, 117
Kaiser Permanente Northwest Region, 105
Kaiser Permanente Portland, 73, 101–5, 109, 110, 112
Kane, N., 156, 157, 159, 160, 162, 177
Kane, R.L., 25, 33, 75
Kane, Rosalie A., 3
  assisted living, 37, 39, 40, 42
  continuum of care, 34
  group residential settings, 27, 28
  health-care reforms, 25
  home-care model, 29–30
  nurse delegation, 36, 37
  nursing homes, 30, 43
  quality of care, 156, 165, 172
Kansas, 35–6
Kanter, J., 272, 278
Kapp, M., 35
Karls, J.M., 234
Katsura, H., 186
Keigher, S., 87, 88
Kemper, Peter, 31, 65, 87, 136
Kingdon, John W., 50, 59, 64, 65
Kinney, G.M., 9
Kinosian, M., 283
Kisker, C.T., 222, 235
Knisley, M., 276, 277
Kodner, D.L., 43
Kohler, L., 236
Koyanagi, C., 282, 283
Kramer, A.M., 107, 172
Krems, S., 196
Kruse, E., 275

labor demand, 160–1
labor force
  in HMOs, 102–4, 112, 114–18
  numbers employed, 1
  restructuring of, 15
  specialization of, 13
labor market, 155–79
labor shortages, 155–6, 163, 164–5
labor supply, 161–2
labor unions, 60, 160
Ladd, Richard, 92
Laguna Research Associates, 77
Lamb, D.M., 274, 275
Lamb, H., 271, 272, 274, 275, 276
LaPlante, Mitchell P., 52
Laxton, C., 162
Lazenby, H., 7
lead-based paint, 190
Leadership Council on Aging, 57
Leaf, P., 271, 278
Leake, B., 275
Lefley, H., 284
legal specialization, 144
Lehman, A.F., 274
Lesseig, D., 281

Lester, D.G., 235
Leutz, W., 73
Leventhal, J.M., 227
Levine, I., 271, 272, 276
Levine, P., 221
Levit, K.R., 7, 10, 11
Lewin-VHI, 10, 142
Lewis-Idema, D., 26
licensed practical nurses (LPNs), 155, 159, 161, 165, 182n
  wages, 169, 170
Lie, S.O., 235
life care communities, 199
life insurance, 140
Light, E., 275
Lindstrom, B., 236
Linkins, K., 7, 8, 9
Linn, L.S., 275
Linsk, N., 88
Litvak, S., 25, 26, 159
Litwak, E., 85
Liu, Korbin, 12, 137
Livingston, J., 276
local government sponsored agencies, 157
Lombardi, T., 163, 165, 166
long-term care
  definition of, 135–6
  number of dependants, 136
Long-Term Care Campaign, 56–7, 62
Long-Term Care Management, 54
Long-Term Care Policy Co-ordinating Council (LTCPCC), 162
Louis Harris & Associates, 151
Lusky, K., 272
Lutterman, T., 281
Lux, L.J., 27
Lycan, D., 272, 274
Lyon, S.M., 38

MacAdam, M., 156, 159, 164, 166, 167, 175
MacLeod, R.J., 274
Macrosystems, Inc., 196
Magaziner, Ira, 62
Maine, 81
managed care systems *see* Health Maintenance Organizations
Manton, K.G., 12, 137, 161
Maple, B., 158
Maraldo, P., 162
Marion Merrill Dow, 8, 158, 159, 162, 169, 170, 172, 183n
marital relations, 226–7
market growth, 6–9, 10
Marmor, Theodore R., 7, 10, 67
Maryland, 81
Massachusetts, 166
Massachusetts Rate Setting Commission, 162
Master, R., 79, 90
Masters Program in Policy Studies, 200
Mathematica Policy Research, Inc., 185
McBride, Timothy D., 136

McCall, N., 77
McCarthy, J., 277
McFarlane, W.R., 273
McKetty, C.C., 16
McKinlay, J., 185
McKinney Act (1987), 196, 197, 203, 207
McKnew, L.B., 44
McKusick, D.R., 155, 158
McManus, M., 223, 224
McRae, J., 272, 274
Mechanic, D.
  integrated care, 72
  mentally ill, 271, 272, 274, 277, 278, 283, 285, 286
Medicaid
  aide training, 167
  chronically ill children, 227, 231–4, 235
  Community Medical Alliance, 79
  concern over legal issues, 144
  differences of consensus over, 58
  eligibility requirements, 143, 144
  Florida Frail Elderly Option, 77
  future financial options, 145, 148–9
  home health care expenditure, 142
  impact on labor market, 161, 164
  influence of policy changes, 5–6
  integrated care financing, 72
  legislation to reduce growth of, 90
  mentally ill, 272, 280, 281–2, 283
  Minnesota LTCOP, 77–8
  nursing homes, 52, 56, 141, 143, 144
  PACE model, 75, 76
  payment to informal caregivers, 88
  personal assistance services, 26–7
  personnel issues, 116
  policy changes, 5–6
  service gaps, 53
  SHMOs, 74, 113
  as source of payment, 11, 54
  state concerns over, 60, 231, 232–4
  waiver program, 28, 33–4, 232–3, 235
Medicare
  benefit examination, 43–4
  costs per visit charge, 169–71, 172, 182n
  demand for (1960s), 101
  DME growth, 13
  financing of home care for elderly, 26, 100, 227
  flexible service packages, 173–4
  for-profit HHAs, 6–7
  future cuts, 2
  future financial options, 149
  and HMOs, 100, 104, 105–7, 108–9, 110, 112
  home health aide training, 102, 167
  home health care expenditure, 142
  increased home visits, 9
  influence of policy changes, 5–6, 11, 18
  informal care support, 86
  integrated care financing, 72
  labor market, 161, 164, 177
  labor personnel regulations, 174, 175
  legislation to reduce growth of, 90
  licensed practical nurses, 165
  mentally ill, 272, 280, 282, 283
  Minnesota LTCOP, 77–8
  nursing home expenditure, 141
  PACE model, 75, 76
  personnel issues, 116
  policy changes, 5–6
  prospective payment system (PPS), 6, 9, 10, 16, 173–4
  regulatory changes, 10, 11
  skilled services definition, 111
  Social HMOs, 112–14
  as source of payment, 10–11
  trade associations monitoring of, 60
Medicare Catastrophic Coverage Act (1988), 58, 147
Medicare Plus II Program, 112
medication management, 36–7
Megbolugbe, I., 195
Menke, T., 161, 162
mental health authorities, 280
mental health professional education, 284
mental institutions, 269, 270, 281
mentally ill, 136, 269–87
  case management, 277, 278, 282, 283
  costs of, 273, 274
  financing, 272, 280–3, 285
  home-care benefits, 273–4
  home-care components, 271–3
  housing, 188, 196–8, 270, 272, 275–7, 285
  integrated care, 84, 272, 273, 275, 277–80, 285
mentally retarded, 136
  integrated care, 72, 83, 84, 94
  integrated care Arizona, 76–7
  interest groups, 59
Mezrich, M., 205
Michigan, 176, 278
Milbank Memorial Fund, ix, 2
Milbank Quarterly, ix
Miller, I.S., 86
Miller, M., 272
Miller, N., 8, 175
Miller, N.A., 33
Mills, P., 273
Milstein, B., 204, 205
Milstray, S., 270
Mindel, C., 185
Minneapolis, 73, 110, 112
Minnesota, 36, 88–9
Minnesota Long-Term Care Option Project (LTCOP), 77–8, 89
Mitchell, George, 62
Moderate Rehabilitation Program for Single-Room Occupancy, 197
Mollica, R.L., 27
monitoring, 123–4, 127, 128
Moon, Marilyn, 137

Morgan, A., 275
Morgenstern, N., 107
Morlock, L.L., 18
Morrissey, J., 271, 272, 276, 280
Morse, G., 272, 274, 275
Moscovice, I., 86
Moynihan, Daniel Patrick, 62
multifacility systems, 7, 171
Mundinger, M.O., 17
Murray, Thomas H., 58, 65
myelodysplasia, 223

National Academy for State Health Policy, 78
National Affordable Housing Act (1990), 207
National Aging Human Resource Institute, 157
National Association of Home Care (NAHC), 8, 10, 11, 60, 61, 165
National Association of Housing and Redevelopment Officials, 189
National Association of State Mental Health Program Directors, 276
National Channeling Demonstration project, 86, 122, 210
National Chronic Care Consortium (NCCC), 79, 91
National Council of State Boards of Nursing, 37
National Expenditure Survey (1987), 142
National Governors Association, 211, 232
National Health Interview Survey, 210, 224
National Home and Hospice Care Survey (NHHCS), 158
National Housing Act, 189
National Long-Term Care Survey, 75, 210
National Medical Care Utilization and Expenditure Survey (NMCUES), 223
National Medical Expenditures Survey (NMES), 10
National Social HMO Research Consortium Data Center, 112
National Survey of Home and Hospice Care, 8
neighbourhood conditions, 201–2, 209–10
Nelson, G., 277
Neu, C.R., 9
New Construction (NC) programs, 193, 194
New York
 ACCESS Program, 124
 Chelsea Village Home-Care Program, 187
 Elderplan, 73, 112
 labor unions, 160
 medication management, 36
 persons with AIDS, 246–50, 258
 work life improvements, 166
Newacheck, P.W., 220, 223, 224, 229
Newcomer, R.J., 73, 74
Newman, Sandra J., 189, 205, 210
 homeless persons, 197

housing and the elderly, 187–8, 194, 196, 199
housing and the mentally ill, 188, 196
housing finance, 192
neighbourhood conditions, 202
Newschaffer, C., 178
Newton, N., 272
"niche" providers, 13
Noelker, S.L., 85, 185, 187
non-profit HHAs, 5–6, 7, 8, 14, 157, 159
Norway, 236
nurse assistants, 115
nurse delegation, 34–7, 41
nurses
 dominant role of, 115
 enhancement of skills, 117
 persons with AIDS, 254–7, 261, 263
 role in assisted living schemes, 42
 see also licensed practical nurses (LPNs); registered nurses (RGs)
nursing boards, 40
nursing home affiliated agencies, 157
nursing homes, 1, 49
 admission thresholds, 34
 attempts to limit growth of, 143
 care plans, 30
 concept of home, 29
 cost-effectiveness of, 31–2
 costs of, 52, 54, 137, 146–7, 150
 discrimination process, 37
 employee earnings, 167–9, 170
 expenditure, 141, 142–3, 158
 financing of, 144, 152n
 future of, 43
 government role, 146
 home-care reform debate, 60
 integrated state programs, 82–3
 likelihood of financial assistance, 143
 lobbying pressure, 39
 long-term care work group options, 47
 Medicaid, 52, 56, 141, 143, 144
 mentally ill, 281
 nursing care, 32–3
 public disenchantment with, 54
 public policy support for, 52
 use-reduction goals, 121–2, 124, 125, 129, 130
 workweek, 158, 159, 182n
Nyman, J., 123

occupational therapists, 115, 155, 161, 182n
O'Connor, C., 36, 37
Office of the Assistant Secretary for Planning and Evaluation, 90
Ohio, 278, 281
Older Americans Act (1978), 6
Older Women's League (OWL), 56–7, 58
Olfson, M., 273, 274
ombudsmen, 40
Omnibus Budget Reconciliation Act (OBRA), 6, 74

Omnibus Reconciliation Act (1980), 6
Omnibus Reconciliation Act (1987), 166–7
On Lok, 33, 75, 76, 124
oral medication, 36–7
Oregon
  assisted living, 28, 34, 39
  informal care support, 86
  integrated care, 79, 80, 81, 92
  nurse delegation, 35
  SHMOs, 73
Oregon Health Sciences University, 117
out-of-pocket payments, 11, 54, 137, 142
Outlook 2000, 159

PACE Demonstrations *see* Programs of All-Inclusive Care for the Elderly
parent support groups, 235
Parker, M., 105–7
Parlocha, P., 272
patients
  benefit potential of, 126
  goals of, 123
Pawalek, J.E., 31
Pawlson, L. Gregory, 51, 64
payment sources, 10–11, 54
Pelletier, L., 282
Pendleton, S., 82–3
Pennsylvania, 89
Pepper, Claude, 62
Pepper Commission (1990), 51, 61, 63, 66, 136, 147
Perozek, Maria, 137
Perrin, James M., 3–4, 220, 227, 230, 232, 234, 235, 238
personal assistant services (PAS), 24–7, 41
personal care aides, 115
Peterson, Mark A., 50, 53, 62
pharmaceutical industries, 17
pharmacy boards, 40
physical functioning, 123, 125
physical therapists, 115, 155, 159, 161, 162, 182n
physical therapy aides, 115
physicians
  involvement of, 127, 129
  persons with AIDS, 263–4, 265–6
Pierce, P.M., 235
Polich, C., 105–7
policy goals, 121–5
political context, 47–67
Pope, A.M., 220
Pope, G., 161, 162
population dynamics, 12, 52
Possidente, S., 274
postacute home care, 49, 66, 145
preadmission screening programs (PAS), 82, 93
Preferred Provider Organizations (PPOs), 229
private insurance payments
  chronically ill children, 227, 228–30
  development of, 56, 59–60, 139–41, 145, 146–7, 148
  as source of payment, 11, 54, 142, 152n
privatization, 14
Program in Assertive Community Treatment (PACT), 278–9, 286
Program Review Bureau, 176
Programs of All-Inclusive Care for the Elderly (PACE Demonstrations), 1, 33, 75–6, 89–90, 175
Projects for Assistance in Transition to Homelessness (PATH), 197–8
proprietary agencies, 7, 8, 14
public attitudes and values, 50, 54–6, 65, 150–2
public HHAs
  decline of (1972–86), 6, 14
  Medicare participation, 5–6
public housing authorities (PHAs), 194, 201, 276
Pynoos, Jon, 59, 186, 206, 209

quality of care, 13, 29, 127
  effect of housing on, 187
  links to labor force work life, 156, 165–7, 172, 173, 178
  state concern over, 38
quality of work life, 156, 162, 165–7, 172, 173, 178

R.L. Associates, 54
Raftery, T., 278
Randolph, F., 270
Rango, Nicholas, 246
rationalization, 14
Reagan, Ronald, 6, 48
recuperative care, 145
Red Cross, 249
Redfoot, D.L., 37, 206, 211
Redick, R., 280, 281, 282
reform *see* home-care reform
registered nurses (RGs), 155, 159, 161, 162, 182n
  wages, 169, 170
rehabilitation-related industries, 17
Reinhard, Susan, 4
renal dialysis, 13
renal disease patients, 6
residential care *see* nursing homes
respite-care programs, 235
Retail, Wholesale Department Store Union, 160
retirement communities, 2, 34, 139, 140
retirement planning, 137, 138
Rhode Island, 278
Rice, Thomas, 137
Ridgway, P., 270, 273
Riley, T., 78, 159
risk adjustment, 91–2
risk assessment, 124–5, 127, 128, 129
risk-based payment methods, 174–5, 178

Index   303

Ritchie, F., 272
Rivlin, Alice M., 52, 59, 63
Robert Wood Johnson Foundation, 95, 148, 193, 207, 208, 280
Rochefort, D., 283
Rosen, S., 18
Rosenbaum, S., 228
Rosenbaum, Walter A., 56
Ruben, R.J., 227

Sabatino, C.P., 25
Sabbeth, B.F., 227
Salkever, D., 224, 225, 270, 282, 283, 285
San Francisco
  On Lok, 33, 75, 76, 124
  people with AIDS, 258
Sandorf, J., 198
Sangl, G., 187
Sangl, J.A., 10
Sapienza, A., 156, 159, 160, 162, 177
Sappenfield, W., 219
Saucier, P., 78
savings, 137–8
Saward, E., 103
Scallett, L.J., 285
Scandinavia, 225, 236
Scanlon, William, 137, 199
Scharer, L., 187, 200, 201, 202
Schinner, A., 283
schizophrenia, 274
Schlenker, R., 173, 174
Schlesinger, M., 7, 10, 72
Schnare, A., 194, 202
Schoenman, J., 178
schools, 226
Seling, M., 271
Senior Care Action Network (SCAN Health Plan), 73, 112
Senior Companion Program, 88
Seniors Plus, 73, 112
Service Employees' International Union (SEIU), 160
Shanks, J., 274
Sharfstein, S., 281
Shaughnessy, P., 172, 173, 174
Shayne, M.W., 220, 234
Shelter Plus Care Program, 198, 207, 209
Shen, J.K., 75
Shortell, S., 18
Silverman, H.A., 10, 161, 164
Silvestri, G., 155, 182n
Simon-Rusinowitz, Lori, 59, 83
SIPP, 84
Skwara, K., 9, 10, 170, 171, 173, 174, 175, 183n
Sloan, K., 206, 211
Smith, P.S., 221
Smith-Barusch, A., 86
Smithey, R.W., 7, 10
Smyth-Staruch, K., 223
Snapp, David, 182n

Social Health Maintenance Organizations (SHMO), 1, 73–5, 76, 89–90, 108, 111–14, 118, 174
Social Security Act, 5, 6
Social Security Administration, 231–2
social service workers, 115, 159
social services, 14–15, 16, 107
Somers, Anne R., 140
Somers, S., 276
South Carolina, 124
special rent adjustment (SRA), 194
spinal cord injuries, 90, 92
Spohn, P.H., 9, 11
Srebnick, D., 276
Stallard, E., 12
Staruch, K.S., 225
Stasny, P., 273
state governments
  assisted living, 38–40
  chronically ill children, 222
  funding of mentally ill, 280–2
  home-care reform debate, 60
  impact on labor market, 163, 164
  informal care system, 86
  integrated care, 76–84, 89, 92–4
  IP programs, 159, 176
  Medicaid program, 60, 231, 232–4
  PACT teams, 278, 279
  payment to informal caregivers, 88–9, 94–5
  work life improvements, 166
Stein, L., 270, 272, 273, 274, 278, 285
Stein, R.E.K., 232
Steinfeld, E., 190
Stoline, A., 281
Stone, Robyn I., 3, 65, 87, 136, 156, 166, 167
Strahan, G.W., 8, 158
Straw, Margret K., 54, 55
stress, 226–7
Struyk, R., 186, 189
substance abuse, 197, 198
  mentally ill, 279
  persons with AIDS, 248, 252, 258, 259, 266
Substantial Rehabilitation (SR) programs, 193, 194
Sullivan v. *Zebley*, 231
Supplementary Security Income (SSI) program, 231–2, 239
Supportive Housing Demonstration Program (SHDP), 197
Supportive Housing Program, 197
supportive services, 14–15, 16, 107, 192–4, 197–8
Supportive Services in Senior Housing demonstration program, 193, 208
Surpin, R., 165, 166
Sussman, M., 187
Suzman, R., 161
Swan, J.H., 6, 7, 13, 14, 16, 17, 171

Sweden, 236
Szasz, A., 156, 158, 164, 165, 171

Tanzman, B., 276
Tarlov, A.R., 220
task definition, 123–5
Taube, C., 270, 272, 273, 274, 278, 282, 283, 285
Tauber, C.M., 12
tax credits, 148
tax incentives, 138
taxation, 150–2
Taylor, W.R., 220
technological advances, 6, 12–14, 50, 63–4, 161
  and chronically ill children, 220
  and persons with AIDS, 256–7
Tennstedt, S., 185
Test, M.A., 270, 273, 274
Texas, 35
Thobaben, M., 272
Thomas, S., 186
Thompson, K., 271, 278
Thorp, E.K., 227
Thyen, Ute, 3–4
Torres-Gil, Fernando, 58, 59
Torrey, E.F., 271, 272, 273, 285
trade associations, 60–1
training, 123, 124–5, 127, 128, 129
  for AIDS staff, 255
  for home health aides, 102, 166–7
Trimbath, M., 282
tuberculosis, 257, 262, 266
Turner, M., 203

uncertified agencies, 7, 8, 13
United Domestic Workers' Union, 160
University of California San Francisco, 73–4, 75
University of Minnesota, 75
Urban Systems Research and Engineering, 196
US CBO, 59
US Congress, 54
US General Accounting Office, 10, 34, 35, 161, 223
US Special Committee on Aging, 12

Vermont, 82
Villanueva, A.M., 6
Villers/Families USA, 56–7
Visiting Nurse Association of America, 61
Visiting Nurse Service of New York (VNSNY), ix–x, 2
  and AIDS, 249–50, 256, 263
visiting nursing service agencies, 8, 114, 157, 158, 159
Vladeck, Bruce C., 44, 53, 56, 62, 175

wages, 162, 167–9, 170
Waldo, D.R., 7, 155, 158
Walker, B., 206
Wan, T., 185
Washington, 34, 35
Weicher, J., 190
Weil, M., 234
Weiman, D., 275
Weisbrod, B., 273
Weissert, W.G., 3, 31, 85, 172, 178, 195
Weitzman, M., 220
West, J., 221
Wiener, Joshua M., 52, 59, 63, 85
Wildfire, J.B., 27
Wilson, K.B., 27, 28, 37, 40, 42
Winship, C., 18
Wisconsin
  assisted living, 34
  funding for mentally ill, 282
  informal care support, 86
  integrated care, 81, 92, 94
  PACT teams, 278
Wisconsin Community Options Program (COP), 80, 84, 93
Witheridge, T., 272, 273, 284
Wolff, N., 274
women
  and AIDS, 246, 248, 258–9
Wood, M., 275
work life improvements see quality of work life
workforce see labor force
Wysong, J.A., 237

Yankelovich, Daniel, 54, 55
young disabled
  growth in numbers of, 53
  informal care of, 84
  integrated care, 72, 76–7, 83–4
  interest groups, 58, 59, 93
  public attitude to, 54, 56

Zachau-Christiansen, Bengt, 225
Zais, J.P., 189
Zedlewski, Sheila Rafferty, 136
Zipple, A., 273
Zukas, H., 26